Introduction to Sound

Acoustics for the Hearing
and Speech Sciences

Third Edition

Textbook Series
Series Editor: M.N. Hegde

Introduction to Sound

Acoustics for the Hearing and Speech Sciences

THIRD EDITION

Charles E. Speaks, Ph.D.

Professor
Department of Communication Disorders
University of Minnesota
Minneapolis, Minnesota

THOMSON

DELMAR LEARNING

**Introduction to Sound
Acoustics for the Hearing and Speech Sciences 3E
Charles E. Speaks**

**Vice President,
Health Care Business Unit:**
William Brottmiller

Executive Director:
Cathy L. Esperti

Acquisitions Editor:
Kalen Conerly

Marketing Director:
Jennifer McAvey

Production Director:
Carolyn Miller

Library of Congress
Cataloging-in-Publication Data

Speaks, Charles E.
    Introduction to sound: acoustics for the hearing and speech sciences / by Charles E. Speaks. - 3rd ed
    p.   cm.
    Includes bibliographical references and index.
    ISBN 1-56593-979-4
    1. Sound. 2. Audiology.
    3. Speech therapy.
    I. Title.
QC225.15.S64   1999
534--dc21   98-29577
                              CIP

NOTICE TO THE READER

Contents

Preface to the First Edition

This book was written to *teach* the fundamental concepts of acoustics, particularly to those who are interested in the discipline of the speech-language-hearing sciences. Readers who are thoroughly grounded in mathematics and physics should be able to move through the various topics quickly. Those who are less comfortable with basic concepts of physics, or with mathematics beyond elementary algebra, will require more careful study of some of the concepts, but ultimately the concepts should be understood.

Students of the speech-language-hearing sciences must have a thorough understanding of the elements of acoustics before they can successfully embark on more advanced study of both normal and disordered human communication. At the University of Minnesota, for example, students in the Department of Communication Disorders who pursue an undergraduate degree must complete a five-credit course in acoustics, which is *prerequisite* to registration in more advanced courses such as Speech Science, Hearing Science, Hearing Loss and Audiometry, Noise and Humankind, Cleft Palate: Oral-Facial Anomalies and Speech, and Voice Disorders. Treatment of the fundamental concepts of acoustics with 2 or 3 weeks of lectures in the context of a broader course such as "speech and hearing science" or "introduction to audiology" cannot, in our opinion, do justice to the topic or serve students well.

There are many aspects of sound that might interest readers other than students in the speech-language-hearing sciences. Why is a "sonic boom" created when an airplane exceeds the speed of sound? Why is a foghorn designed to emit a low-pitched sound instead of a high-pitched whistle? If you are hunting in the woods, why is your distant prey more likely to hear you if it is downwind from you? How do "whispering galleries" work? In what ways do echoes off a canyon wall behave like billiard balls bouncing off rails of the billiard table? When you contemplate purchasing a stereo system, what does the salesperson mean by terms such as frequency response, noise floor, dynamic range, signal-to-noise ratio, decibels, percentage harmonic distortion, and so on? The answers to these and other questions are sprinkled throughout the text.

In the opening sentence, the word "teach" was emphasized because the fundamental goal is to *teach* the important elements of acoustics, not just present the topics. Two examples should suffice. First, some readers will not know, or will have forgotten, what is meant by "antilog$_{10}$ 2." However, everyone will certainly know that $10^2 = 100$. To understand the *concept* of antilogarithms, then, one needs only to realize that "antilog$_{10}$2 = ?" is exactly the same as asking, "what is 10^2?" Once the concept is understood, all that remains is to learn the simple steps for solving antilog problems that are computationally, but not conceptually, more difficult. Second, learning of several concepts in acoustics, the decibel for example, can be enhanced by solving problems. For that reason, the accompanying *Course Notes and Workbook for Introduction to Sound* includes nearly 400 practice problems that are followed by *answers and explanations* of how the correct answers were obtained.

The organization of the topics in the book reflects a combination of both logic and personal preference. For example, the concepts of antilogarithms and logarithms must be understood before one can study decibels, and it is difficult to imagine how one can understand complex sound waves without first mastering the concept of sinusoidal wave motion. The location of other topics within the book reflects the author's preference for teaching. Some might prefer, for example, to begin by reading about "fundamental and derived physical quantities" and "proportionality" from Chapter 1 and "scientific notation" from Chapter 3. Those topics, and some others, should be treated as free-standing modules to be addressed when the reader or teacher elects.

Preface to the Second Edition

The second edition of *Introduction to Sound* retains the singular purpose to *teach* the fundamental concepts of acoustics to students in the speech-language-hearing sciences. To help achieve that objective, this edition differs from its predecessor in three principal ways. **Practice Problems** and **Answers to Practice Problems** have been added for Chapters 1, 5, 7, and 8, and a new set of problems and answers has been added to Chapter 2.

A new section entitled **Frequently Misunderstood Concepts** has been appended to Chapters 1, 2, 4, 5, 6, and 8. An analysis of answers to examination questions by approximately 275 students over the past 3 years led to a distressing realization. Although the mean score was a satisfactory 80%, a few questions were missed consistently by more than half of the students. For example, in response to the question, "An increase in sound pressure by a factor of 4:1 corresponds to an increase by how many decibels?" many students responded with 12 dB SPL or 12 dB IL rather than just 12 dB. The purpose of these new sections, therefore, is to call specific attention to the kinds of mistakes that previous students have made and to attempt further clarification of the basic concepts that had been misunderstood.

Finally, several faculty and student users identified a few errors that appeared in the first edition, and every effort has been made to correct them. I thank them all, and particular appreciation is expressed to Sid Bacon at Arizona State University and Peter Narins at UCLA for their helpful suggestions.

Preface to the Third Edition

The third edition of *Introduction to Sound* continues to retain the singular purpose to *teach* the fundamental concepts of acoustics to students in speech-language-hearing sciences. This edition differs from its predecessors, however, both substantively and cosmetically.

The principal changes are:

- Point-by-point construction of a sine wave is demonstrated by calculating sin θ at 11° intervals from 0° to 360° and then plotting the results (Chapter 2);
- Wave equations are used to explain why *particle displacement* must be 180° out of phase with *particle acceleration*, a relation that is seldom intuitively obvious (Chapter 2);
- A table of common logs has been added (Chapter 3);
- The *preferred center frequencies* for constant percentage bandwidth filters are listed, and the reasons for their selection are explained (Chapter 6);
- The "Summary of an Experiment on the Cat" has been deleted (Chapter 7);
- The universality of the inverse square law to physical phenomena other than sound is described (Chapter 8);
- The concepts of *constructive* and *destructive interference* are introduced in a discussion of standing waves (Chapter 8);
- The relation between *displacement* nodes and antinodes and *pressure* nodes and antinodes in consideration of standing waves in acoustic tubes is explained (Chapter 8);
- The higher modes of vibration of strings, and the commonalities between vibration of a string and the standing waves in tubes closed at both ends, are explained (Chapter 8);
- The discussion of sound *absorption* has been expanded to include differences in absorption coefficients as a function of frequency and among common absorbing materials (Chapter 8);
- The discussion of *total absorption*, including the *sabine* and *metric sabine*, has been expanded (Chapter 8);
- The relation between *absorption* and *reverberation time* has been elaborated to show their practical application to optimal and substandard room acoustics (Chapter 8);
- Fourteen equations have been added to the *Alphabetical Listing of Selected Equations*;
- *All illustrations* have been newly prepared with common formatting, several illustrations have been recomposed to achieve greater clarity, some new illustrations have been prepared, and careful attention has been paid to ensure that all figures are "mathematically correct" (all chapters);

- *Practice Problems* and *Answers to Practice Problems* have been moved to a newly created *Course Notes and Workbook for Introduction to Sound*, which will be accompanied by *printed copies of several hundred PowerPoint slides* that some faculty might choose to use in their classes; and
- A concerted effort has been made to ensure that "nuisance errors" have been virtually eliminated.

In all instances, the modifications, additions, and deletions were driven by a single force: the change must promise to enhance teaching and improve comprehension of the fundamental concepts of acoustics.

Acknowledgments

Any list of persons who should be acknowledged would be woefully incomplete, but the contributions of some must be recognized. One group is my own mentors, including Francis Flynn, Edward Penson, Robert Bilger, Gordon Peterson, Martin Schultz, and James Jerger. The second and equally important group is former students, both undergraduate and graduate.

I express my sincere appreciation to Bob Bilger, David Fabry, Larry Feth, Ted Glattke, Ray Kent, Dianne Van Tasell, and Dix Ward for their careful reading of a manuscript for the first edition and for their excellent suggestions for improvement. Edward Carney provided valuable consultation and assistance to aid in the preparation of many of the technically difficult illustrations for the third edition. Several of the illustrations were created with PLT, plotting software from the Communications Engineering Laboratory, Boys Town National Research Hospital (BTNRH). The software is free and may be obtained from the BTNRH web site—www.boystown.org.

Monica Ray Zobitz worked diligently and creatively to prepare most of the illustrations using CorelDraw. Her editorial assistance with, and substantive contributions to, the final manuscript were invaluable. Angie, Sadanand, Marie, Sandy, and others at Singular Publishing Group are marvelous professionals, and I am particularly grateful to Angie for suggesting the selective use of blue screen to enliven many of the illustrations.

Finally, I wish to thank Nancy Niccum for her encouragement and patience, and Nancy, Brandon, and Jeffrey for the time that could not be devoted to them.

The Nature of Sound Waves

What is sound? One can hardly resist referring to a question that often is posed in high school science courses. "If a tree falls in a forest and no one is around to hear it, is there sound?" Put in more modern terms, "If the Muzak system in the elevator is turned on, but there are no passengers, is there sound?"

Albers (1970) stated that sound "in the strict sense, is a compressional wave that produces a sensation in the human ear" (p. 36). We need not worry for the moment what Albers meant by a "compressional wave," but his reference to producing a "sensation of hearing" deserves comment. When "sensation of hearing" is included in the definition of sound, we emphasize *psychological* attributes of sound: pitch, loudness, and timbre. In other words, from a psychological point of view, "sound is what we hear."

We certainly are aware of the many "sounds" around us—sounds such as human speech, the barking of a dog, the crying of an infant, the cooing of a dove or of a "significant other," music of all forms, thunder, traffic noises, and the exhilarating roar of water cascading down the side of a mountain. A psychological approach to defining sound might have an intuitive appeal because it might seem that it would be easy to understand the *physical events* that characterize sound by reference to the psychological sensations or feelings that are associated with the myriad of sounds that we experience daily.

An alternative is to define sound from a *physical* perspective. In this case, sound is defined by reference to properties of the *source* of the event that we call "sound" and to properties of a *medium* in which, or along which, sound is transmitted. When *physical* properties of sound are emphasized, sound is considered to exist *even if the receiver is absent or is not functional*. In other words, sound does exist even if no one is in the forest or if the elevator is empty. To understand the nature of sound, we must identify and describe the physical characteristics of the events that take place among the trees or within the high-rise building.

Many things can serve as a source of sound: vocal folds; the strings of a piano, guitar, or violin; the membrane on a drum; the bars of a xylophone; the metal plates of cymbals; the whistle; the tapping of heel and toe in dance; and so on. We shall see that there is one principal prerequisite for a body to be a source of sound—it must be able to vibrate. If a body is to be set into vibratory motion, it must have the physical properties of **mass** and **elasticity**, and all bodies in nature possess both of those two properties to some degree.

When something happens to those potential sources *that causes them to be set into vibratory motion, or oscillation*, sound occurs, and the sound that is created can then be transmitted from the source through or along some medium. Air is probably the most common medium that we are likely to encounter. But, as we shall see, other molecular structures such as, for example, water, wires, strings, or steel rails also can transmit sound. Because all molecular structures have some finite **mass** and **elasticity**, all are capable of being both a source of sound and a medium for its transmission. Of course, some structures will be more effective sources or more effective transmitters than others.

Although the properties that permit a structure to be a source of sound are essentially identical to the properties that permit a medium to transmit sound, it is convenient to describe the properties of the transmitting medium and the properties of the source separately.

■ PROPERTIES OF THE TRANSMITTING MEDIUM

Consider the medium of air. Air consists of approximately 400 billion billion (4×10^{20}) molecules per cubic inch (in.). In the quiescent state (before a source of sound has been energized), the molecules are in random motion and are moving at speeds that average nearly 940 miles per hour (mph), which corresponds to 1,500 kilometers per hour (kph). During that random motion they maintain some *average distance* from one another, which allows us to envision the molecules as being distributed fairly evenly throughout the air space.

The billions upon billions of molecules exert a pressure on whatever they come in contact with. When, for example, the random motion causes the air molecules to impinge on the human eardrum (or any other structure), pressure is exerted on the drum. Interestingly, as we shall see later, that does not produce a sensation of "hearing" sound. At sea level that pressure, which also is called "atmospheric pressure," amounts to about 14.7 pounds (lb) per square in., and 14.7 lb/in.^{2} in the English measurement system is equivalent to approximately 100,000 newtons (N) per square meter (N/m^2) or 1,000,000 dynes per square centimeter (dynes/cm^2) in the metric system. The N/m^2 and dyne/cm^2 as measures of pressure will be defined later when the concepts of both force and pressure are developed more fully.

To conceptualize the pressure in air, consider the cylindrical tube shown in Figure 1–1, which has a cross-sectional area equal to 1 in.^{2} and extends from sea level to a height of 25 miles. At sea level, in the quiescent state, there is a pressure acting downward that amounts to approximately 14.7 lb/in.^{2}. At 10 miles above sea level, the pressure is reduced to about 1.57 lb/in.^{2}, and at the height of 25 miles it is only a negligible 0.039 lb/in.^{2}.

Air, and all other bodies that can serve to transmit sound, is characterized by two important physical properties: **mass** and **elasticity**.

Mass

By **mass** we mean *the amount of matter that is present*. Air is gaseous matter, but the definition of mass also holds for the two other forms of matter: liquids and solids.

Mass Contrasted with Weight

Mass is often confused with **weight**, and it is important to distinguish between them. Whereas **mass** refers to the quantity of matter

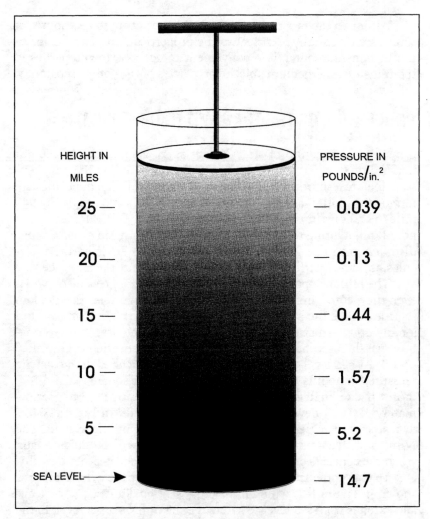

Figure 1–1. A cylindrical tube with a cross-sectional area of 1 in.^{2} that reflects how **pressure** and **density** in an air medium vary with height above sea level.

present, **weight** refers to *the attractive gravitational force exerted on a mass by the earth*. For example, a person is said to weigh 160 lb because the earth attracts the person with a force of 160 lb. However, if the person is flown to the moon, the same amount of matter will be present, but because of the lessened gravitational pull, the weight will only amount to about 27 lb because the force of gravity is only about one-sixth as great on the moon as it is on earth. The weight of an object *is directly proportional to its mass*, but weight and mass are simply different concepts. **Weight** is a force, whereas **mass** is the quantity of matter present.

Although it might be hard to imagine, air has weight as well as mass. A cubic meter of air weighs about 1.3 kilograms (kg), and the air in a classroom with the dimensions of $9 \times 12 \times 4$ m weighs about

560 kg. For those who are not yet comfortable with meters and kilo-grams, a cubic yard (yd) of air weighs 35.1 ounces (oz), and the air in a classroom with the dimensions of $30 \times 40 \times 12$ feet (ft) weighs about 1,170 lb. From that we might conclude that professors who deliver long lectures in a classroom of that size are truly "throwing a lot of weight around."

Mass and Density

It is also useful to distinguish between **mass** and **density**. Look again at the cylindrical tube filled with air in Figure 1–1. Notice that the air molecules are shown to be crowded together very closely (dark-ened regions) near the bottom of the tube, whereas they are rather far apart (lighter regions) in the higher portions of the tube. This occurs because of the pull of gravity.

Because of the force of gravity, the molecules of the atmosphere accumulate near the surface of the earth. There exists, therefore, a downward force or pressure (the distinction between force and pres-sure will be made subsequently) and the molecules are compressed into a smaller volume. The volume near the bottom of the tube is more densely packed, and when a greater number of molecules is compressed into a volume of a certain size, the **density** is increased.

Density (ρ) is *the amount of mass per unit volume*. For example, if we exert a force that causes a volume of 1 cubic in. of air to contain 800 billion billion (8×10^{20}) molecules instead of 400 billion billion (4×10^{20}), the density—the mass per unit volume—would double. It is easy to see in Figure 1–1 that *the amount of mass per unit volume in the cylinder decreases with increasing height above sea level.*

It might be difficult to imagine the different densities associated with the invisible molecules in volumes of air, but there are more visible examples that should serve to make the distinction between mass and density clear. Imagine a grocery bag with a volume of 0.06 cubic meter (about 2 cubic ft [2 ft³]) that is filled with 50 loosely crumpled sheets of newspaper. If you now pack the paper more tight-ly until the same amount of paper (50 sheets) occupies only half of the bag's volume (0.03 cubic meters [0.03 m³]; about 1 cubic ft [1 ft³]), the same amount of matter is present—the **mass**—but the matter will be packed into a smaller volume. After compression, the amount of mass per cubic meter—the **density**—has doubled.

With respect to the first property of a transmitting medium, it is useful to refer to both the **mass** of a medium and to the **density** of a medium, a quantity derived from mass. We shall subsequently explain more explicitly what is meant by "a quantity that is *derived from another quantity.*"

Elasticity (E)

The second property of a transmitting medium is **elasticity**. All mat-ter, whether gaseous, liquid, or solid, undergoes distortion of either shape or volume or both when a force is applied to it. Moreover, all matter is characterized by the tendency to "recover" from that distortion. The property that enables recovery from distortion to either shape or volume is called **elasticity**. We shall see subsequently that elasticity is more properly defined as *the ability to resist changes in shape or volume* rather than the ability to recover from such changes.

Imagine a weight attached to a spring that is suspended from the ceiling. When the spring is stretched and then released, it returns to its original unstretched position (and beyond, but that will be the subject of a later topic), unless it has been "overloaded." By "overloaded" we mean that the original stretching of the spring was sufficient to exceed what is called its **elastic limit**. If the applied force exceeds the elastic limit, deformation is permanent. If the applied force exceeds the elastic limit by a sufficient amount, the object breaks.

A portable radio has a spring that holds the battery in place. If you remove the spring, you can verify that it is relatively easy to stretch it so far that it will not "spring back" when released. Its elastic limit was exceeded. In some forms of matter, the elastic limit is very small. In other forms of matter, such as tempered steel, the elastic limit is very large. The elastic limit of air is so very large that it need not concern us.

With air, the concept of elasticity can mean *the tendency of a volume of air to return to its former volume after compression.* Return again to the air-filled cylinder in Figure 1–1. We know that air molecules are present, that they are in random motion, that—on the average—they are equidistant from one another, and that the density of the air is greater near the bottom of the tube.

Suppose we now insert a plunger into the cylinder and push downward. All of the molecules that were present in the full length of the tube will now be crowded into a smaller space; the **density** is increased. When the plunger is removed, the air molecules return to their former "position," or more appropriately, the air volume resumes the density that existed before compression. The density of the air is said to be *restored*, and the restoring force is called **elasticity**.

■ PROPERTIES OF THE SOUND SOURCE

Let us turn now from a discussion of transmitting media to a consideration of bodies that can serve as a source of sound. We will be concerned with the same two properties that characterized the transmitting medium: **mass** (or density) and **elasticity**.

Vibratory Motion of a Tuning Fork

One object that can serve as a source of sound is a tuning fork, as shown in Figure 1–2. The tuning fork is a U-shaped metal bar. The prongs, or tines, of the fork have **mass** (a quantity of matter is present) and they also possess the restoring force of **elasticity**. Because of

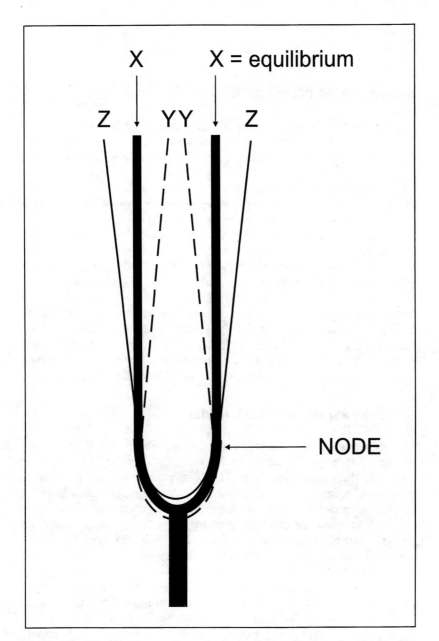

Figure 1–2. The vibratory pattern of a tuning fork, a U-shaped metal bar with the properties of **mass** and **elasticity**. Once struck, the tines move from **X** (equilibrium), to **Y** (maximum displacement in one direction), back to **X**, to **Z** (maximum displacement in the other direction), and back to **X** to complete one **cycle** of vibration.

their elasticity, the tines of the fork will return to their former position after they have been displaced. This can be best illustrated by striking the fork gently with a soft hammer. The tines will be set into

vibration, which takes the form of each tine moving back and forth—the two tines will always move in opposite directions.[1]

Displacement From Equilibrium

Imagine a microscopic view of the pattern of vibration of the two tines. The position of the fork before a force is applied is called its *equilibrium position*, and the heavy solid lines labeled **X** in Figure 1–2 show equilibrium for the fork. When the hammer strikes the fork, a force is applied that causes the tines to be displaced from equilibrium. The force causes both tines to move inward toward positions **Y**, which are shown with the dashed lines.

The amplitude of displacement is proportional to the magnitude of force applied. In other words, the harder we strike the fork with the hammer, the greater the amplitude of displacement from equilibrium. Upon reaching maximum points of displacement inward, *the tines' motion is momentarily halted*, and then, because of the restoring force of elasticity, the tines return toward equilibrium, **X**. Motion does not cease after the tines have returned to positions **X** by the restoring force of elasticity. Instead, the tines continue to move through equilibrium toward maximum displacement in the opposite direction, which is shown by the thin solid lines labeled **Z**.

Newton's First Law of Motion: Inertia

The reason that the tines continue to move beyond equilibrium to a maximum outward displacement (**Z**) is explained by the first of Sir Isaac Newton's three laws of motion: *All bodies remain at rest or in a state of uniform motion unless another force acts in opposition.* In other words, the tines (and stem) move through and beyond the positions of equilibrium until a reaction, or restoring, force *stops* such motion. The property that Newton's first law addressed is called **inertia**, and his first law can be stated differently as *the tendency of a body in motion to remain in motion, and the tendency of a body at rest to stay at rest.*

The amount of **inertia** that an object has is directly proportional to the **mass** of the object. In fact, we may think of mass, the quantity of matter present, as a *measure of inertia*. Thus, a massive object such as a steel ball with a circumference of 1 meter has considerable inertia in comparison with the more negligible mass and inertia of a ping-pong ball. Because of the large inertia of the steel ball, a large force is required to start it in motion, to stop its motion, or to change the direction of its motion. In contrast, a ping-pong ball can easily be set into motion, its motion can easily be stopped, and the direction of its motion can easily be changed.

Vibratory Motion

We have seen, then, that the fork was displaced (toward **Y**) by application of an external force, and that the magnitude of displacement was proportional to the force applied. Next, we saw that the restoring force of **elasticity** (F_r) caused the tines to return toward equilibrium (**X**), and an **inertial force** (F_i) caused the tines to move *through equilibrium* toward maximum displacement in the opposite direction (**Z**). The process continues as the restoring force of elasticity returns the tines back toward equilibrium (**X**), the force of inertia causes the tines to be displaced beyond equilibrium (**Y**), and so on.

Because of the interaction of the two opposing forces, **elasticity** (an elastic restoring force, F_r) and **inertia** (an inertial force, F_i), the tines of the fork continue to move to and fro, and the fork is set into **vibration**. It is convenient to refer to displacement in one direction as positive (+) and displacement in the opposite direction as negative (−); the designation of which direction is positive and which is negative is arbitrary.

Vibratory motion consists of back and forth movement of a body that has **mass** and **elasticity**, and because all bodies are characterized by some finite amount of mass and elasticity, all are capable of being set into vibratory motion. The back and forth motion occurs as the result of two opposing forces: **inertial force** (F_i) and **elastic restoring force** (F_r).

Newton's Third Law of Motion: Reaction Forces

The fact that two forces are operating rather than one is consistent with Newton's third law of motion, which states: *with every force there must be associated an equal reaction force of opposite direction.* A hammer, on striking a nail, exerts a force on the nail. The nail exerts an equal, but opposite, force on the hammer to cause a rapid deceleration of its movement.

Another example of a reaction force can be observed by pushing your hand against the edge of a desk. You are exerting a force on the desk. You should notice, though, that the shape of your hand has been distorted, and that distortion occurs because of the reaction force exerted on your hand by the desk. The reaction force exerted on your hand occurs because the desk is elastic. All solid materials possess some degree of elasticity, and because of their elasticity they can exert forces on other objects.

Newton's third law tells us that *a force cannot exist alone*, which is why it is impossible to have a one-person tug of war. A more familiar, but distressing analogy, is to consider why a car gets stuck in the snow. Because of the slippery snow, we cannot develop sufficient frictional force to "push the car out." It is stuck, and even a powerful engine might not alter that unhappy state. Instead, we must develop sufficient traction by spreading a substance, such as sand, or by digging down to the earth so that the "push of the ground" causes the car to move.

In terms of the tuning fork, after the original force was applied to cause the tines to be displaced, the tines moved in one direction due to the force of inertia, and the movement continued in that direction until the **inertial force** ($\mathbf{F_i}$) was overcome by the **elastic restoring force** ($\mathbf{F_r}$). In other words, *elasticity serves as the "reaction force" to inertia.*

An important feature of the vibratory motion of a tuning fork (and of other sources of sound) is that *we do not need constant reapplication of the external force* that produced the initial displacement from equilibrium. The opposing forces of inertia and elasticity sustain the movement of the fork much as one push of a child's swing in the park is sufficient to keep the child swinging for some time. Movement of the tines from equilibrium to maximum displacement in one direction, back to equilibrium, to maximum displacement in the opposite direction, and finally back to equilibrium is called one **cycle** of vibration. Many such cycles of vibration will occur before the vibratory motion is finally stopped, and then we must strike it again to achieve additional vibration.

■ SOUND SOURCE ACTING ON A MEDIUM

We have seen that **mass** and **elasticity** are the two critical properties of both the source of sound and of the medium that transmits sound. Next, let us place the tuning fork in a medium such as air, apply an external force to cause the tines to be displaced, and see how the moving tines affect the surrounding air medium.

Those effects are illustrated in Figure 1–3. The rows, from top to bottom, represent discrete positions of the tines of the tuning fork and of individual air molecules at various moments in time during vibratory movement: equilibrium, maximum displacement (+), equilibrium, maximum displacement in the opposite direction (−), equilibrium, and so on. Each column, from left to right, shows the position of a single air molecule.

Movement of Air Particles

In the top row the molecules are shown to be equidistant from one another before they are energized by the moving tines. Imagine, then, that the tuning fork has been vibrating to and fro for some time and that, with considerable license, it is possible to visualize the effects of the moving tines on the air molecules, one by one, over time.

The vibratory motion of the fork exerts a force on molecule **A**. In Row 2, we see that molecule **A** is displaced from equilibrium to some maximum displacement that is proportional to the magnitude of force applied. The molecule has also been set into vibratory motion and it moves back and forth (from row to row) about its position of equilibrium—because of the opposing **inertial forces** ($\mathbf{F_i}$) and **elastic restoring forces** ($\mathbf{F_r}$)—in the same way that was described for tuning fork tines.

The movement of molecule **A**, in turn, exerts a force on molecule **B**, causing it to commence vibratory motion, and this applica-

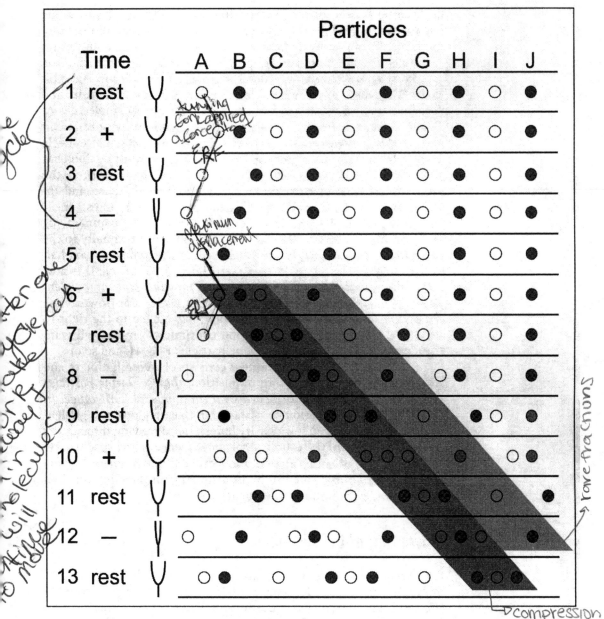

Figure 1–3. Displacement of individual air particles due to the vibratory motion of a tuning fork. Each particle moves back and forth over an infinitesimally small distance about its average position. The darker shaded area traces a compression moving to the right over time, and the lighter shaded area traces a rarefaction, also moving to the right over time.

tion of forces is spread from molecule to molecule (from column to column) much as you see when you flick the first of a long row of standing dominoes.

Figure 1–3 enables us to make a distinction between **particle movement** and **wave propagation**. Look at the molecule, or particle, in Column A as it moves through three **cycles** of vibration from the top row to the bottom row. Particle **A** and, in turn, each of the other particles, simply oscillate to and fro about their average equilibrium positions. *The medium is not displaced over an appreciable distance.*

Next look at the darker shaded area of the figure. In row six, molecule **A** is maximally displaced to the right, **B** is at equilibrium, and **C** is maximally displaced to the left. As a consequence, molecules **A**, **B**, and **C** are crowded closely together; *that region in space is now in a state of high **density***, a state called **compression**. One-quarter cycle later (row seven), the region of high **density**, or **compression**, has moved to the right to involve particles **B**, **C**, and **D**. Over time, the **compression** continues to move rightward through space and involves particles **C**, **D**, and **E**, then particles **D**, **E**, and **F**, and so on.

Now look at the lighter shaded area of the figure, commencing with column D and row six. Particle **C** has moved maximally to the left, particle **D** is at equilibrium, and particle **E** has moved maximally to the right. The region in space associated with particle **D** is now thinned, or rarefied; *that region in space is now in a state of low **density***, a state called **rarefaction**. One-quarter cycle later (row seven), the region of low **density**, or **rarefaction**, has moved to the right to particle **E**. Over time, the **rarefaction** continues to move rightward through space to locations involving particles **F**, **G**, **H**, and so on.

In summary, **particle movement** consists of an oscillation to and fro about the average equilibrium position; *the oscillating particles in the medium are not displaced over an appreciable distance.* In contrast, **wave propagation** consists of alternate regions of **high density (compressions)** and **low density (rarefactions)** moving through the medium away from the source. As a consequence, some specified region in space that is in a state of **rarefaction** at one moment in time (e.g., column D, row six) will be in a state of **compression** one-half cycle later (e.g., column D, row eight).

Movement of the Air Mass

Recall that in air there are approximately 400 billion billion (4×10^{20}) molecules per cubic in. It therefore makes more sense to talk about the effects of tine movement on the surrounding **air mass** rather than on just a single molecule. This is illustrated in Figure 1–4. The outward movement of the tines toward a positive (+) displacement causes the surrounding air molecules to be crowded, or condensed, or compressed as the force of displacement is passed from molecule to molecule. In other words, there is an increase in **density** of the air because the force of the moving tines causes the molecules to be compressed into a smaller volume. This **compression**, or **condensation**, phase of sound is shown by the darkened bands in Figure 1–4.

As the tines return toward equilibrium because of the elasticity of the fork, the force on the surrounding medium is relieved, and the air molecules also return toward their position of equilibrium. This results in a thinning of the molecules in the sense that they are now

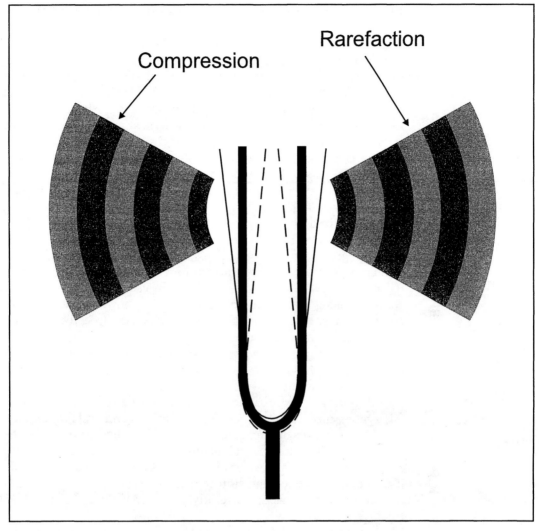

Figure 1–4. Alternate regions of **compression** (darker shading) and **rarefaction** (lighter shading) move outward through an air mass because of the vibratory motion of a tuning fork.

less crowded and the medium is therefore characterized by less density. This **rarefaction** phase of sound is shown in Figure 1–4 by the lightened bands.

As we look at the air mass at points farther and farther from the tuning fork, we see that there are alternate regions in which the molecules are crowded together with an increase in density of the air space (**compression**) and regions in which the molecules are thinned with a decrease in density of the air space (**rarefaction**). These alternate regions of compression and rarefaction are caused by the effects of the moving tines being passed from region to region of the air.

Displacement of the Air Medium and Wave Motion

It is important to emphasize again that *the medium is not displaced over any appreciable distance during this process*. An individual molecule is displaced only over a very small distance. What is moving through the air space is a "wave of disturbance." Alternate regions of increased and decreased density move through the air medium. If we could take a microscopic look at just one region of the air to see how its density changes over time, we would see that its volume is characterized by alternately increased and decreased density. The increased density of one region, in turn, is followed by an increased density of the next region, and so on. Thus, a region characterized by compression in Figure 1–4 at one moment in time will be characterized by rarefaction a brief moment later in time.

In a very elastic medium, such as air, sound is characterized by the *propagation of density changes* through the medium. Although changes in density are propagated through the medium, the individual molecules are not permanently displaced. Think again of the domino analogy. A single domino does not move far—it just falls down. But a wave of disturbance moving along the long row of dominoes should be clearly visible.

An easy way to see wave motion is to observe "the wave" that in recent years has become so popular at many sporting events. The individual spectators move back and forth and, if sober, are not displaced from their seats. If the movements of the spectators are properly synchronized, a "wave" can be seen to move around the stadium.

The properly synchronized flashing of light bulbs can create the same image. The entrance and marquee of some theaters contain long rows of light bulbs that can be alternately illuminated and turned off. If all the lights flash on and off together, we see no "wave." If the electrician times their flashing carefully, however, a "wave" can be seen to move along the row of lights.

In this discussion of properties of both the sound source and the transmitting medium, we have referred to certain physical quantities such as **mass, density, force, pressure, displacement,** and so on. Before we consider the characteristics of sound further, it will be useful to review these and other physical quantities in greater detail.

FUNDAMENTAL PHYSICAL QUANTITIES

There are three **fundamental quantities** in physics: **length, mass,** and **time**. All other quantities can be described in terms of these three, which is to say that quantities other than length, mass, and time are **derived quantities**. To specify the value, or magnitude, of each fundamental quantity, we can use either of two units of measure. One is the English system, and the other is the metric system.

There are two versions of the metric system: the **MKS** and **cgs** systems. With the **MKS** metric system, length is measured in meters (m), mass is measured in kilograms (kg), and time is measured in seconds (s). With the **cgs** metric system, length is measured in centimeters (cm), mass is measured in grams (g), and time is measured in seconds (s).

The English **fps** system is more cumbersome. With this system, length is measured in feet (ft), mass is measured in pounds (p)—although the pound actually is a measure of gravitational force rather than mass—and time is still measured in seconds (s).

We will describe the three fundamental quantities and their derivatives primarily by reference to the metric system. The **MKS** metric system has become the system of choice in physics. The **cgs** system, however, appears in much of the literature that has been written over the decades and we must, therefore, be familiar with both systems and be able to move back and forth between them. Both metric systems will be used throughout this text, but the emphasis will be on the **MKS** system. Only on rare occasions will we persist with reference to the **fps** system.

Length

Length is simply a measure of distance, which is *the extent of spatial separation between any two points*. To determine the magnitude of distance, we select a unit of measure such as the meter (the **MKS** system), and through the process of measurement, we determine how many times this unit (the meter) is contained in a given distance. To measure the length of a board, we select a meterstick (or a yardstick in the **fps** system) and determine how many times the meterstick can be contained over the length of the board.

For many years the meter was defined arbitrarily. In the late 1700s, for example, the meter was defined as 1/10,000,000 of the distance from the equator to the North Pole along the surface of the earth. But confirming that distance proved to be virtually impossible as well as hazardous. New definitions emerged in 1889 and again in 1960. Finally, in 1983 the 46-member General Conference on Weights and Measures met in Paris and agreed to define the meter relative to another of the three fundamental physical quantities—**time**. The speed of light is 299,792,458 meters per second (m/s), and one meter is now defined as the distance traveled by light in a vacuum during 1/299,792,458 of a second.

When we compare the old definition with the new one by showing the relation between meters and inches, it might seem that the change in definition is trivial; 1 m used to equal *about* 39.37 in., but as of 1983, 1 m equals *exactly* 39.37007874 in.; all additional decimal values beyond the 8th decimal equal zero. This seemingly small difference actually is fairly important, at least to the physicist. Previously, 1 in. equaled *approximately* 2.54 cm, but now 1 in. corresponds to *exactly* 2.54 cm and 1 ft now equals *exactly* 0.3048 m. More importantly, the new definition accomplishes a goal that physicists had sought for a long time; the physical quantity **time**, which is the most accurately measured of the three fundamental quantities, is now used to define another physical quantity, **length**.

The metric system, either **MKS** or **cgs**, is very convenient for describing multiples or submultiples of the standard unit of length. All are expressed as multiples of ten (.001, .01, .1, 1, 10, 100, 1,000, and so on). A centimeter (cm) is 1 one-hundredth (.01) of a meter (m), a millimeter (mm) is 1 one-thousandth (.001) of a meter and one-tenth (0.1) of a centimeter, and a kilometer (km) corresponds to 1,000 m. That is why the metric system is less cumbersome than the English system where you must divide by 12 to convert inches to feet; by 3 to convert feet to yards; by 5,280 to convert feet to miles; by 1,760 to convert yards to miles; and so on. Only the submultiples of the inch (1/2, 1/4, 1/8, 1/16, 1/32, 1/64, and so on) possess reasonable regularity.

Mass

Mass, as we discussed previously, is a property of all matter and can be defined as the quantity of matter present. When we use the word "quantity," we mean simply that there is an observable property than can be measured or in some way specified numerically. Recall, also, that it is important to distinguish between **mass** and **weight**. The unit of measure of mass is the kilogram in the **MKS** system and the gram in the **cgs** system. A kilogram is defined as the mass of a cylinder of platinum housed at the International Bureau of Weights and Measures, and a gram is 1/1,000 of a kilogram.

The concept of **mass** is tied inextricably to the concept of **inertia** and the word, mass, is sometimes used to refer to how much inertia a body has. The greater the mass of an object, the greater its inertia.

Time

Time might be the physical quantity that is most easily and accurately measured, but it is also a quantity that is difficult to define in a way that has any intuitive appeal. Daniloff, Schuckers, and Feth (1980), for example, said:

> It is difficult to define *time* without saying that it is that quantity we measure in seconds, minutes, or hours. Any physical event that recurs on a regular basis can be used to mark off equal intervals of time. Thus, the period required for one complete revolution of the earth is identified as one day. (p. 75)

Because a solar day is divided into 24 hours (hr), an hour into 60 min, and a minute into 60 s, each day has 86,400 s. That led to the concept that the second is 1/86,400 of a solar day.

■ DERIVED PHYSICAL QUANTITIES

By a **derived quantity** we simply mean a quantity that is expressed as either a quotient, or a product, of the fundamental quantities or of fundamental and derived quantities. For example, length is a fundamental physical quantity. On the other hand, the *area* of a rectangle is given by the product of two measures of length (usually referred to as the "length" times the "width"), and area, therefore, is a derived physical quantity. Derived quantities of interest in the study of sound include **displacement (x)**, **velocity (c)**, **acceleration (a)**, **force (F)**, and **pressure (p)**.

Displacement (x)

Displacement (x) is defined as *a change in position,* and it is specified by calculating the distance from a reference, or starting position, to a new, or ending position. It is important to note that displacement actually involves two concepts: **distance** and **direction**. A body moves over a certain **distance**, but, for a given distance, the body can move in any number of **directions**. Thus, *to specify displacement we must account for both the direction moved and the distance moved.*

Quantities that are specified by both *magnitude and direction* are called **vector quantities**, or just **vectors**. Consider the examples shown in Figure 1–5. Starting points are shown by an **x** and ending points by an **o**. The length of the line represents the magnitude of distance moved, and the direction the arrow points represents the direc-

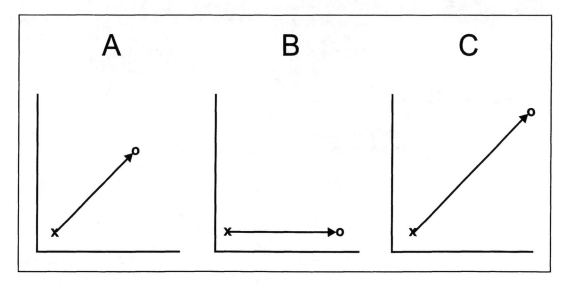

Figure 1–5. Explanation of vector quantities in which the *length* of each line represents the **magnitude of displacement** (distance moved) and the *direction* of the arrow represents the **direction of displacement**.

tion moved. Thus, **A** and **B** have different displacements, because the movement occurred in different directions, even though both are shown to have moved the same distance. Correspondingly, **A** and **C** have different displacements because they occurred over different distances, even though the movements occurred in the same direction. Finally, **B** and **C** have different displacements because their movements are characterized both by different directions and different distances.

Quantities such as **mass, time, energy,** and so forth are specified only by reference to magnitude; they have no direction associated with them. They are called **scalar quantities**, or just **scalars**. The distinction between scalars and vectors is particularly important when we wish to add or subtract the values of some particular quantity. When the quantities are scalars, simple algebraic addition or subtraction is sufficient. **Time** is a scalar. If the time required to travel from point **a** to point **b** is 1 s, and the time required to travel from point **b** to point **c** is 1.5 s, then algebraic addition tells us that the time required to travel from **a** to **c** must be 2.5 s. When the quantities are vectors, we must use methods of vector analysis rather than algebraic addition or subtraction.

Velocity (c)

Velocity (c), probably from the Latin word "celeritas" for quickness, swiftness, or speed, refers to *the amount of displacement per unit time*. Velocity also is a vector quantity because specification of displacement per unit time must incorporate a specification of both the distance moved and the direction moved. Thus, displacement is accomplished during some period of time. If we divide displacement by the time required to complete the displacement, we calculate the **average velocity** of the body that was displaced.

If a motorcycle travels in a northwesterly direction for a distance of 180 kilometers (km), or 112 miles, in 2 hr, the average velocity of travel is 90 kph (56 mph). We are accustomed to think of **speed** rather than velocity in such cases, but speed and velocity are not always equal. Speed corresponds to velocity *when direction is not considered*; speed has only magnitude (a **scalar**), whereas velocity (a **vector**) has both magnitude and direction.

It is easy to understand the distinction between speed and velocity if you imagine you are paddling a canoe across a lake. As you cross the lake, suppose there is no wind and the surface of the water is glassy. You simply aim toward your desired destination and paddle. By the time you are ready to return, suppose a strong wind has come up that is blowing at right angles to your intended path. Now it will be necessary to compensate for the wind by aiming your canoe in a direction different from where you want to end up.

Figure 1–6 illustrates the difference between the speed and velocity of the canoe during the windy condition. Let **x** be the starting point. The length of line S_1 shows the speed with which the canoe is moving in one direction, and the length of line S_2 shows the

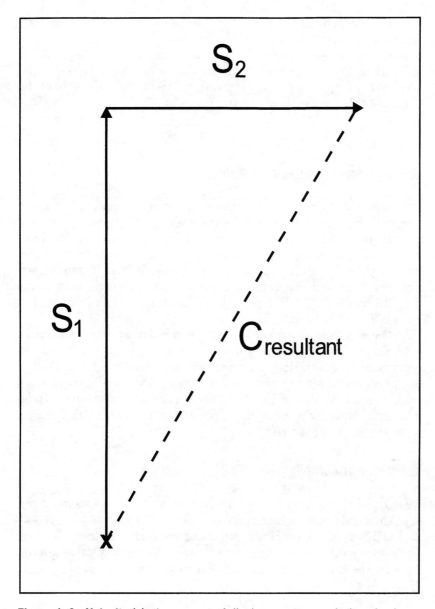

Figure 1–6. Velocity (c), the amount of displacement per unit time, is shown as a vector quantity in relation to the speed of movement in two directions (**S₁** and **S₂**) at right angles to each other.

speed with which the canoe is moving at right angles to the first direction because of the wind. Each of those speeds is given by the simple formula:

$$s = \frac{d}{t}$$

Equation 1.1

where **s** = average speed, **d** = distance, and **t** = time.

The dashed line **c** represents the **resultant velocity**, and its length is greater than the lengths of either of the two lines representing speed alone. We could calculate the value of the resultant velocity by the use of the Pythagorean theorem, which states that the square of the hypotenuse in a right triangle is equal to the sum of the squares of the two sides of the triangle. Thus,

Equation 1.2

$$c_{resultant} = \sqrt{S_1^2 + S_2^2}.$$

Average and Instantaneous Velocity

We previously mentioned the concept of **average velocity**. The motorcycle moved with an average velocity of 90 kph (56 mph), but the rate of movement surely must have varied during the 2-hr trip. To incorporate variability in rate of movement into an understanding of velocity, we distinguish between average velocity and **instantaneous velocity**. Instantaneous velocity is the velocity that is measured over an infinitesimally small time interval, perhaps an interval as small as a millionth or billionth of a second.

The distinction between **average velocity** and **instantaneous velocity** applies also to **speed**. For example, if a car is driven 80 km (approximately 50 miles) in 1 hr, its **average speed** is 80 kph. During the period of travel, the **instantaneous speed**, the speed measured for such a small interval of time that the speed can be considered to be a constant during the interval, might vary over a considerable range from moment to moment.

Summary of Velocity

Velocity (either average or instantaneous), then, is displacement per unit time and it can be expressed in a myriad of ways: meters per second (**MKS** system), centimeters per second (**cgs** system), miles per hour, feet per day, or whatever (**fps** system). We simply calculate the ratio of the measure of displacement to the measure of time with Equation 1.1.

Acceleration (a)

Velocity is defined as *the amount of displacement per unit time.* That is the same as saying that velocity is *the time-rate of displacement.* Just as velocity is the time-rate of displacement, **acceleration** (**a**) is *the time-rate change in velocity.* Acceleration also is a vector quantity; hence a change of velocity in one direction is not the same as a change of velocity in another direction. The magnitude might change, the direction might change, or both might change.

Although it might at first seem strange, an automobile traveling at a constant **speed** around a circular path is undergoing acceleration. If we think about it for a moment, though, it makes sense. The speed might not vary, but the *direction* of motion is constantly changing. If the direction is changing, the velocity must also be changing because the concept of velocity incorporates both speed and direction. Finally, then, if the velocity changes, acceleration must have occurred, because acceleration is the time-rate change in velocity.

If velocity increases, acceleration is said to be "positive," and if velocity decreases, acceleration is said to be "negative." Negative acceleration, of course, is commonly called *deceleration*. Acceleration (**a**) is given by:

$$a = \frac{\Delta c}{t},$$

Equation 1.3

where $\Delta c = c_2 - c_1$.

If a car travels at a velocity of 10 m/s (c_1) and then is accelerated to a velocity of 30 m/s (c_2), and if that change is accomplished in 5 s, acceleration equals 4 m/s/s, which usually is written as 4 m/s^2:

$$a = \frac{(30 - 10)}{5} = 4 \text{ m/s/s} = 4 \text{ m/s}^2.$$

Force (F)

Force (F) is simply a *push* or a *pull*, and is given by *the product of mass* (**m**) *and acceleration* (**a**):

$$F = ma.$$

Equation 1.4

Equation 1.4 is Newton's second law of motion, although his law originally was stated as: *The acceleration of an object is directly proportional to the net force applied to the object and inversely proportional to the object's mass.* Thus, Newton's second law expressed symbolically was $a = F/m$. When both sides of Newton's original equation are multiplied by the mass (**m**), we obtain Equation 1.4, which is the more familiar form of Newton's second law.

An equally correct way to state Newton's second law of motion is that *the net force applied to an object is equal to the mass of the object multiplied by its acceleration.* A force is required to accelerate an object because the object has **mass**, and the object therefore has **inertia**. The inertia of the object serves to oppose a change in motion, and therefore a **force** must be applied to overcome the **inertia**.

Consequences of Applying a Force

Force can produce two consequences that are particularly important for gaining an understanding of both sound sources and sound transmission. First, a force can cause matter to be *distorted*. If a spring is stretched by a pulling force or compressed by a pushing force, the spring is distorted. When the force that produced the distortion is removed, the spring will return to its original condition because of elasticity unless, of course, the force that caused the distortion was sufficiently large that the elastic limit of the spring was exceeded. Second, a force also can cause matter to be *accelerated*. Therefore, we can define **force** not only as a *push* or a *pull*, but also as *that which imparts acceleration to a mass*.

Force as a Vector Quantity

Force also is a vector quantity, and therefore we must specify not only the *magnitude* of force but also the *direction* of force. In other words, it *does* matter whether the force is acting to the left or the right or upward or downward in space. Almost without exception, a force of some magnitude pushing on a body from a southerly direction produces no effect in an easterly direction; the exception will be addressed under the section "The Pendulum: An Example of Slow-Motion Vibration."

Because force is a vector quantity, we must be careful when we speak of the "addition of forces." If we have two forces of exactly the same magnitude acting on the same body, the resultant force will not necessarily have twice the magnitude of one of the forces alone. The resultant force could, in fact, be zero if the equal forces acted from exactly opposite directions, and in that case the body remains at equilibrium. If two people simultaneously apply equal forces to a swinging door, but from opposite directions, the door will not move.

With respect to hearing, you might have reasoned that there is a pressure (the distinction between pressure and force will be made in a moment) of 100,000 N/m^2 (1,000,000 dynes/cm^2) impinging on your eardrums. Fortunately, your eardrums (tympanic membranes) will not "cave in" under this pressure because there is an equal air pressure in your middle ear cavity that produces a force on the eardrums from the opposite direction. That works well, of course, until something happens to reduce the pressure on the outside of the drum such as when you are in an airplane that climbs to 40,000 ft or so. When you feel the pain that results from the differential pressure on the two sides of the eardrum, you might elect to yawn or chew gum. That opens a tube (eustachian tube) that leads from the back of your mouth to the middle ear cavity and restores the pressure to the same value that exists outside the drum.

It is important to remember that a resultant force is not simply the algebraic sum of the two forces. Force is a vector quantity, and vector summation is required to calculate the resultant force. If the two forces operate at right angles to one another, the resultant force could be solved by use of the Pythagorean theorem in the same way that it was used for determining the resultant velocity in Figure 1–6.

Units of Measure for Force

With the **MKS** system, the unit of measure of force is the **newton (N)** in honor of Sir Isaac Newton who first defined force in his second law of motion (Equation 1.4). One **newton** is defined as *the force required to accelerate a mass of 1 kg from a velocity of 0 m/s to a velocity of 1 m/s in 1 s.* In other words, when the mass of 1 kg is stationary, it has a velocity of 0 m/s. If you wish to accelerate that mass so that it will move with a velocity of 1 m/s, and if you wish to accomplish that change in velocity in 1 s, a force must be applied, and the value of that force is defined as 1 N.

With the **cgs** system, the unit of measure of force is the **dyne**. The definition of force in the **cgs** system is equivalent to that described above for the **MKS** system, but the units are changed from kilograms to grams and from meters to centimeters. Thus, one **dyne** is defined as *the force required to accelerate a mass of 1 gram (g) from a velocity of 0 cm/s to a velocity of 1 cm/s in 1 s.* One newton (**MKS**) corresponds to 100,000 dynes (**cgs**).

Pressure (p)

In the study of sound we will not be particularly concerned with measuring, for example, the force exerted by one molecule on another. Instead, we want to determine the sum of many such small forces that act on some surface—the eardrum, for example. To do this we will concern ourselves with *the amount of force per unit area*, which is the **pressure (p)**, as shown in Equation 1.5:

$$p = \frac{F}{A},$$

Equation 1.5

where **F** = the force applied and **A** = area.

Suppose we have a force of 1 N applied uniformly to a surface area of 100 m^2 (100 square meters) such as is shown in Figure 1–7. We could calculate with Equation 1.5 that the pressure, the amount of force per unit area, is 0.01 N/m^2.

Units of Measure for Pressure

Because force is measured in **newtons (MKS)** or **dynes (cgs)**, and because pressure is the amount of force per unit area, the unit of measure of pressure is the **newton per square meter (N/m^2)** in the **MKS** system and the **dyne per square centimeter (dyne/cm^2)** in the **cgs** system. A pressure of 1 N/m^2 in the **MKS** system corresponds to how many dynes/cm^2 in the **cgs** system?

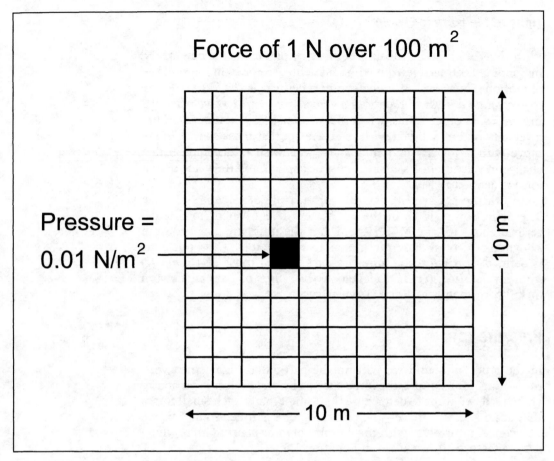

Figure 1–7. A **force** of 1 newton (N) distributed uniformly over an area of 100 m² produces a **pressure**, the amount of force per unit area, of 0.01 N/m².

$$1 \text{ N} = 100,000 \text{ dynes}$$

and

$$1 \text{ m} = 100 \text{ cm}.$$

Therefore, $1 \text{ N/m}^2 = 100,000 \text{ dynes/m}^2$

$$= \frac{100,000 \text{ dynes}}{10,000 \text{ cm}^2},$$

and,

Equation 1.6 $1 \text{ N/m}^2 = 10 \text{ dynes/cm}^2.$

An alternative to the newton per square meter with the **MKS** system is the **pascal (Pa)**. The relations among these three units of measure for pressure are:

Equation 1.7 $1 \text{ Pa} = 1 \text{ N/m}^2 = 10 \text{ dynes/cm}^2.$

VIBRATORY MOTION OF A SPRING-MASS SYSTEM

Now that the fundamental and derived physical quantities have been defined, we can examine the nature of vibratory motion in a different, but more complete, way by reference to a spring-mass system shown in Figure 1–8. One end of a spring is attached to a rigid structure such as a wall, and the other end is attached to a mass that lies on a nearly frictionless surface. An arrow points toward a displacement scale. In panel A of the figure, the arrow points to "0" (equilibrium) on the scale. The mass is at equilibrium because the net force acting on the spring-mass system is zero; hence, there is no motion.

Characteristics of a Spring

A spring is highly elastic. Because of its elasticity, the spring can be displaced from equilibrium either by moving the mass to the left, which *compresses* the spring, or by moving the mass to the right, which *extends*, or *stretches*, the spring. When the spring is compressed, as is shown in panel B of Figure 1–8, the mass is displaced from equilibrium and the arrow in panel B points toward a "−" value on the displacement scale. When the spring is stretched, the mass is displaced from equilibrium in the opposite direction, and the arrow in panel C points toward a "+" value on the displacement scale.

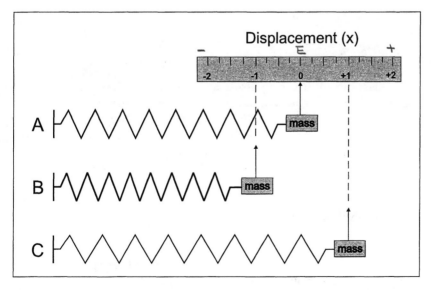

Figure 1–8. A spring-mass system with one end of the spring attached to a rigid structure. In panel A, the spring is in equilibrium, which corresponds to "0" on the displacement scale. In panel B, the spring is compressed, and the mass has moved to "−1" on the displacement scale. In panel C, the spring is stretched (extended), and the mass has moved to "+1" on the displacement scale.

Regardless of whether the spring is compressed or extended, the restoring force of elasticity *opposes* the force that acts to deform the spring. The more the spring is compressed, the greater will be the force required to accomplish additional compression because of the restoring force of elasticity. Stated differently, the magnitude of the restoring force (F_r) of elasticity is directly proportional to the magnitude of the spring's displacement (x), which is called Hooke's law in honor of Robert Hooke who published his observation in the late 1600s. Hooke's law is expressed as:

Equation 1.8
$$F_r = -kx$$

where F_r is the restoring force of elasticity,

x is the magnitude of displacement of the spring, and

k is a spring constant.

The minus sign in Equation 1.8 serves to remind us that the direction of the restoring force is opposite the direction of the displacement.

Stiffness

Although all springs are elastic, some springs require a greater force than others to be either compressed or extended because of differences among springs in **stiffness**. **Stiffness** is the spring constant (k) in Equation 1.8. In other words, the stiffer the spring, the greater the value of k, and the greater the force that is required to compress or stretch the spring some given distance.

Compliance

The elasticity of a spring also can be quantified by a measure of a spring's **compliance**. **Compliance** is inversely related to stiffness, which means that springs with relatively little stiffness are characterized by relatively large compliance. As compliance increases, the force required to compress or stretch the spring decreases. Hence, compliant springs can be displaced from equilibrium more easily than stiff springs.

Vibratory Motion of the System

If the mass in Figure 1–8 is moved to the left and then released, *the system will be set into vibration*. Its motion will be similar in most respects to the motion of the tuning fork that was illustrated in Figure 1–2. The arrow will pass through equilibrium toward a maximum displacement to the left (" – " on the displacement scale) as the spring becomes progressively more compressed. When the restoring force of elasticity (F_r) *overcomes the inertial force* (F_i), *motion is momentarily halted*, and then the direction of motion of the system is reversed. The system then passes through equilibrium toward a maximum displacement to the right ("+" on the displacement scale) as the spring becomes progressively more stretched, and so on.

We shall see in Chapter 2 that the spring-mass system, the tuning fork, and any vibrating system for which the magnitude of the restoring force is directly proportional to the displacement ($F_r \propto x$) are engaged in what is called **simple harmonic**, or **sinusoidal**, **motion**.

■ THE PENDULUM: AN EXAMPLE OF SLOW MOTION VIBRATION

We previously discussed the vibratory motion of the tuning fork and the vibratory motion of air molecules that was occasioned by the motion of the fork. Because the movement of the fork is too rapid to see—and, of course, we certainly cannot see the air molecules, let alone discern how rapidly they are moving—the concept of vibratory motion might be difficult to grasp. We can, however, achieve a more intuitive understanding of vibratory motion by examining the characteristics of a slow-moving vibratory system such as the pendulum shown in Figure 1–9.

The pendulum is shown to be in equilibrium when the bob is at point **X**. Next, let us displace the pendulum to point **Y** and then release it. The pendulum, of course, will return toward equilibrium **X**. It does not stop when it reaches equilibrium, but rather it contin-

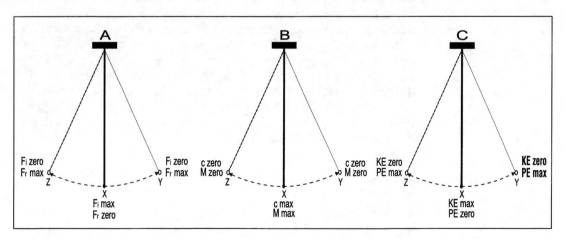

Figure 1–9. Vibratory motion of a pendulum moving from maximum displacement in one direction, through equilibrium, to maximum displacement in the opposite direction, and back to equilibrium. Panel A shows that the inertial force (F_i) is zero at maximum displacement and maximal at equilibrium, whereas the elastic restoring force (F_r) is maximal at maximum displacement and zero at equilibrium. Panel B shows that velocity (c) and momentum (M) are zero at maximum displacement and are maximal at equilibrium. Panel C shows that potential energy (PE) is maximal at maximum displacement and zero at equilibrium, whereas kinetic energy (KE) is maximal at equilibrium and zero at maximum displacement.

ues on toward a maximal displacement in the other direction **Z**. Upon reaching maximal displacement, it will again return toward and beyond the position of equilibrium **X**, and so on. In other words, the motion of the pendulum appears to be very similar to what we saw previously for the tuning fork. Each engages in *vibratory motion*.

In essence, the same kinds of opposing forces that governed the motion of the tuning fork are responsible for the motion of the pendulum, with one important exception. When the pendulum or tuning fork tines are maximally displaced in either direction, they return toward equilibrium because of a **restoring force (F_r)**. With the tuning fork in Figure 1-2 and the spring-mass system in Figure 1–8, the restoring force is **elasticity**. With the pendulum in panel A of Figure 1–9, the restoring force is **gravity**. With this exception in mind, we see that the pendulum is restored to equilibrium from maximal displacement because of the restoring force of gravity, and it moves beyond its position of equilibrium toward maximal displacement because of **inertia (F_i)**.

The pendulum continues to move toward maximal displacement until the restoring force of gravity (F_r) overcomes the force of inertia (F_i). At the point of maximal displacement, the inertial value is zero, the restoring force of gravity is maximal, *and motion is momentarily halted*. As the pendulum then moves back toward equilibrium, the restoring force of gravity diminishes and the force of inertia increases. When the pendulum reaches equilibrium, the net force of gravity on the motion is zero and the force of inertia is maximal, which results in the continuation of motion toward a new displacement in the opposite direction.

When the concept of **force** as a vector quantity was introduced, we stated that "it *does* matter whether the force is acting to the left or the right or upward or downward in space. Almost without exception, a force of some magnitude pushing on a body from a southerly direction produces no effect in an easterly direction." The vibratory motion of the pendulum is an exception. We will consider the downward-acting gravitational force to be in a "southerly" direction, and the path of excursion of the pendulum to be in an "easterly-westerly" direction. In this circumstance, it is clear that the force of gravity in a southerly direction *does affect* the vibratory motion that takes place in an easterly-westerly direction.

Momentum

As we continue to think of the opposing forces that result in vibratory motion, it will be convenient to substitute the effect of **momentum** for the force of inertia. **Momentum (M)** is defined as *the product of mass (m) and velocity (c)*, as shown in Equation 1.9:

Equation 1.9
$$M = mc.$$

Thus, **momentum** is directly proportional to both **mass** (the amount of matter present) and **velocity** (the time-rate of displacement); as either mass or velocity increases, momentum increases. A large car traveling with the same velocity as a smaller car has greater momentum because of its greater **mass**. Similarly, if two cars have identical mass, momentum is greater for the car traveling with the greater **velocity**. With respect to the moving pendulum, we see in panel B of Figure 1–9 that momentum is maximal and the net force acting on the pendulum is zero when the pendulum is at (passing through) equilibrium. At maximal displacement in either direction, momentum is zero and the force of gravity is maximal.

Why does the pendulum gain momentum as it moves toward equilibrium? In Equation 1.9, examine the two quantities that determine momentum, and then recall the discussion of fundamental and derived physical quantities. Momentum of the pendulum does not change because of a change in **mass**—the quantity of matter present remains the same. It follows, therefore, that momentum must change because of a change in **velocity**. In other words, as the pendulum moves from maximum displacement toward equilibrium, momentum increases because the velocity of motion increases. In summary, at maximum displacement, *where motion is momentarily halted*, both **M** and **c** are zero. As the pendulum passes through equilibrium, both **M** and **c** are maximal.

The Energy Principle

Movement of the pendulum, as well as that of other matter set into vibratory motion, also can be described by the **energy principle**. According to the **law of conservation of energy**, any system that can do work (such as the pendulum, the tuning fork, the spring-mass system, or any other body that can be set into vibratory motion) must receive a supply of energy from somewhere.

What is energy? **Energy** is an abstract concept that refers to something that can produce a *change* in matter such as, for example, displacement of a mass, distortion of the shape of solid matter, expansion of gases, and so forth. When a change in matter occurs, **work** has been done, and **energy** is *a measure of the capacity to do work*. One way to distinguish between energy and work is to realize that **energy** is something that a body *possesses*, whereas **work** is something that a body *does*.

Work

Work is accomplished only when *a **force** succeeds in moving the body that the force acts upon*, and the quantity of work that is accomplished is given by *the product of the magnitude of force applied and the distance moved*:

$$W = Fd,$$ **Equation 1.10**

where **F** = the force applied and **d** = the distance moved.

If a force does not give rise to motion, no work has been done. The act of pushing against a cement wall with a force of 50 N accomplishes no work unless, miraculously, the wall is moved through some distance.

With the **MKS** system, force is expressed in newtons and distance is expressed in meters. The unit of measure of **work** in the **MKS** system is the **joule**. One joule of work is accomplished if a force of 1 N acts through a distance of 1 m (1 joule = 1 N × 1 m). In the **cgs** system, the unit of measure of **work** is the **erg** (1 erg = 1 dyne × 1 cm). To relate the two units of measure of **work**, 1 joule = 10,000,000 ergs:

$$1 \text{ N} = 100,000 \ (10^5) \text{ dynes,}$$

and $$1 \text{ m} = 100 \ (10^2) \text{ cm.}$$

Therefore, $$1 \text{ joule} = 100,000 \ (10^5) \text{ dynes} \times 100 \ (10^2) \text{ cm}$$
$$= 10,000,000 \ (10^7) \text{ ergs}$$

Transformation of Energy

As we stated before, energy cannot be depleted, but rather it is transformed from one form to another, or it is transferred from one place to another. If you wind the spring on an old fashioned clock, the spring gains energy as it is wound. In turn, it loses energy as it does work on the clock. If you pull the trigger on a rifle, exploding gases do work on the bullet, which gives energy to the bullet. When the bullet strikes an object, it does work on the object and loses energy.

Return now to the pendulum shown in panel C of Figure 1–9. When the pendulum is raised from equilibrium to maximum displacement, the pendulum gains **potential energy (PE)**, which is a form of *stored energy*. In the case of the pendulum, potential energy can be thought of as *an energy of position*, and it sometimes is called **gravitational potential energy**; it has potential energy because of the gravitational attraction of the earth.

The potential energy associated with the pendulum in its raised position is transferred, or converted, to *an energy of motion* when released, which is called **kinetic energy (KE)**. When the pendulum reaches the equilibrium position, potential energy is zero and kinetic energy is maximal. As the pendulum continues to move beyond equilibrium to maximum displacement, kinetic energy is converted to potential energy, and at maximum displacement, kinetic energy is zero and potential energy is maximal.

At all points during the excursion, the sum of **PE** and **KE** *remains constant*, and that defines the **total energy** in accordance with the **law of conservation of energy**. According to that law, energy can be transformed from one kind to another, but energy is never created or destroyed—the total energy remains a constant.

Frictional Resistance

In the case of the pendulum, the tuning fork, and the spring-mass system discussed earlier, we have proceeded as if vibratory motion continues indefinitely. Actually, that is not the case because of *opposition to motion by the force of **friction***. Because **friction** opposes, or resists, motion, it serves to limit velocity of motion. As the pendulum swings along its path, friction at the point of suspension and friction on the bob of the pendulum due to air resistance cause energy to be *transformed* from **kinetic energy** to **thermal energy** (heat). Because of the opposing force of friction, the amplitude of each excursion of the pendulum is less than the amplitude of the previous excursion.

In Chapter 2 we will refer to this diminishing amplitude as **damping**, or **damped vibration**. Resistance to motion attributable to friction, which sometimes is called **frictional resistance**, or just **resistance**, is analogous to electrical resistance, which serves to oppose, or impede, the flow of electrical current in an electrical circuit. We will return to the concept of **transfer of energy** when we discuss sound wave propagation.

Characteristics of Pendular Motion

There are two important characteristics of the vibratory motion of the pendulum, **amplitude** and **frequency**.

Amplitude

The first characteristic is **amplitude** of displacement. Amplitude of displacement, a derived physical quantity, is *a vector quantity that incorporates both magnitude and direction of displacement*. The amplitude of displacement of the pendulum is proportional to the force applied.

Frequency

The second characteristic is **frequency** of vibratory motion. We noted earlier that when the tines of a tuning fork move from equilibrium to maximum displacement (+), back through equilibrium (0), to maximum displacement in the opposite direction (−), and finally back to equilibrium (0), we have completed one **cycle** of vibration. The same is true with the pendulum. Movement from **X** to **Y** to **X** to **Z** and back to **X** in Figure 1–9 defines one cycle of pendular vibration. **Frequency (f)** refers to *the rate of vibratory motion, that is, the number of cycles completed per second* (**cps**). Thus, if the pendulum completes four cycles each second, **f** = 4 cps. If the rate of motion were increased so that 25 cycles are completed each second, then **f** = 25 cps.

The unit of measure for frequency has been changed from **cycles per second (cps)** to **hertz (Hz)** to honor Henrich Hertz, a German physicist. Conversion between **cps** and **Hz** is simple: 1 **Hz** = 1 **cps**. Thus, for the two examples mentioned above, **f** = 4 Hz (4 cps) and **f** = 25 Hz (25 cps).

Frequency is the number of *cycles per second*. We also can calculate the number of *seconds per cycle*, that is, *the amount of time required to complete just **one cycle***. That defines the **period (T)** of vibration. Thus, if the pendulum completes 4 cycles of vibration in 1 s (**f** = 4 Hz), then 1 cycle must be completed in 1/4 s. Similarly, if **f** = 25 Hz, one cycle must be completed in 1/25 s. For those two examples, we say that the period (**T**) is 1/4 (.25) s and 1/25 (.04) s.

You might already have noticed that conversion from frequency to period or from period to frequency is fairly simple:

Equation 1.11

$$T = \frac{1}{f}$$

and

Equation 1.12

$$f = \frac{1}{T}.$$

Thus, if **f** = 4, **T** = 1/4 (.25), and if **T** = .25, **f** = 1/.25 = 4. When we divide 1 by some number, we are *taking the reciprocal of that number*. Thus, we say that period is the reciprocal of frequency and that frequency is the reciprocal of period.

Frequency and **amplitude** are independent characteristics of pendular motion (the value of one does not depend on the value of the other), but **frequency** and **period** are not independent.[2] The value of one completely determines the value of the other.

Determinants of Frequency of Vibration for a Pendulum

What properties of the pendulum determine the **period** and **frequency** of vibration? It is tempting to think that you might increase the frequency (and thereby decrease the period) if a greater force were applied. Recall, however, that the magnitude of force applied determines the magnitude of displacement, hence, the amplitude of vibration.

If you recall the child's swing, you should realize that the swing moves at the same rate no matter how hard you push. It can be displaced farther in response to a greater force, but it will not move with a greater frequency. The more experienced child, however, learns that you can swing faster (with greater vibratory frequency) by looping the rope around the supporting structure a few times. When that is done, the swing (or pendulum) is shorter, and the *length* of the pendulum is the principal determinant of frequency of pendular vibration.

The equation for the period (T) of the pendulum is:

Equation 1.13

$$T = 2\pi\sqrt{\frac{L}{G}},$$

where **L** = length and **G** = gravitational force.

Thus the **period** of pendular vibration *is directly proportional to the square root of the length*, which means that as length increases, period increases, and as length decreases, period decreases. But, because frequency and period are inversely related, we see that **frequency** *is inversely related to the square root of the length*. That, of course, is what we learned from the child who shortened the length of the rope in order to "swing" more rapidly.

The dependence of frequency of vibration of a pendulum on length was first discovered by Galileo when he observed the swing of lamps hanging in the cathedral at Pisa. The frequency of swing of the lamps never changed. Gravity, of course, is a constant in the equation with a value of 9.8 m/s^2 or 980 (more precisely, 981.456) cm/s^2. Those values are the metric equivalents of 32.2 ft per s per s (32.2 ft/s^2) in the **fps** system of measurement.

We have discussed two principal characteristics of pendular vibration. The first is **amplitude**, which is directly proportional to the force applied. The second is **frequency**, which is inversely proportional to the length of the pendulum, and frequency is the reciprocal of the period. The concepts of amplitude and frequency will be used subsequently to help define characteristics of vibratory motion in general, not just the movement of the pendulum.

■ PROPORTIONALITY

It might be helpful to elaborate on what is meant by **inversely proportional** and **directly proportional**. When **A** is *inversely proportional* to **B**, as **B** decreases **A** increases and, conversely, as **B** increases, **A** decreases. An inverse relation can be stated simply as:

$$A \propto \frac{1}{B},$$

Equation 1.14

which means that **A** is inversely proportional to **B**.

Equations 1.11 and 1.12 that specified the relation of frequency and period were of the form shown in Equation 1.14, which means that frequency and period are inversely related.

When **A** is *directly proportional* to **B**, as **B** increases, **A** increases, and as **B** decreases, **A** decreases. Direct proportionality can be described in the form:

$$A \propto B,$$

Equation 1.15

which means that **A** is directly proportional to **B**.

Consider Equation 1.13 for the period of a pendulum. **L** appeared in the numerator, which means that period and length are directly related, and as we saw previously, period is directly proportional to the square root of length.

It is easy to inspect an equation and know if you are dealing with an inverse or direct relation. To determine if **A** is directly or inversely related to **B**, look at **B** in the equation. If **B** appears in the denominator of the ratio, **A** is *inversely related* to **B**. If **B** appears in the numerator of the ratio, **A** is *directly related* to **B**. What if there is no ratio? If there *appears* to be no ratio because there is no denominator (actually, the denominator has a value of "1"), the proportional relation takes the form shown in Equation 1.15, A $\propto$ B. An example appeared in Equation 1.9, which expressed that momentum (**M**) was directly proportional to both mass (**m**) and velocity (**c**).

■ SOUND WAVE PROPAGATION

Let us return now to a sound wave that results from the vibratory motion of some mass. Suppose a source of sound is energized—a tuning fork, for example, is struck. As shown in Figure 1–4, the action produces a wave of compression that moves through the air medium. As we learned earlier, the individual air molecules move back and forth about their average positions of equilibrium, *but they do not move over a great distance*. In fact, particle displacement is on the order of 0.0000000768 (7.68×10^{-8}) m. Because of the force that was applied to them, the movement of those particles produces alternate regions of increased density (**compression**) and decreased density (**rarefaction**), and it is that disturbance that is propagated through the medium.

In our previous discussion of vibratory motion, we considered the pendulum (an example of slow-motion vibration) because the vibratory movements of the tuning fork are too rapid to see. It might also be helpful to think of waves of compression that can be seen. Imagine that you are sitting on a dock over a lake on a day with the wind so calm that the surface of the water is glassy—the water medium is "in equilibrium." Now, dip a stick in and out of the water one time. What happens? You will see a disturbance (a wave of disturbance) move out from the point where the stick entered the water. Do it again, but this time dip the stick in and out of the water repeatedly at regular intervals, say once every 2 s. Now the wave of disturbance will be repeated, and you will see a series of concentric circles of larger and larger diameter moving away from the center. The water wave is reasonably analogous to the propagation of a sound wave in air, except that the water wave that we see is moving along a two-dimensional surface.

We should agree, then, that there is a wave of disturbance that moves along the surface of the water. But, are the water molecules displaced over any great distance? Place a small cork on the surface of the water and imagine it represents a "water particle." As the wave of disturbance moves outward, the cork will be seen to bob (approximately) up and down. The cork moves over a relatively small distance, but a *wave of disturbance* is propagated through the medium for a considerable distance. The same is true for propagation of sound in air—the propagation of density changes through an elastic medium.

Two events occur at some certain *rate* during sound wave propagation. One is *the rate of vibratory movement* of the air particles (**frequency** of vibratory motion). The second is *the rate with which the disturbance is propagated* through the medium (the **speed** of sound).

Frequency of Vibratory Motion (f)

The rate at which the source of sound vibrates, expressed in hertz (**Hz**), is called the **frequency (f)**. What determines the frequency with which the tuning fork, or any other sound source, will vibrate? *The frequency of vibration of the source of sound is determined by properties of the source.* It does not matter whether the sound wave that results will be propagated through air or water or along a steel rail, and it does not matter what force is applied to the source.

In the case of the tuning fork, the principal factors that determine the frequency of vibration are the density of the metal and the length of the bar. Thus, a single tuning fork that is always characterized by some constant density and length will always vibrate with the same frequency when it is struck. With the pendulum, we learned that length was the principal factor that determined frequency of vibration. We shall see later that the frequency of vibrating strings such as on a piano or guitar depends on the length, mass, and tension of the strings. But, it is important to remember that, as long as nothing happens to alter those characteristics of the source, the frequency of vibration will be the same.

What about the frequency of vibration, to and fro, of the air molecules in response to the vibration of the source? Their frequency depends on, and is the same as, the frequency of vibration of the source. Thus, if the tuning fork vibrates with a frequency of 125 Hz, the air molecules in the medium also vibrate with a frequency of 125 Hz. If we select a new fork that vibrates with a frequency of 250 Hz, because of a different density of the metal and/or a different length of the bar, the frequency of air particle vibration also will be 250 Hz.

Speed of Sound (s)

The vibration of either tuning fork mentioned above, the one with f = 125 Hz or the one with f = 250 Hz, results in a wave of compression that is propagated through the medium. What will determine the **speed** of sound wave propagation?

Whereas the frequency, or rate, of vibration of the source is dependent on characteristics of the source, *the speed of sound wave propagation is dependent on characteristics of the medium.* Thus, the waves of compression that result from the two forks vibrating with different frequencies move through the medium with the same speed.

Common experience tells us that some amount of time is required for a sound wave to reach our ears. We can see the ball leave the tee from a distant golfer before we hear the "crack" of the ball;

we can see the conductor's hands signal the celebrity to commence singing the national anthem at the World Series before we hear the first words; and we can see the flash of lightning long before (we hope) we hear the crash of thunder.

These differences between how soon we "see something" and how soon we "hear something" occur because light and sound travel at different speeds. The speed of light is 299,792,458 m per s (186,282.397 miles per s; a slight change from the value of 186,282.423 that was accepted before the General Conference on Weights and Measures met in Paris in 1983). The speed of sound in air at sea level with a temperature of 0° centigrade (C) is only 331 m per s (1,085.96 ft per s). Thus, the speed of light is almost 1 million times faster than the speed of sound.

The speed of sound in air is given by:

Equation 1.16
$$s = \sqrt{\frac{E}{\rho}},$$

where **E** refers to elasticity and ρ refers to density.

Thus, speed is directly proportional to the square root of the **elasticity (E)** of the medium, which is measured in N/m^2 **(MKS)** or dynes/cm^2 **(cgs)**, and inversely proportional to the square root of the **density** (ρ) of the medium, which normally is measured in kilograms per cubic meter (kg/m^3), but sometimes in grams per cubic centimeter (g/cm^3). The relation between these two alternative expressions is given by:

$$1 \text{ g/cm}^3 = \frac{0.001 \text{ kg}}{(0.01 \text{ m})^3} = 1,000 \text{ kg/m}^3.$$

Generally, we will be interested in the speed of sound waves traveling in air that is warmer than 0° C, and changes in air temperature do affect the speed of sound wave propagation. As the medium warms, the ambient pressure of the medium remains constant, but the expanding gases cause the density of the medium to decrease.

We can reason from Equation 1.16 that the speed of sound increases as temperature increases because an increase in temperature produces a decrease in density, and $s \propto 1/\sqrt{\rho}$. More specifically, the speed of sound increases approximately 0.61 m/s (61 cm/s or 2 ft/s) for each 1° C increase in temperature. For example, if the speed of sound is 331 m/s (33,101 cm/s; 1,086 ft/s) at 0° C, it will increase to 343 m/s (34,320 cm/s; 1,126 ft/s) if the temperature rises to 20° C (68° Fahrenheit).

From Equation 1.16 it is obvious that *the speed of sound in air is independent of the frequency of vibration of the source*, because only characteristics of the medium are included in the equation. Thus, the speeds of two sound waves, one with f = 125 Hz and one with f = 250 Hz, are identical when the waves travel in the same medium.

It also follows that the sound wave that results from a tuning fork vibrating with a frequency of, for example, 500 Hz will be propagated at different speeds in different sound transmission media. In air, the disturbance travels with a speed of about 331 m/s (1,086 ft/s). In water with a temperature of 0° C (if it has not yet frozen), the disturbance from the same vibrating fork travels much faster, about 1,433 m/s (4,702 ft/s). On a steel rail the speed is even greater, about 4,704 m/s (15,434 ft/s).

Does the contrast of speed along steel and speed through air make sense from Equation 1.16? Steel is a little more than 6,000 times as dense as air. If we ignore elasticity, we might conclude that the speed of sound would therefore be less in steel because speed is inversely proportional to the square root of density. We cannot, however, ignore elasticity. In fact, steel is about 1,230,000 times more elastic than air. Thus, counter to our sometimes common intuition, **elasticity** can be thought of as *the ability to resist deformation,* and steel certainly offers a greater resistance to deformation than does air. The contribution of the difference in elasticity between air and steel far outweighs the difference in density. As a result, the speed of sound is approximately 14 times greater in steel than in air ($\sqrt{1,230,000/6000} = 14.3$).

■ TYPES OF WAVE MOTION

We have talked about the nature of wave motion that occurs with a sound wave, and we then drew the analogy of wave motion on the surface of water. Now we wish to describe the characteristics of all wave motion in a little more detail. We say "all wave motion" because wave motion certainly is not confined to sound. The vibrations, or tremors, of buildings or bridges also are examples of wave motion. Another is the pattern that you see if you flick one end of a stretched rope that is fastened at one end to a wall.

The types of waves that result from vibratory motion are classified according to *the direction of vibration of the medium relative to the direction in which the wave is moving.* There are two types of wave motion: **transverse** and **longitudinal**.

Transverse Wave Motion

One type of wave motion is a **transverse wave**. Consider a stretched rope such as that shown in Figure 1–10 with its two ends extending to infinity so that no "reflections" will occur. We have "painted" several dots along the rope at equal intervals that we will refer to as "rope particles." Next, we will flick the rope and, with the aid of a fast camera, periodically "stop the action" and examine the position of each of the particles at different moments in time. If we take a series of such pictures at regular intervals, we will be able to see the course of movement of each of the rope particles from moment to moment. Time progresses from t_0 at the top of the figure to t_5 at the bottom.

The first picture, taken at time zero (t_0), shows the rope stretched—it is at equilibrium. In the second picture (t_1), taken a frac-

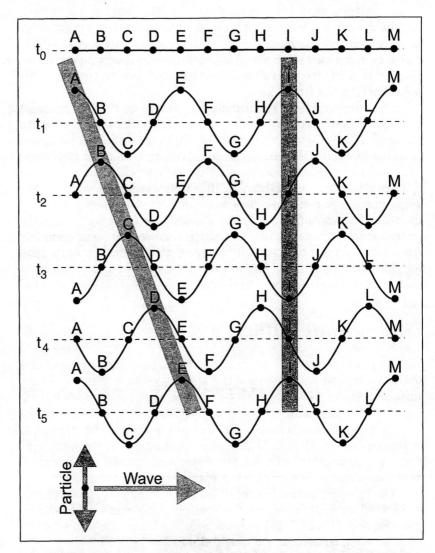

Figure 1–10. Transverse wave motion of a stretched rope. "Particles" (**A** through **M**) painted on the rope move alternately up and down over time (from t_0 through t_5) at right angles to the direction of wave motion from left to right.

tion of a second (one-quarter **cycle**) later, we see that particle **A** moved upward, **B** stayed in place, **C** moved downward, **D** stayed in place, **E** moved upward, **F** stayed in place, and so on. As you move down the rows of the figure, you see that, over time, each particle is moving up and down. Furthermore, each particle is moving up and down *with exactly the same frequency* as every other particle. Consider one cycle of vibration for particle **A**: movement from equilibrium at time zero (t_0) to maximal displacement upward (t_1), to equilibrium (t_2), to maximal displacement downward (t_3), and back to equilibrium (t_4). Every other particle completes one cycle of vibration in exactly the same amount of time. Particle **B**, for example, completes one cycle between t_1 and t_5. Particle **I** behaves like particle **A** and completes one cycle of vibration between t_0 and t_4. The upward and downward displacements of particle **I** are shown by the darker shaded region in the figure.

Look again at the positions of the particles along the rope and you will see peaks occurring at regular intervals from left to right. At t_1 the peaks correspond to particles **A**, **E**, **I**, and **M**. Those peaks are analogous to regions of **compression**, or **high density**, for sound transmitted through air. We also can see valleys from left to right that correspond to points **C**, **G**, and **K**. Those valleys are analogous to regions of **rarefaction**, or **low density**, for sound in air.

As we move through time by looking down the rows, you should note that the locations of the peaks move from left to right (shown by the lighter shaded region in the figure). At t_1, the first peak appeared at **A**, but at t_2 particle **A** has moved downward and particle **B** has moved upward. As a result, the peak that formerly was at **A** (t_1) now has moved toward the right to correspond to point **B**. The same is true for all of the other peaks, and so at t_2 the peaks are located at **B**, **F**, and **J**. Over time, as you move down through time t_5, the peaks have moved from left to right. For now, we won't concern ourselves with what happens when a peak finally moves far enough to the right to reach the imaginary surface to which the rope is attached (at infinity), but that concept will be introduced in Chapter 8.

With the type of wave motion that occurs with the rope in Figure 1–10, the direction of wave movement is from left to right in contrast to the direction of particle movement, which is up and down. That is called transverse wave movement, and a **transverse wave** is defined as one in which *the direction of vibration of the medium is at right angles (90°) to the direction of the wave that is propagated through the medium*. Transverse wave motion is the type of motion that happens, for example, when you pluck the string of a guitar. Another example of (almost) transverse wave motion occurs when you throw a pebble into a pond near to where a cork lies motionless (in equilibrium). A wave of disturbance with peaks and valleys will move out away from where the pebble struck the water. As the wave moves outward, the cork (and the water medium) will bob approximately up and down at right angles to the direction of wave movement.

Longitudinal Wave Motion

The second type of wave motion is a **longitudinal wave**, which is illustrated in Figure 1–11 by a spring-mass system that is lying on a frictionless surface. As with the stretched rope, "individual particles" of the spring are identified with dots and are labeled from **A** through **H**. Time progresses from t_0 at the top of the figure to t_8 at the bottom.

When the spring is in equilibrium (t_0), the dots are spaced at equal intervals. In the next picture (t_1), a short segment of the spring has been compressed and then released. Particle **A** has moved to the

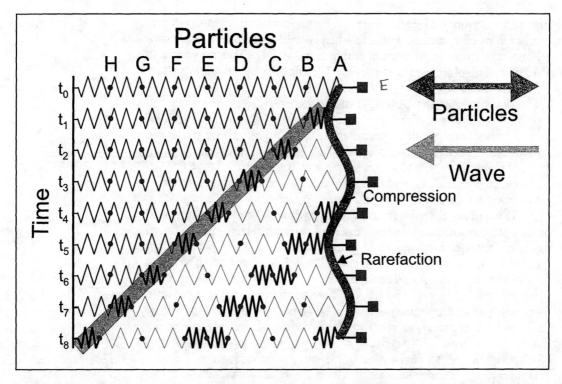

Figure 1–11. Longitudinal wave motion of a spring-mass system lying on a frictionless surface. "Particles" (**A** through **H**) painted on the spring move alternately back and forth from left to right over time (from t_0 through t_8) in the same plane as the wave movement from left to right.

left. From t_0 through t_8, particle **A**—and the mass attached to the spring—can be seen to move to the left and the right (back and forth) through two complete **cycles** of vibration. Each new picture shows the positions of the spring particles at progressively later moments in time, and ultimately each of the particles **B** through **H** undergoes exactly the same motion that was seen for particle **A**. That is to say, each particle vibrates back and forth with exactly the same amplitude and frequency as particle **A**.

Compressions, or **condensations**, are shown by the dots being crowded together (high density) and **rarefactions** are shown when the dots appear far apart (low density). From picture to picture the particles of the spring move back and forth, and the compressions and rarefactions move in the same plane as the particles. This leads us, then, to the definition of a **longitudinal** wave. A **longitudinal wave** is one in which *the direction of particle movement is parallel to the direction of wave propagation*.

■ SOUND WAVES

How should sound waves be classified? Sound waves in air are **longitudinal waves**; *the direction of air particle movement is parallel to* *the direction of wave movement.* In fact, it is not unreasonable to think of the air molecules as small elements of matter attached to each other by springs. This is illustrated in Figure 1–3 in which 10 individual particles are in the columns from left to right and "frozen moments" in time are in the rows from top to bottom. The source of sound is the tuning fork. The first row shows the fork and the medium in equilibrium. Three complete cycles of vibration are shown in the remaining rows. By way of review, we should be able to identify the following aspects of vibratory motion.

1. The tuning fork in Figure 1–3 moves through three cycles of vibration after it is struck by moving from equilibrium, to maximal displacement (+), through equilibrium, to maximal displacement in the opposite direction (−), and back to equilibrium during each **cycle**.

2. Each particle vibrates back and forth relative to its average position of equilibrium, which is shown in the top row of Figure 1–3. The **amplitude** and **period** of vibration of each particle is the same as for every other particle.

3. The individual particles do not vibrate together. That is to say, not all of them simultaneously move to the left or to the right. Rather, they move in a progressive fashion just as we observed in Figure 1–10 for the dots on the stretched rope and in Figure 1–11 for the dots on the spring-mass system. If the dots were members of a marching band, we would say they are "marching out of step with one another." In Chapter 2 we will learn to say that they are "out of phase" with one another.

4. The back and forth movement of the air particles produces a movement, or propagation, of the **compressions** (high density) and **rarefactions** (low density) from left to right in Figure 1–3. During the compression phase, the particles are moving to the right, and during the rarefaction phase, the particles are moving to the left.

5. The individual particles are envisioned to be connected by a spring, which is equivalent to an **elastic bond**, and each particle can be viewed as *exerting a force on the one to the right of it*. By that we mean, during **compression**, each spring pushes the particle to its right forward, whereas during **rarefaction**, the springs or elastic bonds are stretched, which pulls the particle backward.

6. Each particle is doing **work** on the particle in front (to the right) of it. This results in a **transfer of energy** through the medium in the direction in which the wave is traveling.

■ TRANSFER OF ENERGY

We learned previously that the medium itself is not transferred during sound wave propagation; each particle is displaced from equilibrium over only a very small distance. However, **energy** is transferred through the medium in the direction in which the wave is propagated as each particle does work on the one next in line.

The transfer of energy during transmission of sound is exactly the same as in the discussion of the pendulum. In other words, *potential energy is greatest and kinetic energy is least when the molecule is at maximal displacement*. As the particle returns toward equilibrium, potential energy is transformed to kinetic energy. At equilibrium, *kinetic energy is maximal and potential energy is zero*.

Previously, sound in air was said to be *characterized* as *the propagation of density changes through an elastic medium*. It is more correct to *define* sound as *the transfer of energy through an elastic medium*. We learned previously in our discussion of pendular vibration that **friction** serves to limit the velocity of pendular motion. The same thing occurs when sound energy is transferred through a medium such as air. The air mass offers **resistance**, and some of the kinetic energy will be transformed into thermal energy (heat). When that transformation is complete, the sound energy is dissipated, which means that no more useful work can be accomplished because of friction.

The sound waves that we have discussed to this point have come from the vibratory motion of tuning forks, the pendulum, a stretched rope or string, and a spring-mass system. Each of those examples produces the same pattern of wave motion, which is called **simple harmonic motion**. The characteristics of simple harmonic motion will be described in the next chapter.

■ NOTES

1. The stem of the fork will also be set into vibration, but it will move up and down as the tines move back and forth. The fork also has two points, located near to where the metal bars are bent, at which no vibration occurs. Points of no vibration are called **nodes**.
2. Strictly speaking, frequency of pendular vibration is independent of amplitude only if the amplitude is small. For our purposes, however, the influence of amplitude on frequency will be disregarded.

■ FREQUENTLY MISUNDERSTOOD CONCEPTS

1. What happens to the **speed** of **sound wave propagation** in air as the **period** of a sine wave that is propagated through the medium increases?

   The speed of sound wave propagation in air *is unaffected* by changes in the period of the sine wave because **frequency** (and **period**) and **speed** are independent quantities. Speed of sound is determined by properties of the air medium and is given by Equation 1.16:

   $$s = \sqrt{\frac{E}{\rho}},$$

   where **E** refers to elasticity and ρ refers to density.

When the air is characterized by what are called *standard conditions* (0° centigrade and a pressure of 1.013×10^5 N/m^2, the speed of sound is 331 m/s regardless of the **frequency**, hence the **period**, of the sound wave that is propagated through the medium. As the **temperature** of the medium increases, the pressure in the medium remains constant, the gases expand, and the **density** decreases. Because the speed of sound is inversely proportional to the square root of the density, the speed of sound increases by 0.61 m/s for each degree centigrade rise in temperature. Thus, if the temperature were increased to 25° C, the speed of sound wave propagation would increase by 15 m/s (0.61×25) from 331 m/s to 346 m/s (331 + 15).

2. What happens to **potential energy (PE)** as a pendulum swings *away from* equilibrium?

At the precise moment that the pendulum swings *through* equilibrium, **PE** is zero and **KE** is maximal. As the pendulum swings *away from* equilibrium in either direction, **KE**, which is an *energy of motion*, is converted to **PE**. Thus, **PE**, which is a form of *stored energy*, increases.

3. One **newton** in the **MKS** system corresponds to how many **dynes** in the **cgs** system?

The **newton** and **dyne** are units of measure of **force**, and 1 N = 100,000 (10^5) dynes. See Equation 1.6 and review the section on "Units of Measure for Force."

Simple Harmonic Motion

In this chapter the details of vibratory motion will be examined more closely. When we discussed the concept of transfer of energy in Chapter 1, the vibratory motion of air particles was simulated in Figure 1–11 by a spring-mass system. If the mass is pushed to the left to compress the spring, a rightward reaction force results, and if the mass is pulled to the right to extend the spring, a leftward reaction force results. In other words, there is always a restoring force ($\mathbf{F_r}$) to return the mass to equilibrium, and the magnitude of the restoring force is proportional to the change in length of the spring, which we learned is **Hooke's Law** (Equation 1.8, $F_r = -kx$). That means that *the restoring force of elasticity is proportional to the distance that the mass is displaced from equilibrium.*

It follows, therefore, that during the course of the oscillatory motion of the spring-mass system, the magnitude of the restoring force changes over time because the magnitude of displacement changes. As the mass moves toward equilibrium, the restoring force diminishes, and as the mass moves away from equilibrium toward a maximum displacement, the restoring force increases. Because of this buildup and decay of the restoring force, *the mass is accelerated as it moves toward equilibrium and decelerated as it moves away from equilibrium,* which means that the velocity of the mass is constantly changing.

The result is **vibration**, or **oscillation**, of the mass backward and forward that simulates the to and fro vibratory, or oscillatory, motion of the air molecules. One **cycle** of vibration is defined as it was previously: movement from equilibrium to maximal displacement (+), back through equilibrium, to maximal displacement in the opposite direction (−), and back to equilibrium.

■ THE WAVEFORM

It is useful to study a graph that illustrates the nature of this simple vibratory motion by plotting changes in the magnitude, or amplitude, of displacement over time. Rather than designate the starting time as the moment when the mass was released, we will assume that the system has already been set into oscillation, and then plot two cycles of oscillation that commence at the exact moment that the mass in Figure 1–11 passes through equilibrium and heads in the opposite direction. That is analogous to the air molecules in Figure 1–3 being displaced from equilibrium to the right.

Such a plot is shown in Figure 2–1, which displays the **time-domain waveform**, or just **waveform**. This is the kind of result you would obtain if, for example, the path of point **A** for the spring-mass system in Figure 1–11 were traced over time from t_0 to t_8. But, it is important to avoid a serious misinterpretation: *The air mass does not literally undergo an excursion of the type shown in Figure 2–1.* Instead, the air molecules move back and forth just as the spring-mass system moves back and forth, and the wave of disturbance moves through the medium in essentially a straight line. The curved line in the figure is simply a *graphic representation* (i.e., the **waveform**) of what is transpiring.

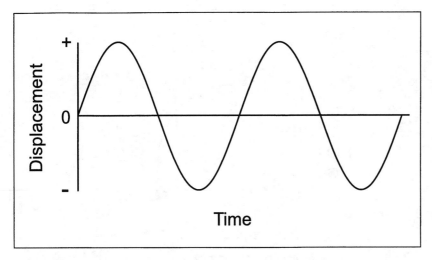

Figure 2–1. Graphic representation of the movement of a spring-mass system over time that was presented in Figure 1–11. The pattern of movement reflects **simple harmonic motion**, which also is called **sinusoidal motion**. This kind of representation is called the **waveform**.

In Figure 2–1, the waveform shows *displacement* as a function of time, but the concept of a waveform is not restricted to a display of changing displacement. Many other quantities (e.g., velocity, acceleration, force, pressure, momentum, and so on) can be shown as a function of time, and they also are waveforms.

■ THE CONCEPT OF SIMPLE HARMONIC MOTION

The type of motion that the spring-mass system (and the air molecule) undergoes is called **simple harmonic motion**, and we shall see subsequently why simple harmonic motion can also be called **sinusoidal motion**. Simple harmonic motion can be represented as *projected uniform circular motion*.

Uniform Circular Motion

What is meant by uniform circular motion? *Uniform circular motion occurs when a body moves around the circumference of a circle at a constant number of degrees of rotation per second.*

Figure 2–2 shows a wheel that is turning counterclockwise. The dot on the wheel moves at a *uniform rate* around the circumference. In this example, one complete revolution of the wheel and, therefore, one complete revolution of the dot, is accomplished in 1 s. Because the dot moves through 360° during one revolution, the wheel turns at a uniform rate of 1° per 1/360 s.

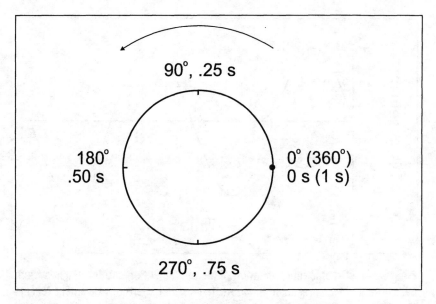

Figure 2–2. A dot moving at a uniform rate around the circumference of a wheel through 360° of rotation in 1 s.

We shall try to develop the concept that the back and forth movement of the mass, or the back and forth movement of the air molecules, is analogous to a point moving around the circumference of a circle at a constant rate. When that is accomplished, we will be able to say that movements of the mass and of the air molecules are examples of **simple harmonic motion**. We will also be able to explain why straight-line, back and forth motion, which also is called **rectilinear motion**, can be pictured to have the same pattern shown in Figure 2–1.

One of the best explanations was provided by Hirsh (1952), and Figure 2–3 is taken from his textbook. A person seated on a Ferris wheel is pointing a flashlight at a wall that is coated with a light-sensitive material. The Ferris wheel starts to move at a constant speed, which means that both the person and the flashlight will move around the circumference of the circle at a constant number of degrees of rotation per second. Thus, the rider undergoes **simple harmonic motion**.

What will the projected image look like when the wall is stationary? It will be a straight line. The upper limit will correspond to the moment in time when the person is at the top of the path of the wheel. The lower limit will correspond to the moment in time when the person is at the bottom of the path. The midpoint of the line will correspond to the starting (equilibrium) position. Thus, *circular motion can be projected as rectilinear (straight-line) motion.* You can demonstrate this for yourself by pointing a flashlight at a wall and then moving the flashlight in a circular motion on a path perpendicular to the wall. The beam of the light will move up and down in a straight line.

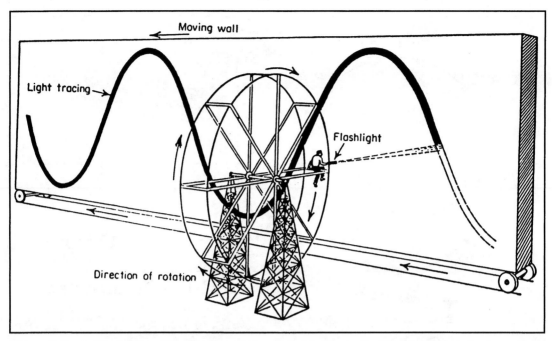

Figure 2–3. An illustration of how a sinusoid is created by the projection of uniform circular motion. From *The measurement of hearing* (p. 20) by I. J. Hirsh, 1952, New York: McGraw-Hill Book Company, Inc. Copyright 1952 by the McGraw-Hill Book Company. Reproduced with permission.

Next, suppose that the wall moves from right to left. The straight-line image that was observed when the wall was stationary will now take the form of the curved line that is shown in Figure 2–3. You can demonstrate this effect for yourself by pointing a flashlight toward a wall and attempting to walk along the wall from left to right at a constant speed as you rotate the flashlight as before. The curved image will result.

Projection of Uniform Circular Motion

In Figure 2–4 the projected circular motion—**simple harmonic motion**—is shown in more detail. The circle at the left of the figure represents the Ferris wheel with the passenger aboard. Point P_0 defines the equilibrium, or starting position, and equilibrium also is labeled as 0°. The person then is set into counterclockwise motion around the circumference of the circle through points P_1, P_2, and so on until the person has moved completely around the circumference. The excursion around the circumference is marked at 45° intervals, and at the end of one complete rotation, the passenger will have passed through 360°.

At the right of Figure 2–4 we show the projection of that circular motion, just as the image of the flashlight beam was projected in Figure 2–3. In this case, the projection displays the **displacement**

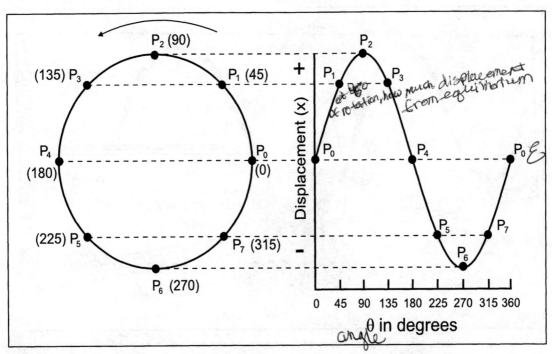

Figure 2–4. Projection of uniform circular motion. The points (**P₀** through **P₇**) on the turning wheel, which is moving at a uniform rate, hence undergoing **simple harmonic motion**, are projected as corresponding points (also **P₀** through **P₇**) on a sinusoidal function. Each point on the sinusoidal function shows the **magnitude of displacement** from the baseline corresponding to that angle of rotation.

waveform (x). The only difference from what was shown in Figure 2–3 is that the "coated wall" has been rotated 90° relative to its position in Figure 2–3 so that the circle and the projection appear in the same two-dimensional plane. The projection (the **waveform**), of course, has exactly the same curved form that it did in Figure 2–3, where it resulted from a flashlight moving with the Ferris wheel.

The waveform in Figure 2–4 also is marked with dots at regular intervals labeled from **P₀** through **P₇**, and the precise location of each of those points on the projection corresponds to the location of the corresponding points on the turning wheel. It is worthwhile to examine the nature of the correspondence in detail, because the relation between circular motion and the form of its projection is fundamental to understanding both simple harmonic motion and sound.

When the passenger is at point **P₀**, the passenger is located on the "baseline," or reference line, and the projection of the beam also lies along the baseline. As the wheel begins to rotate counterclockwise, the passenger—and the projected beam—are displaced upward from the baseline. At 45° (**P₁**) of rotation, the horizontal (dashed) line indicates exactly where the projection would be at this point. That point on the projection also is labeled **P₁**, and it therefore corresponds to 45°. Between 45° and 90°, the passenger travels through the same number of degrees as between 0° and 45°, *but the magnitude of linear dis-*

placement above the baseline is less between 45° and 90° than it was between 0° and 45°. At 90°, of course, the height of the projected curve is at its maximum, which corresponds to the passenger being at the highest point above the baseline.

Between P_2 and P_6 the passenger moves downward, and the projection also moves in a downward, or negative, direction. At P_3 the magnitude of displacement is the same as at P_1, and in a similar vein, P_4 corresponds to P_0 and P_5 corresponds to P_7. The relation between the magnitudes of displacement for P_2 and P_6 also should be apparent. P_2 corresponds to a maximal displacement above baseline (90°) and P_6 corresponds to a maximal and equal magnitude of displacement below baseline (270°). From P_6 through P_0 the passenger is climbing back upward toward the baseline (and so is the projection) to complete one cycle of rotation, which corresponds to 360°.

Notice that the horizontal axis (abscissa) of Figure 2–4 is labeled in degrees. That allows us to specify exactly where the person (**P**) is in the excursion around the wheel at any given moment. Thus, the starting point P_0 corresponds to 0°, P_1 corresponds to 45°, P_2 to 90°, and so on until the passenger returns to the starting point, which corresponds to 360°.

When the passenger reaches the top of the circle, which corresponds to 90° of rotation (1/4 of a cycle), the projection has reached its maximal height in a *positive* (+) direction of displacement. When the passenger has completed exactly half of the circle, which corresponds to 180° of rotation, the projected beam is in exactly the same position that it was at equilibrium, or starting position. Maximal displacement of the beam in a *negative* (−) direction occurs when the person has completed 270° of rotation. Finally, when movement around the circumference of the circle is complete, the person has returned to the starting point, which corresponds to 360° of rotation, and the projection is back to zero displacement.

One rotation of 360° is defined as a **cycle**, and that is identical to our previous definition: one **cycle** corresponds to displacement from equilibrium to maximum, back to equilibrium, to minimum (maximum displacement in the opposite direction), and back to equilibrium. Equilibrium corresponds to 0°, 180°, and 360°; maximum displacement corresponds to 90° (+) and 270° (−).

The projected graph of uniform circular, or simple harmonic, motion shows the magnitude of **displacement** (**x**) as a function of degrees of rotation. The abscissa also could be labeled in units of time. Suppose the wheel rotates with a **frequency** (**f**) of one rotation per second. That means that the **period** of rotation—the time required to complete one cycle of rotation—is 1 s because $T = 1/f$, and $1/1 = 1$. Therefore, 90° (1/4 of the cycle) corresponds to 0.25 s (1/4 of 1 s), 180° to 0.50 s (1/2 of 1 s), and so on. If we increase the frequency to two rotations per second, the period will equal 0.5 s (the time required to complete one cycle of rotation). Now, 90° still corresponds to 1/4 of the excursion and to a maximal amplitude of displacement, but because of the increased frequency, it will correspond to 0.125 s, which is 1/4 of 0.5 s (the time required to complete one cycle).

The Sine Wave

Figure 2–5 is similar to Figure 2–4, but now the projections of three wheels of different sizes are shown. Look at the similarities and differences among the three projections. In all cases, one cycle corresponds to 360°, maximal displacement corresponds to 90° and 270°, and so on. Although maximum positive displacement corresponds to 90° for all three wheels, it is obvious that the largest wheel results in the largest displacement of the projection.

Even though the magnitude of displacement (**x**) varies with the size of the wheel, *the general form, or shape, of the three projections (the three waveforms) is the same.* The next step, then, is to identify the constant feature that characterizes the three projections, which involves determining the **sine of an angle**.

Consider the triangle shown in Figure 2–6. The angle is 45°, the side opposite the angle is labeled **x**, the base is labeled **b**, and the hypotenuse is labeled **r**. The sine of the angle, which is called **sin θ**, equals **x/r**. In other words, if we know the lengths of **x** and **r**, we divide **x** by **r** and the result is called the **sine of the angle**. With the example in the figure, the length of **x** is 10 cm, the length of **b** also is 10 cm, and the length of **r** is 14.14 cm. The ratio of **x** to **r**, **x/r**, is 10/14.14 = 0.707, and 0.707 is the sine of a 45° angle. That is the same as saying that the length of **x** is 70.7% of the length of **r**.

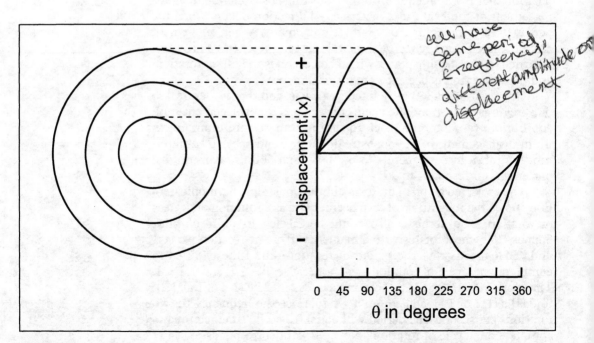

Figure 2–5. Projections of a rotating point on each of three wheels undergoing simple harmonic motion. Because the radii of the wheels are different, the magnitudes of displacement (**x**) of the projections of the three wheels also are different.

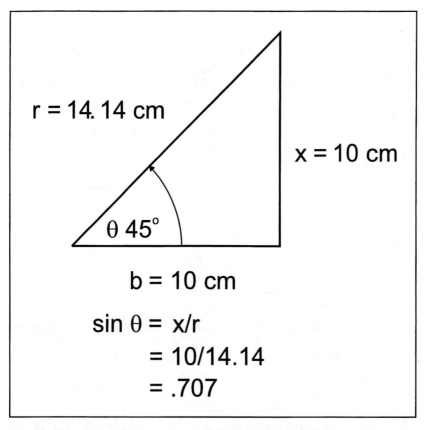

$$r = 14.\,14 \text{ cm}$$

$$x = 10 \text{ cm}$$

$$\theta \ 45°$$

$$b = 10 \text{ cm}$$

$$\sin \theta = x/r$$
$$= 10/14.14$$
$$= .707$$

Figure 2–6. A triangle with angle of 45°, hypotenuse **r**, base **b**, and side **x**. The ratio **x/r** is called the **sine of the angle** (**sin θ**), and the sine of any constant angle such as 45° is a constant, regardless of the absolute magnitudes of **x** and **r**. Thus, for a 45° angle, if **x** = 1.00, **r** must equal 1.414, and the sine of the angle is 0.707. If, for the same angle, **x** = 2.0, **r** must equal 2.828, but the sine of the angle still is 0.707.

For any given angle, the ratio **x/r** (the sine of the angle) is a constant, but, of course, the constant ratio *for other angles* will not necessarily be 0.707. You will see later that sin θ = 0.707 only when the angle is 45° and 135° and −0.707 for 225° and 315°. The sine of other angles is different from 0.707. For example, you can verify with your pocket calculator that the sine of 90° is 1.00, the sine of 270° is −1.00, the sine of 180° and 360° is 0.00, and so forth. In all cases, however, the sine of the angle is given by the ratio of **x** to **r**.

We could have formed other ratios for the triangle as well. For example, the ratio **b/r** is called the **cosine** of the angle, and the ratio **x/b** is called the **tangent** of the angle, and both of those are constants as well *for a given angle*.

Figure 2–7 contains the same three circles that appeared in Figure 2–5, but in Figure 2–7 a triangle with an angle of 45° is placed within each circle. The radius (**r**) of each circle forms the hypotenuse for

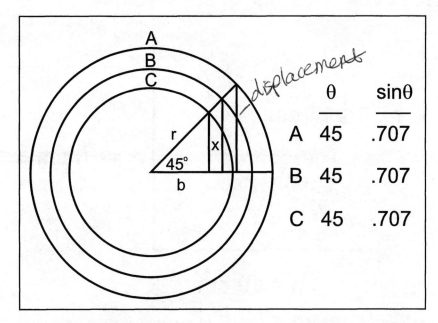

	θ	sinθ
A	45	.707
B	45	.707
C	45	.707

Figure 2–7. Three triangles inserted within the three wheels shown previously in Figure 2–5. Because the circumferences of the three circles are different, the absolute magnitudes of **x**, **b**, and **r** vary, but the sine of the 45° angle, **x/r**, is a constant 0.707 for all three triangles.

the triangle of each circle and, of course, the radius of each circle intersects the circumference of that circle. The length of **r** is different for each of the three circles.

The side of the triangle opposite the angle corresponds to *the magnitude of displacement* (**x**) just as it did in Figure 2–3 where a beam of light was projected from the Ferris wheel. And, finally, the length of **x** and the length the base (**b**) also are different for each of the three circles.

The important point to emphasize is that *the ratio of* **x/r**, *which is the* **sine of the angle**, *is identical for all three triangles* because the angle is constant. For each of the three triangles, **sin** θ = 0.707. In other words, it does not matter what the three lengths are; if the *angle* is 45°, the ratio of the length of **x** to the length of **r** will always be 0.707. As we stated previously, that is the same as saying that the length of **x** will always be 70.7% of the length of **r** when the angle is 45°. In other words, at 45°, the displacement *always* is 70.7% of the maximum displacement that will be achieved at 90°, regardless of the magnitude of the maximum displacement. Thus, for a constant angle, **sin** θ also is a constant.

Fortunately we can use a pocket calculator or published trigonometric tables to find the sine (and cosine and tangent) of any angle rather than calculate it by dividing **x** by **r**. For example, at 90°, **sin** θ = +1.00; at 135°, **sin** θ = 0.707 and it projects to the same height as at 45°; at 180°, **sin** θ = 0.00; and at 270°, which projects to the same height (maximum displacement) as at 90°, but in the opposite direction, **sin** θ = −1.00.

Displacement (x) Represented by sin θ

In Figure 2–8 we have redrawn the three wheels from Figure 2–5, but in this case *the heights of the projections are shown by* **sin** θ *instead of* **x**. Now the three projections are superimposed on one another, because for each angle throughout the cycle, the sine of the angle is a constant. In Figure 2–5 the same three circles produced projections that reached three different maximal heights of displacement. That is because we plotted "absolute displacement" above baseline in Figure 2–5, which was different for the three wheels of different sizes. In Figure 2–8 displacement is represented by **sin** θ, which is a constant for any constant angle. The result is three superimposed curves, which reveals what is constant about uniform circular motion even though that motion can occur along circumferences of different sizes.

Construction of a Sine Wave

Table 2–1 lists the sines of angles (**sin** θ) selected at equal intervals of 11.25° from 0° to 360°, and the function in Figure 2–9 is formed by

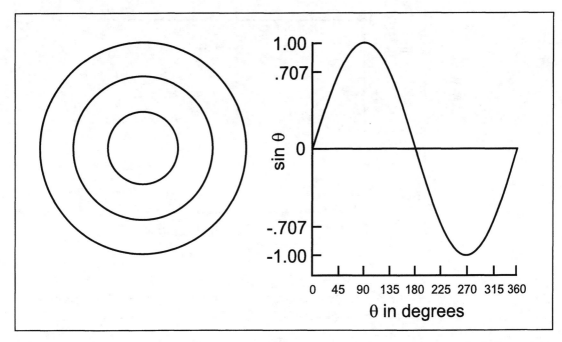

Figure 2–8. Projections of the same three rotating wheels shown previously in Figure 2–5. In Figure 2–5, magnitude of displacement was given by **x**. The ordinate in this figure, however, is the sine of the angle, **sin** θ, as the wheel moves through 360° of rotation. Because the sine of any constant angle is a constant regardless of the absolute magnitude of **x**, a single projection is common to all three wheels.

Table 2–1. Sines of selected angles at 11.25° intervals

θ	sin θ	θ	sin θ	θ	sin θ	θ	sin θ
0.00	0.000						
11.25	.195	101.25	.981	191.25	−.195	281.25	−.981
22.50	.383	112.50	.924	202.50	−.383	292.50	−.924
33.75	.556	123.75	.831	213.75	−.556	303.75	−.831
45.00	.707	135.00	.707	225.00	−.707	315.00	−.707
56.25	.831	146.25	.556	236.25	−.831	326.25	−.556
67.50	.924	157.50	.383	247.50	−.924	337.50	−.383
78.75	.981	168.75	.195	258.75	−.981	348.75	−.195
90.00	1.000	180.00	.000	270.00	−1.000	360.00	0.000

Figure 2–9. Construction of a sine wave is accomplished by plotting **sin** θ for 33 angles selected at equal intervals of 11.25° from 0° to 360°.

plotting **sin** θ as a function of θ in degrees from the entries in Table 2–1: θ = 0°, sin θ = 0; θ = 11.25°, sin θ = .195; . . . ; θ = 45°, sin θ = .707; . . . ; θ = 90°, sin θ = 1.0; . . . ; θ = 135°, sin θ = .707; . . . ; θ = 180°, sin θ = 0;

. . . ; θ = 270°, sin θ = −1.0; and so on. It should be apparent that those 33 *discrete* points in Figure 2–9 are forming a sinusoidal function. If an infinite number of such points were displayed, a *continuous* sinusoidal waveform would be constructed.

Summary of Sinusoidal Motion

We have seen that the *common element* in all of the projections of simple harmonic, or uniform circular, motion is *the sine of the angle.* For any constant angle, regardless of the size of the triangle, the sine of that angle is the constant. In other words, each of the three wheels in Figure 2–8 achieved 38.3% of maximum displacement at 22.5° (sin 22.5° = 0.383), 70.7% at 45° (sin 45° = 0.707), 100% at 90° (sin 90° = 1.00), and so on. It is for that reason that **simple harmonic motion** also can be called **sinusoidal motion**, and the projection, or graph, of simple harmonic, or sinusoidal, motion is called a **sine wave**, a **sinusoidal wave**, or just a **sinusoid**.

Movement around the circumference of a circle at a constant number of degrees of rotation per second (uniform circular motion) is called **simple harmonic**, or **sinusoidal, motion** and the projection, or graph, of sinusoidal motion is called a **sinusoidal wave**. You should notice, however, that movement of the spring-mass system in Figure 1–11 was rectilinear (back and forth in a straight line), not circular, and the movement of the air particles in Figure 1–3 also was back and forth, not circular. In spite of that seemingly significant difference, we still represented the back and forth motions as being sinusoidal in form in Figure 2–1, even though it was not labeled a sine wave at that time.

Rectilinear Motion Represented as Uniform Circular Motion

The task that remains, then, is to explain how back and forth motion of air particles can be *represented as uniform circular motion.* To do this we appeal again to an explanation provided by Hirsh (1952), which is illustrated in Figure 2–10. At the left of the figure is a wheel to which a rod is attached. The rod is connected to a piston, which is housed in a piston chamber in a way characteristic of the old-fashioned steam engine.

The point where the piston is attached to the wheel is labeled **90°**. The wheel is now set into clockwise (it could be counterclockwise as well) rotation at a uniform rate, which also can be called a **uniform angular velocity**. Thus, the point on the wheel where the piston rod is attached to the rim will undergo simple harmonic motion. What happens to the piston in the chamber? As the wheel turns, the piston rod will cause the piston in the chamber to move back and forth.

The position of the piston at the point of equilibrium is labeled 0°. When the wheel has rotated to the 90° angle, the piston has

Figure 2–10. The relation between linear back and forth movement and uniform circular motion in the understanding of sinusoidal motion. The wheel, turning clockwise, causes the piston in the chamber to move *back and forth*. Each position of the piston can be identified in degrees that correspond to the angle of rotation of the wheel. The chamber is connected to a balloon by a tube. Because of the changing air pressure in the chamber, tube, and balloon, the balloon acts as a pulsating sphere and produces a **spherical sound wave**. **Compressions** and **rarefactions** move outward through the medium in all directions as an increasing larger sphere that, in a two-dimensional representation, appears as increasingly larger concentric circles. Adapted from *The measurement of hearing* (p. 22) by I. J. Hirsh, 1952, New York: McGraw-Hill Book Company, Inc. Copyright 1952 by the McGraw-Hill Book Company, Inc. Reproduced with permission.

moved maximally rightward and that position also is labeled 90°. When the wheel has reached 180°, the piston has returned to its position of equilibrium, which also is labeled 180°. The piston has moved maximally leftward when the wheel reaches 270°, and therefore maximal displacement of the piston to the left is labeled as 270°. Finally, when the wheel has completed one full cycle, the piston is returned to equilibrium (360°). The important point is that the wheel is engaged in uniform circular motion, but the piston is engaged in rectilinear (straight-line) motion. Thus, with a simple "mechanical translation," we can label points along a rectilinear excursion in degrees in a way that corresponds exactly to points along a circular excursion.

Simple Harmonic Motion and Sound Waves

To achieve sound from the motion observed in Figure 2–10, we rely on the rest of the apparatus that is shown. At the right of the piston chamber there is an opening to a tube that leads to a balloon. The balloon acts as a pulsating sphere and produces a spherical wave—one in which the condensations and rarefactions move outward from the center of the source in all directions as increasingly larger concentric circles.

When the wheel and piston are motionless, the balloon remains partially inflated, which we shall call equilibrium. When the wheel moves clockwise to 90°, the piston is displaced maximally to the right, which in turn forces air up the tube and causes the balloon to be inflated. As the wheel continues to turn, the piston moves back and forth, and alternately it causes the balloon to move from inflated, to equilibrium, to deflated, to equilibrium, and so on.

One cycle of the wheel's movement corresponds to one cycle of the piston's movement, and each, in turn, corresponds to one cycle of movement of the balloon. Each cycle, whether it be that of the wheel in uniform circular motion or the piston in rectilinear motion, comprises 360°.

When the balloon surface expands outward because air is forced up the tube, a force is applied to the air molecules just as that which occurred with the movement of the tuning fork. Thus, the circular motion of the wheel and the straight-line movements of the piston cause the inward and outward movements of the balloon surface, which affect the air medium in the same way that occurred with the vibratory motion of the fork. The result is increases (**compression**) and decreases (**rarefaction**) in density that are propagated through the elastic medium. Sound has been created.

If the back and forth movements of the piston are simple translations of the circular motion of the wheel, then we also should be able to label the sound wave in degrees if we perform a simple translation. We know that 90° corresponds to the wheel having moved 1/4 of the way through its cycle and to the piston having moved 1/4 of the way through its cycle. When the piston has completed 1/4 of a cycle, it is maximally displaced, and air is forced up the tube to inflate the balloon. Thus, maximal outward displacement of the balloon also corresponds to 90°. Finally, maximal outward displacement of the balloon produces a condensation in the air medium, and maximal condensation, therefore, occurs at 90°. Similarly, maximal rarefaction corresponds to 270°.

■ DIMENSIONS OF THE SINE WAVE

When we previously discussed the vibratory motion of the tuning fork and the pendulum, factors such as amplitude, frequency, and period were mentioned. Those are called "dimensions" of the sound wave. In this section, these, and other dimensions, will be considered in greater detail.

Amplitude

The first dimension is **amplitude**, which is a measure of the strength, or magnitude, of the sound wave. In most of the examples that will be cited, use of the term amplitude will refer specifically to the **sound pressure**. The top waveform in Figure 2–11, which is adapted from

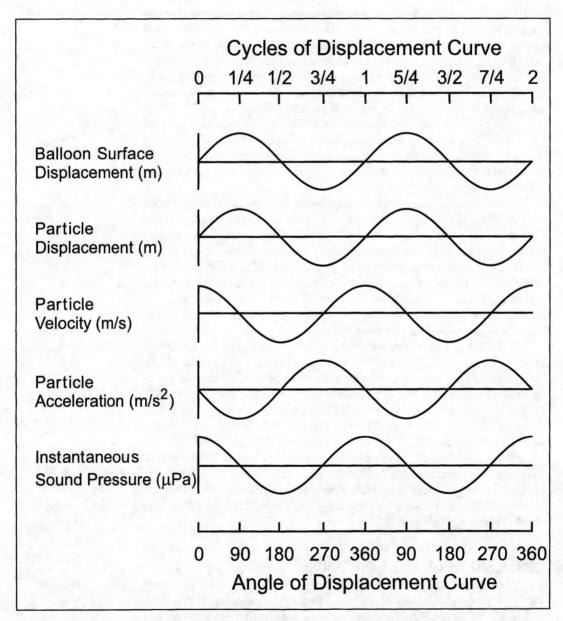

Figure 2–11. Sinusoidal functions that show the relations among **displacement**, **velocity**, **acceleration**, and **sound pressure** as measures of one dimension of sine waves: **amplitude**. Adapted from *The measurement of hearing* (p. 24) by I. J. Hirsh, 1952, New York: McGraw-Hill Book Company, Inc. Copyright 1952 by McGraw-Hill Book Company, Inc. Reproduced with permission.

Hirsh (1952), represents the inward and outward movements of the balloon surface that were caused by the turning wheel and moving piston shown in Figure 2–10. The balloon surface is displaced sinusoidally over time, but of course our interest is in the sinusoidal wave that results, not the source of the wave (displacement of the balloon surface).

As the balloon moves outward, air molecules immediately adjacent to the balloon surface are pushed outward from their resting position. As more and more molecules are pushed outward, there is an increased number of molecules per unit space—they are crowded together—which results in an *increased density* (**compression**). As the balloon begins to deflate, the molecules move back toward their original position, but there are fewer molecules in the immediate surface area of the balloon. That, of course, is the region of *decreased density* (**rarefaction**).

In the second waveform of Figure 2–11 the movement, or displacement, of a single air molecule (particle displacement as a function of time) is shown. The individual particle is displaced sinusoidally over time. Stated differently, the **amplitude of displacement** varies sinusoidally over time, and maximum amplitude of displacement corresponds to 90° (+) and 270° (−). The magnitude of particle displacement, however, would indeed be difficult to measure.

The difficulty of measurement can be overcome by considering some of the derived quantities that were described in Chapter 1. The particles can be said to move with some speed, but we also know that because the *direction* of movement is changing, the **velocity** of particle displacement must also be changing because the concept of velocity incorporates both magnitude of displacement and direction.

The third curve in Figure 2–11 shows the particle velocity waveform, and we can see that the magnitude of particle velocity also is changing sinusoidally over time. It is important to note that *the particle velocity waveform is shifted relative to the particle displacement waveform*. This can be understood by recalling the previous discussion on pendular oscillation.

When displacement is maximal, velocity is zero and motion is momentarily halted. When displacement is zero (when the body is moving through equilibrium), velocity is maximal. This relation between displacement and velocity is preserved in Figure 2–11. Particle velocity is at maximum when particle displacement is zero, and particle velocity is zero when displacement is maximal (when displacement corresponds to 90° and 270°).[1] Thus, we see that the amplitude of simple harmonic motion can be described by reference to either particle displacement or to particle velocity.

If particle velocity is changing, then the particle must be undergoing acceleration, either positive or negative. The fourth curve in the figure shows the particle acceleration waveform. *Acceleration is greatest when displacement is maximal.* As was noted in the introduction to Chapter 2, the particle is accelerated as it moves from maximum displacement toward equilibrium, and it is decelerated as it moves away from equilibrium toward maximum displacement.

The particle acceleration waveform in Figure 2–11 is shifted relative to both the particle displacement waveform and the particle velocity waveform.[2] The relations among particle displacement, particle velocity, and particle acceleration are as follows:

1. Particle velocity *leads* particle displacement by 90° (when x = 0°, c = 90°);
2. Particle acceleration *leads* particle velocity by 90° (when c = 90°, a = 180°); and
3. Particle acceleration, therefore, *leads* particle displacement by 180° (when x = 0°, a = 180°).

Why must acceleration lead displacement by 180°? First, Equation 1.4 (Newton's second law of motion) stated that force equals the product of mass and acceleration:

$$F_i = ma.$$

Second, Equation 1.8 (Hooke's law) stated that the elastic restoring force is directly proportional to the magnitude of displacement:

$$F_r = -kx.$$

In sinusoidal motion, therefore, we have two opposing forces, an inertial force (F_i) and an elastic restoring force (F_r). Third, Newton's third law of motion informed us that with every force there must be an *equal* reaction force of *opposite* direction.

Newton's third law, expressed as a wave equation, is:

Equation 2.1 $F_i = F_r,$ and therefore

Equation 2.2 $ma = -kx.$

There are two constants, **m (mass)** and **–k (stiffness)**, and two variables, **a (acceleration)** and **x (displacement)** in Equation 2.2. As we saw in Figure 2–11, the two variables, **a** and **x**, vary sinusoidally over time. Finally, to satisfy Newton's third law of motion ($F_i = F_r$), the two variables, **a** and **x**, *must* be opposite one another.

Recall that atmospheric pressure amounts to 100,000 **Pa (N/m^2)** at sea level. As the balloon surface moves outward and inward, the number of molecules per unit volume (density of the medium) changes over time, and **pressure** in the medium is related to the density of the medium. Thus, there will be changes in air pressure that also occur sinusoidally over time. Those changes in pressure take the form of alternate increases and decreases *relative to the resting pressure of 100,000 Pa.*

The pressure waveform is shown at the bottom of Figure 2–11. It reveals that the instantaneous sound pressures also vary sinusoidally. Moreover, we can see that the pressure waveform "mirrors" the particle velocity waveform, and that both are shifted by 90° relative to the particle displacement waveform. Thus, the pressure waveform *leads* the particle displacement waveform by 90° (when x = 0°, p = 90°).

Figure 2–12 shows two sinusoidal waveforms that display sound pressure as a function of time. The amplitude of wave **A** at 90° is 2 Pa and the amplitude of wave **B** at 90° is 4 Pa. It should be apparent that each sine wave's "pressure" is really many different values of instantaneous pressure that vary sinusoidally over time. In fact, the pressure is only 2 Pa for wave **A** when particle displacement is zero. (See Figure 2–11 for a review of that relation.)

We will consider, therefore, various alternative metrics that can be used *to express the amplitude of the sine wave*. Although the same metrics will be used in Chapter 5 to express the amplitude of sound waves that are not sinusoidal, such as speech or music, the equations that we will associate with each metric in this chapter *apply only to the sine wave*. Different equations will be required when we subsequently encounter "complex" waves—that is, waves that are not sinusoidal.

Figure 2–12. Sinusoidal distribution of instantaneous sound pressure for two sound waves of identical frequency that differ in **amplitude**.

Instantaneous Amplitude (a)

By **instantaneous** amplitude (**a**) we mean *the amplitude of the waveform at some specified instant in time, or at some specified angle of rotation.* Thus, in Figure 2–12, the amplitude of wave **A** is 0 Pa at 0°, 2 Pa at 90°, and as we shall see later, the amplitude is 1.414 Pa at 45°, because at 45° the displacement always is 70.7% of maximum (sin 45° = 0.707), and 70.7% of 2 = 1.414.

There are instances in which **instantaneous amplitude** is quite useful, but not generally so, and it never makes sense to specify the instantaneous amplitude without also specifying the corresponding angle of rotation, or moment in time, at which the measurement was taken. Of course, nothing is accomplished by calculating the **mean instantaneous amplitude** of a sine wave, because for every positive instantaneous amplitude there is a corresponding—and exactly equal —negative instantaneous amplitude. Therefore, *the mean instantaneous amplitude of sine waves normally will be zero* (unless what is called a "direct current, or dc, bias" exists).

Maximum Amplitude (A)

The **maximum** amplitude (**A**), which is sometimes called the "peak amplitude (**P**)," is *the instantaneous amplitude that corresponds to 90° (or 270°)*. Thus, wave **A** in Figure 2–12 has a maximum, or peak, amplitude of 2 Pa and wave **B** has a maximum amplitude of 4 Pa.

Peak-Peak Amplitude

The **peak-peak** amplitude *is the absolute (not algebraic) difference between the maximum amplitude at 90° and 270°.* Thus,

Equation 2.3   Peak-to-Peak = 2P.

For the two sine waves in Figure 2–12, the peak-to-peak values are 4 Pa for Wave **A** and 8 Pa for Wave **B**.

Root-Mean-Square Amplitude (rms)

The **root-mean-square** amplitude (**rms**) is probably the most common metric that will be encountered for expressing the amplitude of sine waves, but it often seems difficult to achieve an intuitive grasp of what **rms** means. We can achieve an *approximate* understanding of **rms amplitude** by defining it as *the standard deviation of all the instantaneous amplitudes in a sine wave.*

Recall that if we calculate the mean or average of instantaneous amplitudes or pressures, the result is zero (unless there is a dc bias). The standard deviation, however, is the square root of the mean of the squared deviations of the instantaneous pressures about their mean of zero. When we square the deviations, we remove the algebraic sign (all values become positive) and the problem is solved.

In Figure 2–13 we show one sinusoidal waveform, and with some statistical hazard, we will sample only six of the infinite number of instantaneous amplitudes: +2.0, +4.0, and +2.0 during the positive half of the cycle, and −2.0, −4.0, and −2.0 during the negative half of the cycle. Table 2–2 summarizes the steps that are taken to calculate the standard deviation of any set of numbers (X). In this case, the set of numbers is the six instantaneous amplitudes.

In the calculation, we see that the sum (ΣX) and the mean ($\Sigma X/N$) of the instantaneous amplitudes are 0.0 (left column). In the second column, the mean of 0.0 is subtracted from each instantaneous amplitude in the first column. Thus, the numbers in the second column are *deviations of the instantaneous amplitudes from the mean of 0.0*. In the third column, each deviation is squared. At the bottom of the third column we see that the sum of the squared deviations ($\Sigma[X - \bar{X}]^2$) is 48.0.

The next computation shows that the mean of the squared deviations ($\Sigma[X - \bar{X}]^2/N$) is 8.0. In statistics, that value is called the variance (σ^2) of the distribution of the six numbers (X). The final computation yields the square root of the mean of the squared deviations

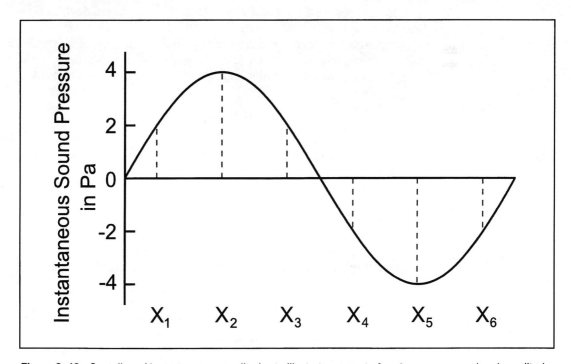

Figure 2–13. Sampling of instantaneous amplitudes to illustrate concept of **root-mean-square (rms)** amplitude.

Table 2–2. Procedures for calculating the standard deviation.

X	X − X̄	(X − X̄)²
2.0	2.0	4.0
4.0	4.0	16.0
2.0	2.0	4.0
−2.0	−2.0	4.0
−4.0	−4.0	16.0
−2.0	−2.0	4.0

$\Sigma X = 0.0$ $\Sigma(X - \bar{X})^2 = 48.0$

$\dfrac{\Sigma X}{N} = 0.0$

$$\sigma^2 = \frac{\Sigma(X - \bar{X})^2}{N} = 8.0 \text{ (ms)}$$

$$\sigma = \sqrt{\frac{\Sigma(X - \bar{X})^2}{N}} = 2.828 \text{ (rms)}$$

$(\sqrt{\Sigma[X - \bar{X}]^2 / N})$, which in statistics is called the standard deviation (σ). For this particular sine wave, the value is 2.828. This is one origin of the name **root mean square (rms)**. It is the square *root* (**r**) of the *mean* (**m**) of the *squared* (**s**) deviations of the instantaneous pressures; hence, it is the **rms pressure**.

In practice we do not actually calculate the standard deviation of instantaneous amplitudes, which would be a feat of considerable accomplishment because there are an infinite number of them. In fact, with the use of Equation 2.4, the **rms amplitude** *of a sine wave* can be determined from knowledge of the maximum amplitude (**A**):

Equation 2.4
$$\text{rms} = \frac{A}{\sqrt{2}}.$$

Because the square root of 2 is a constant equal to 1.414, Equation 2.4 can be rewritten as:

Equation 2.5
$$\text{rms} = \frac{A}{(1.414)}.$$

Finally, because you can either divide by a number *or multiply by the reciprocal of that number*, Equation 2.5 can be changed to read:

$$\text{rms} = A\left(\frac{1}{1.414}\right)$$

Equation 2.6
$$= A(.707),$$

because 0.707 is the reciprocal of 1.414.

Thus, to calculate the **rms** amplitude *of a sine wave*, either divide the maximum amplitude by 1.414 (Equation 2.5) or multiply the maximum amplitude by 0.707 (Equation 2.6).[3] What is the unit of measure? The unit of measure of **instantaneous sound pressure** is the pascal. Similarly, the unit of measure of **rms sound pressure** is the pascal. Thus, the **rms pressures** of the two sine waves in Figure 2–12 are 1.414 Pa for wave **A** and 2.828 Pa for wave **B**.

Mean Square Amplitude

Mean square sound pressure relates to **rms** sound pressure as the variance (σ^2) in statistics relates to the standard deviation (σ). Thus, the variance equals the standard deviation squared and mean square sound pressure equals the rms pressure squared.

$$\text{Because rms} = \frac{A}{\sqrt{2}},$$

$$\text{and because mean square} = \text{rms}^2,$$

$$\text{mean square} = \frac{A^2}{2}.$$ **Equation 2.7**

Mean square amplitude has some utility for those who are concerned with measurements in mechanical dynamics, but it is not likely to be encountered as a useful metric for acoustics in the speech and hearing literature. It was presented here only to complete the picture of statistical-acoustical equivalents.

Full-Wave Rectified Average Amplitude (FW_avg)

Before we consider the equation for the **full-wave rectified average** (**FW_avg**), it might be useful to discuss briefly what is meant by **rectification**. When you connect some electronic device, such as a cassette tape deck, into an electrical wall outlet, the recorder receives a sinusoidally alternating electrical current that looks just like (i.e. has the same shape of waveform) the acoustical sine waves we have described. It is called an *alternating* electrical current because during half of its cycle the current is flowing in one direction (+), and during the other half of its cycle the current is flowing in the opposite direction (−). The frequency of that electrical current is exactly 60 Hz (in the United States), which means it has a period of 0.0167 s (T = 1/f).

The waveform at the top of Figure 2–14 shows the sinusoidal electrical current that is directed to a cassette player. A problem arises because the player cannot function with the alternating current that the power company provides. It must have a direct current, which is current that flows in only one direction, such as you get from a battery. Thus, the alternating electrical current shown at the top of Figure 2–14 must be converted into direct current such as is shown by the second function in Figure 2–14.

We need not explain all of the steps that are required to accomplish the conversion from alternating to direct current, but the first

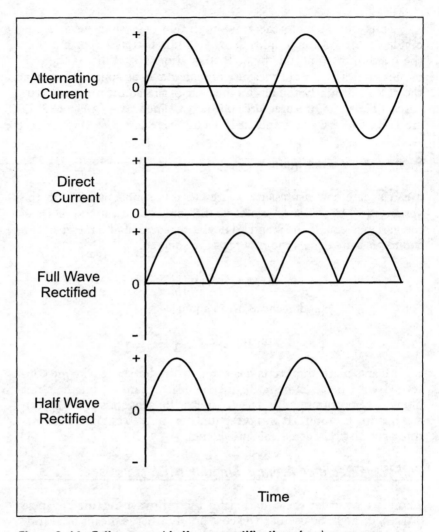

Figure 2–14. Full-wave and **half-wave rectification** of a sine wave.

step is important for us. In the third function of the figure, the negative half of each cycle has been "flipped" to become positive. That process is called **full-wave rectification**. We learned previously that it makes no sense to calculate the arithmetic mean of the instantaneous amplitudes of the sinusoid because we would obtain precisely the same answer, zero, for all sinusoids regardless of differences in their maximum sound pressure unless a dc bias exists. That circumstance no longer exists with the full-wave rectified sinusoid shown in the figure; all of the instantaneous amplitudes are now positive. Suppose, therefore, that we *calculate the arithmetic mean of all of the instantaneous amplitudes in the rectified wave*. That defines the **full-wave rectified average (FW_{avg})**.

Fortunately, we do not have to perform such a computation. Instead we can use Equation 2.8:

$$FW_{avg} = \frac{2A}{\pi}$$

$$= \frac{2A}{3.1416} \quad \text{(substituting the value of } \pi)$$

$$= A(.636) \quad \text{(dividing 2 by 3.1416).} \qquad \textbf{Equation 2.8}$$

Thus, we see that the **FW**$_{avg}$ is almost two-thirds as large as the maximum sound pressure, whereas the **rms** is approximately 70% as large as the maximum pressure.

Half-Wave Rectified Average Amplitude (HW$_{avg}$)

The last metric we will consider is the **half-wave rectified average** (**HW$_{avg}$**). In **half-wave rectification**, the negative half of each cycle is eliminated rather than flipped to become positive. The bottom function of Figure 2–14 shows the result. It should be obvious that the average of the instantaneous amplitudes that remain will be exactly half of what was obtained when we calculated the full-wave rectified average. Thus,

$$HW_{avg} = \frac{A}{\pi} \qquad \text{(rather than } \frac{2A}{\pi})$$

$$= \frac{A}{3.1416}$$

$$= A(.318) \text{ (taking the reciprocal of 3.1416).} \qquad \textbf{Equation 2.9}$$

The **FW$_{avg}$** is almost two-thirds (63.6%) as large as the maximum sound pressure, and because **HW$_{avg}$** = 0.5 **FW$_{avg}$**, the **HW$_{avg}$** is almost one-third (31.8%) as large as the maximum sound pressure.

Comparisons Among Metrics. The waveform at the top of Figure 2–15 represents a sinusoidal wave that has a maximum amplitude of 4 Pa. Thus, the instantaneous amplitudes vary sinusoidally from a minimum value of −4 Pa to a maximum value of +4 Pa. The lower portion of the figure shows the **rms** (Equation 2.6), **mean square** (Equation 2.7), **FW$_{avg}$** (Equation 2.8), and **HW$_{avg}$** (Equation 2.9).

It is important to note that whereas the instantaneous amplitudes vary sinusoidally over time, the other metrics are described by straight lines that remain horizontal to the baseline. They do not vary. Suppose we could direct the sinusoid to some kind of measuring instrument that has an indicating meter, or needle, like you might have seen on the VU meter of some tape recorders. If the measuring instrument had been designed to respond to the instantaneous pressure, it would move back and forth about some average value at a rate corresponding to the frequency of the sinusoid. If the instrument had been designed to respond to any of the other measures of amplitude, the needle would remain perfectly stationary—*those values remain constant over time because each is time-averaged.*

Figure 2–15. Comparison of **mean square, root-mean-square, full-wave rectified average,** and **half-wave rectified average** measures of amplitude of a sine wave.

Frequency (f) and Period (T)

The second dimension of the sinusoidal wave is the **frequency (f)** and its reciprocal the **period (T)**. As we learned earlier, frequency is defined as *the rate, in hertz, at which a sinusoid repeats itself*. Period is defined as *the amount of time, in seconds, that is required for a sinusoid to complete one cycle*.

Consider the two sinusoids that are shown in Figure 2–16. Wave **X** has a period of .001 s, which means that the frequency is 1000 Hz (see Equation 1.12). Wave **Y**, on the other hand, has a period of .0005 s,

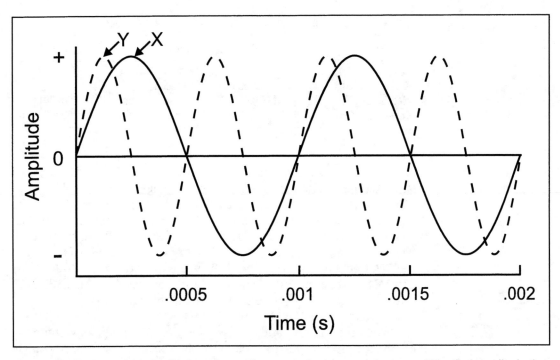

Figure 2–16. Sinusoidal distribution of sound pressure for two sound waves of identical amplitude that differ in **frequency**.

and thus its frequency is 2000 Hz. The inverse relation between frequency and period should be apparent. As frequency is doubled (from 1000 Hz to 2000 Hz), period is halved (from .001 s to .0005 s).

You might observe that we have to resort to rather cumbersome numbers when the frequency is very large or the period is very small. Suppose, for example, that the frequency were 2,345,129 Hz. If that seems cumbersome to write, think about its period (0.0000004264 s). We can partially avoid such cumbersome expressions by using multiples of **hertz** for frequency and submultiples of **second** for period. The various alternatives that are commonly used to describe both frequency and period are shown in Table 2–3.

We can see from Table 2–3 that 1 kilohertz (1 kHz) = 1000 Hz, that 1 Megahertz (1 MHz) = 1,000,000 Hz, that 1 MHz also = 1000 kHz, and so on. For period, a ms is 0.001 (one-thousandth) s, a μs is 0.000001 (one-millionth) s, and so on.

Those multipliers are encountered frequently. Consider your AM radio dial. The AM tuner is designed to receive radio signals with frequencies that range from 550 kHz to 1600 kHz. Thus, if you set your dial to 1560, that means the tuner is adjusted to receive a signal with a frequency of 1560 kHz. (If you happen to be driving [very] near to where the Walhonding and Tuscarawas rivers join to form the Muskingum river, you will be tuned to station WTNS in Coshocton, OH.) Suppose, instead, that you set your FM tuner to 91.2. That doesn't mean 91.2 Hz, but rather 91.2 MHz, which is equivalent to

Table 2–3. Standard units of measure for frequency and period

Frequency		Multiplier	Period		Multiplier
Hertz	(Hz)	1	second	(s)	1
Kilohertz	(kHz)	1,000	millisecond	(ms)	.001
Megahertz	(MHz)	1,000,000	microsecond	(μs)	.000001
Gigahertz	(GHz)	1,000,000,000	nanosecond	(ns)	.000000001

91,200,000 Hz. The FM tuner covers the range from 88 MHz to 108 MHz, and it is more convenient to label the dial in megahertz than hertz.

The tuner on your television set receives frequencies that are both below and above the range of frequencies for FM radio stations. VHF (very-high-frequency) tuners range from 54 MHz to 88 MHz (below the FM frequencies) for channels 2 through 6, but from 174 MHz to 216 MHz (above the FM frequencies) for channels 7 through 13. UHF (ultra-high-frequency) tuners lie in a much higher frequency range that extends from 470 MHz to 890 MHz.

In Equations 1.11 and 1.12, we learned that frequency and period are reciprocally related. Thus, to determine period from knowledge of frequency, you simply calculate the reciprocal of frequency ($1/f$) and, correspondingly, to determine frequency from knowledge of period, you calculate the reciprocal of period ($1/T$). If frequency is expressed in hertz and you take the reciprocal, *period will be expressed in seconds*. If frequency is expressed in kilohertz rather than hertz, when you calculate the reciprocal, *the result for period will be in milliseconds*, not seconds. Similarly the reciprocal of frequency in megahertz will be *period in microseconds*.

Suppose that the frequency of a sinusoid is 2 kHz, but you want to express the corresponding period in *seconds rather than milliseconds*. You must proceed in either of two ways. You can convert 2 kHz to hertz by multiplying by 1000 (see Table 2–3), and the reciprocal of 2000 Hz is .0005 s. Alternatively, you can calculate the reciprocal of 2 kHz, which is 0.5 ms, and then convert 0.5 ms to seconds by multiplying by 0.001 (see Table 2–3). The answer, of course, is the same—0.0005 s.

Determinants of Frequency

We learned earlier that the frequency with which a source of sound vibrates is governed by *properties of the source of sound*. Specifically, the frequency of vibration of some simple harmonic oscillator, such as a spring-mass system, depends on the **mass** and **stiffness** of the system.

The frequency with which that system oscillates is called the **natural frequency (f_{nat})** of the system. The **natural frequency** is inversely proportional to the square root of the **mass** (frequency decreases as mass increases) and directly proportional to the square root of the **stiffness** (frequency increases as stiffness increases). For different sources of sound, different properties must be considered. We know, for example, that vibratory frequency of a pendulum depends almost entirely on its length (Equation 1.13). What about the string or wire on a guitar, violin, or piano? In that case, the frequency of vibration depends on the **length, cross-sectional mass**, and **tension** of the string, and the relation of each of those three factors to *the frequency of a vibrating string* is shown in Equation 2.10:

$$f = \frac{1}{2L}\sqrt{\frac{t}{m}},$$ **Equation 2.10**

where **L** = length, **t** = tension, and **m** = cross-sectional mass.

We can see that the frequency of vibration of a string increases (1) as length decreases (inversely proportional to twice the length), (2) as tension increases (directly proportional to the square root of tension), or (3) as mass decreases (inversely proportional to the square root of mass). This makes sense if you think about the wires on a piano. Tones of lower frequency are produced by longer and more massive wires (inverse relations). To increase the frequency of vibration of any of the wires, you increase the tension—the same process that you go through when you "tune" any stringed instrument such as a guitar. We will learn subsequently that the vibratory pattern of the string or wire is more complex than has just been described. The string actually vibrates at many frequencies simultaneously. Thus, Equation 2.10 applies to only the lowest frequency of vibration, which is called the **fundamental frequency**.

The equation for the lowest frequency of vibration for a string is particularly important for those who are interested in voice production, because the frequency of vibration of the vocal folds depends mainly on the length, cross-sectional mass, and tension of the folds. The nature of the proportionalities (direct or inverse) for vocal fold vibration is the same as we just learned for a string.

The natural frequency for other sources of sound depends on different characteristics. The frequency of a drum's membrane, for example, is directly related to the *tension* of the membrane, but inversely related to its *radius, thickness, and density*. The equations for calculating frequency of vibration of sources such as stretched membranes, bars, and the like, however, are beyond the scope of this book. In all cases, however, the unifying concept is that f_{nat} *is directly proportional to the square root of the stiffness and indirectly proportional to the square root of the mass.*

Angular Velocity (ω)

There are occasions in which it is useful to describe frequency by reference to what is called **angular velocity** (ω) rather than hertz. Before we attempt to define angular velocity, let us consider some alternative ways that *could* be used to express frequency, *although they have not been adopted*. We learned earlier that back and forth vibration is analogous to a point on a turning wheel moving about the circumference of a circle. Consider the circle shown at the left of Figure 2–17. If a reference point moves completely around the circumference of a circle, it has completed 360° of rotation. If the 360° rotation is accomplished in 1 s, f = 1 Hz, and if the rotation is accomplished in 1 ms, f = 1000 Hz or 1 kHz.

Suppose, instead, that the unit of measure for frequency were *degrees of rotation per second* rather than hertz. If that were the case, we would say that f = "360° per s" in the first case and f = "360,000° per s" in the second. Frequency has *not* been described in that way, but it would be perfectly valid. Of course, it would often result in frequency being described by rather large numbers.

We could try a different approach such as that illustrated in the middle circle in the figure. We might reason that because one cycle consists of *four quarter cycles* (each of which corresponds to 90°), f = 360° per s could be expressed as f = "*4 quarter cycles per s*" (dividing 360 by 90), and f = 360,000° per s could be expressed as f = "*4000 quarter cycles per s*." With either of these approaches, the full circle of 360° is simply divided into some number of equal segments—360 equal segments to arrive at "degrees per second," and four equal segments to arrive at "quarter cycles per second."

It turns out, of course, that no one has described frequency by dividing the circle into either 360 equal parts, or four equal parts. Instead, *the circle is divided into 6.2832 parts of equal size.* Why 6.2832 parts? One cycle equals 360°, and 360° corresponds to 2π radians, which equals 6.2832 radians (2 × 3.1416). For the circle shown at the right of Figure 2–17, we show one of the 6.2832 possible segments, and it has been drawn to equal 1 radian.

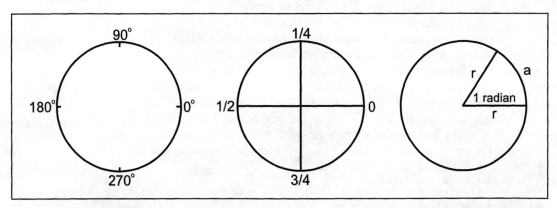

Figure 2–17. An explanation of **angular velocity** in which a point moves around the circumference of a circle. At the left, the frequency of rotation of the point is represented in "degrees per s" because the circle is divided into 360 equal parts. At the middle, frequency of rotation is represented in "quarter cycles per s" because the same circle is divided into only 4 equal parts, rather than 360. At the right, frequency of rotation is represented in "2π radians per s" because the same circle is divided into 6.2832 equal parts, where 6.2832 equals 2π. See text for an explanation of a radian.

You might read in a geometry textbook that a radian is equal to the angle subtended by an arc whose length is equal to the radius. Stated differently, *an angle equals a radian when the intersection of the two sides of the angle with the circumference yields an arc whose length is exactly equal to the length of the radius.* For the angle shown in Figure 2–17, the two sides of the angle are both of equal length and both are equal to the radius (**r**). An arc (**a**) is formed by the intersection of those two radii with the circumference, and the length of the arc **a** equals the length of the radius **r**.

Any circle has 360°, and for any circle there are exactly 2π radians. Because π equals 3.1416, any circle therefore has 6.2832 (2 × 3.1416) radians, and 1 radian corresponds to 57.3° (360° divided by 2π). Another way to conceptualize what is meant by radians is to imagine that we "snip" a circle and then "unroll" it. *Regardless of the size of the circle that we unroll,* the length of the line that we are left with will be *exactly* (to four decimal places) 6.2832 times the length of the radius of the circle, or 3.1416 times the length of the diameter of the circle.

How can radians be used to express frequency? When we used degrees to express frequency, we said that one cycle = 360°, and therefore 1 Hz (cps) corresponds to 360° per s. Because one cycle = 2π radians, 360° per s corresponds to 2π radians per s. *When frequency is expressed in radians per s, the unit of measure is called the **angular velocity** (ω).*

Equation 2.11 shows the relation between angular velocity and frequency:

$$\omega = 2\pi f,$$

Equation 2.11

which means that to determine angular velocity in radians per second, you simply multiply frequency in hertz by 2π. Thus, if f = 1 Hz, ω = 6.28 rps (radians per s), if f = 100 Hz, ω = 628 rps, and if f = 1 kHz, ω = 6280 rps. In practice, angular velocity is not often used in this way. It will be useful to keep angular velocity in mind, however, when we describe the third dimension of the sine wave—**phase**.

Phase

Consider the wheel shown in Figure 2–18. This time we have four reference points (A, B, C, and D) rather than one. In terms of the Ferris wheel analogy, four people are seated at 90° intervals, and each is aiming a flashlight at the same wall. The wheel is turning in a counterclockwise direction and the sinusoidal projections from the four sources are shown at the right of the figure. Note, also, that the degrees of rotation that have been used to label the abscissa refer to the course of travel of person **A**, where 0° is the starting point, 90° is 1/4 of the way around the circle, and so on.

The four curves cannot be superimposed on one another, of course, because the passengers are seated at different locations around the cir-

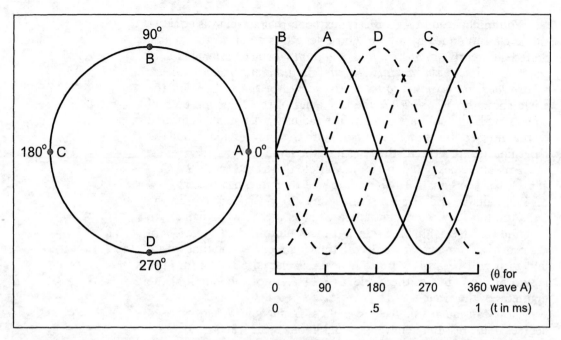

Figure 2–18. An explanation of **starting phase**. At the left, four reference points (A, B, C, and D) are located at different angles: 0°, 90°, 180°, and 270°. When the wheel commences to turn, each point rotates around the circumference with the same amplitude and frequency as the other points. Projections of the sinusoidal motions of the four different points are shown at the right. The only difference among the four functions is the angle of rotation at t_0, which is the **starting phase**.

cumference of the wheel. In fact, we could specify their relative positions by reference to degrees of separation. Thus, **B** *leads* **A** (**B** ahead of **A**) by 90°, **C** leads **B** by 90°, **C** leads **A** by 180°, and so on. Just as the position of the passengers could be described in degrees, so could the differences among the four sinusoidal projections. Curve **B** *leads* **A** by 90°, or we could say that curve **A** *lags* curve **B** by 90°; either is perfectly acceptable.

It is important to remember that all four sinusoids in Figure 2–18 *have exactly the same frequency and exactly the same amplitude.* That must be the case in this example because there is only one wheel with a fixed circumference (determinant of amplitude), and the rate at which the wheel turns (determinant of frequency) will result in all four reference points rotating with the same frequency.

Starting Phase

Even though the four curves in the figure have the same amplitude and frequency, they obviously are different and the difference is in what is called the **starting phase**. Wave **B** *starts* at 90°, whereas wave **A** *starts* at 0°, wave **C** *starts* at 180°, and wave **D** *starts* at 270°. By **starting phase** we mean *the displacement, in degrees, at the instant* *the vibration, or rotation, begins.* The four curves in the figure all have different starting phases.

Phase Angle: Instantaneous Phase

We can also speak of **phase angle**, or **instantaneous phase**, and in this case similarities or differences in frequency are irrelevant. With starting phase, we referred to what can be called **time zero**, a reference time where displacement commenced. The **phase angle**, also called the **instantaneous phase**, is *the angle of rotation at any specified moment in time.* Thus, at t = 0.5 ms in Figure 2–18 the **phase angles** are 180° for **A**, 270° for **B**, 360° for **C**, and 90° for **D**. **D** has a starting phase of 270° and therefore leads **A** by 270°, and that separation will always remain because **D** and **A** rotate with the same frequency. This contrasts with what we saw in Figure 2–16, which displayed two sine waves with different frequencies.

When the frequencies are different, the two waves will move in and out of phase rather than maintain a constant phase separation, even though the starting phases of the two waves happen to be the same. We will capitalize on this concept in Chapter 8 when the phenomenon of **beats** is described.

Phase angles also can be described in radians rather than degrees. Recall that a circle has 360° and 2π radians. The relation between these two for describing phase angle is shown in Figure 2–19. If 360° corresponds to 2π radians, then 0° = 0 radians, 90° = $\pi/2$ radians (1/4 of 2π), 180° = π radians (1/2 of 2π), and 270° = $3\pi/2$ radians (3/4 of 2π).

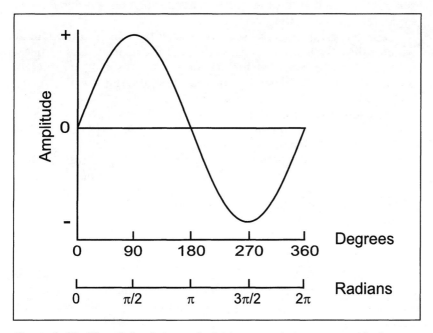

Figure 2–19. The relation between **instantaneous phase** expressed in **degrees** and in **radians**.

Another Application of Radians

Those who elect to study **psychoacoustics**, a branch of science that is concerned with *psychological correlates* of the physical dimensions of sound waves, will almost certainly encounter instances in which phase angle is described in radians. Imagine the following experiment. A sinusoid is presented to a listener who is wearing a pair of earphones. The signal is delivered simultaneously to both ears. Thus, the frequency and the amplitude of the signal are the same in both ears.

Suppose that in one portion of the experiment the *starting phase* of the signal is exactly the same in the left ear as in the right ear. The two signals are said to be *in phase* because there is no difference in phase angle. That condition could be called S_0, which means that the *difference* in phase angle of the signals (S) between the two ears is 0 radians.

In a second portion of the experiment, suppose that the starting phase of the signal in the left ear is 0°, but the starting phase of the signal in the right ear is 180°. Curves **A** and **C** in Figure 2–18 are examples of this condition. The two signals are obviously out of phase by exactly 180°. Because 180° corresponds to π radians, that circumstance can be called S_π (see Figure 2–19).

Wavelength (λ)

The final dimension of the sinusoidal wave is the **wavelength** (λ). In the course of our discussion of sound to this point, we have described two quantities that are measured *by reference to time*. One quantity is **frequency (f)**, which was described as the rate at which the sinusoid repeats itself and is measured in hertz. Frequency is determined by characteristics of the sound source.

The second quantity is **speed of sound (s)**, which is the rate at which a disturbance is propagated through the medium and is measured in feet per second (**fps**), meters per second (**MKS**), or centimeters per second (**cgs**). The elasticity and density of the transmitting medium determine propagation speed.

The fourth and final dimension of the sine wave shows the relation between the two quantities, frequency and propagation speed; it is called the **wavelength** (λ). Wavelength can be defined as *the distance traveled by a sine wave during one period of vibration*, or as *the distance between two identical points (identical phase angles) on two adjacent cycles*. Wavelength is directly proportional to the speed of sound and inversely proportional to frequency, as is shown by Equation 2.12:

Equation 2.12
$$\lambda = \frac{s}{f},$$

where λ is wavelength in meters,

f is frequency in hertz,

and

s is the speed of sound in meters per second.

Consider the examples shown in Figure 2–20 where two sinusoids (f = 1100 Hz and f = 550 Hz) travel in two different media, air and water. Look first at the wave with f = 1100 Hz traveling in air. Its period (1/f) is 0.9 ms. After 1 s has elapsed, the wave will have traveled 340 m (assuming the speed of sound is 340 m/s). Therefore, during just *one period* it will have traveled only 1/1,100 of that distance, which is 0.3 m. That is the distance traveled during one period, which is a definition of wavelength, and that is the answer we would obtain with Equation 2.12: $\lambda = 340/1,100 = 0.3$ m.

Compare that outcome with what we would obtain if f = 550 Hz in air. The speed of sound is still 340 m/s, which means that the sinusoid will still travel 340 m in 1 s. The period now, however, is 1.8 ms. During that 1.8 ms (one period), the wave will travel 0.6 m.

What happens when the same sine waves are propagated through water? For convenience, we will treat the speed of sound in water as if it were four times the speed in air (1,360 m/s), which is a reasonable approximation. When f = 1100 Hz, the wave will travel 1,360 meters in 1 s, the period is still 0.9 ms, and the distance traveled during 1 period will be four times as great (1.2 meters). If f = 550 Hz, the wavelength will be increased from 0.6 m in air to 2.4 m in water. Thus, we see that wavelength is directly proportional to the speed of sound and inversely proportional to its frequency.

The period of most sound waves that are likely to be encountered is typically very small. For example, the period of the vocal fold wave during vowel production by an average adult male is only about 10 ms and the period for the average adult female is just a little over 4 ms. The wavelengths of those sounds in air, however, are relatively large—about 1.5 m (5 ft) for the female and about 3.4 m (11 ft) for the male. In other words, one complete cycle of vibration will span a distance of about 1.5 m for the vowel produced by the female and 3.4 m for the vowel produced by the male. Will a sound of lower frequency (and longer wavelength) travel through the air medium faster than a sound of higher frequency (and shorter wavelength)? No! Speed of sound is governed by properties of the medium, and frequency of vibration is governed by properties of the source. Wavelength simply shows the relation between those two quantities: **s** and **f**.

■ DAMPING

When the vibratory motions of, for example, a simple spring-mass system were presented in Chapter 1, and when sine waves were described in this chapter, each cycle of (sinusoidal) motion was represented as being identical in every respect to every other cycle. That representation is appropriate when the sine wave is conceptualized from a strictly mathematical perspective, and *when there is no opposition to motion*. Oscillating systems, however, do encounter opposition to motion in the form of **friction**, or **frictional resistance**, and **friction** serves to limit **velocity**.

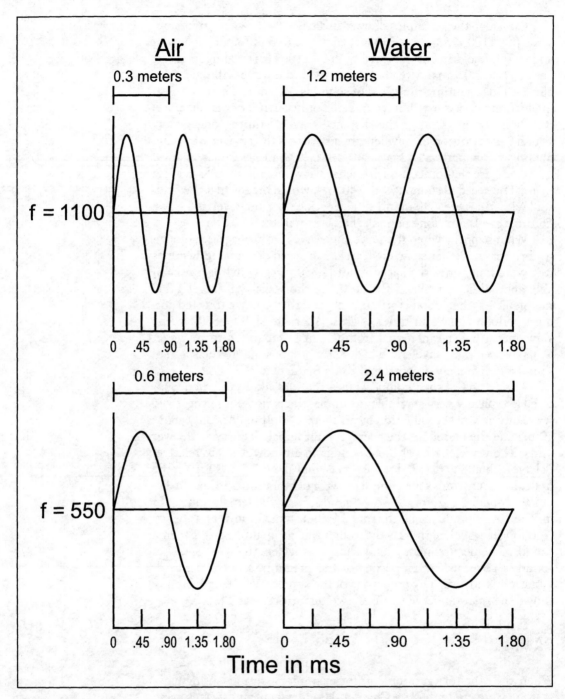

Figure 2–20. An illustration of the dependence of **wavelength** on both frequency and speed of sound wave propagation. Comparison of the two functions within a column (left for air; right for water) shows how wavelength varies with frequency when speed of propagation is held constant. Comparison of the two functions within a row (top for 1100 Hz; bottom for 550 Hz) shows how wavelength varies with speed of propagation when frequency is held constant.

Review of Simple Harmonic Motion

When amplitude of vibration diminishes over time, the oscillations, or vibrations, are **damped**. To further our understanding of damping, it will be helpful to review and expand on some of the characteristics of vibratory motion described previously.

A spring-mass system, or other simple harmonic oscillator, vibrates sinusoidally. In Figure 2–21 we see that the amplitude of **displacement** (dashed line) of the system varies sinusoidally over time. In accordance with Hooke's law, the restoring force of **elasticity** also varies sinusoidally over time. The magnitude of the restoring force of elasticity is directly proportional to the magnitude of displacement. Elasticity is *in phase* with displacement; hence, the sinusoidally varying elastic force is shown by the same dashed line that is used to describe displacement.

Velocity (solid line) also changes sinusoidally over time, and as you recall, velocity *leads* displacement by 90°. Also recall that, whereas velocity leads displacement by 90°, velocity *lags* **acceleration** (dotted line) by 90°, and acceleration is 180° degrees out of phase with displacement. As the mass of the system moves from maximum displacement toward equilibrium, the velocity of motion increases, and the system gains **momentum**.

Because **momentum** is given by the product of **mass** and **velocity** (**M = mc**; Equation 1.9), momentum is directly proportional to

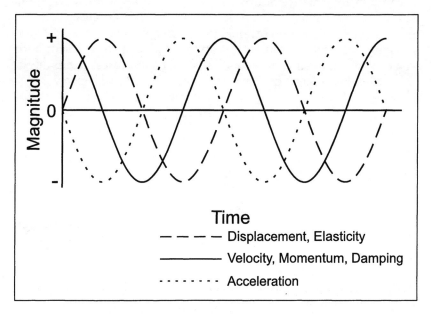

Figure 2–21. The relations among sinusoidal waveforms for **displacement, elasticity, velocity, momentum, damping (frictional resistance),** and **acceleration.**

velocity of motion. Momentum also varies sinusoidally over time, and momentum is *in phase* with velocity. Thus, momentum is shown by the same solid line that is used to represent velocity. Because momentum is in phase with velocity, elasticity is in phase with displacement, and velocity *leads* displacement by 90°, we can see that momentum also *leads* the restoring force of elasticity by 90°. Therefore, momentum is greatest when velocity is greatest, velocity is greatest when displacement is zero (i.e., when the vibrating mass is passing through equilibrium), and the force of elasticity is zero when displacement is zero.

Effects of Friction on Vibratory Motion

Once energy is imparted to an object, vibratory motion would continue indefinitely with no decrement in amplitude over time if there were no opposition to motion. Because **frictional resistance** serves to limit velocity, however, vibratory motion will not continue indefinitely.

The amplitude of vibration of the mass diminishes over time, and the vibrations are therefore **damped**. The same is true of the child's swing in the park, and of all other forms of vibratory motion. One push is sufficient to cause the swing and child to move to and fro, but because of friction, the amplitude of each successive excursion (displacement) is slightly less than the amplitude of the previous excursion; **damping** has occurred.

Damping occurs because of the **resistance** of the air medium and because of internal friction within an oscillating system. Damping also varies sinusoidally as a function of time, and because frictional resistance is directly proportional to velocity, damping is represented in Figure 2–21 by the same solid line that is used to represent both velocity and momentum. Thus, as velocity increases, damping increases because kinetic energy is transformed to thermal energy (heat). Because of the loss of energy due to damping, free vibrations do not continue indefinitely, and the amplitude of vibration diminishes over time.

The Magnitude of Damping

How long will the vibrations of a damped system continue? We learned earlier that the magnitude of the *initial* displacement of the mass depends on the magnitude of force applied. It should make sense, therefore, that the duration of vibratory motion depends on *the amount of damping present* relative to *the magnitude of the force applied*. Thus, the duration of vibrations is directly proportional to the force applied and inversely proportional to damping.

Different vibratory systems are characterized by different amounts of damping. In systems that are **low damped**, the vibrations last for a relatively long time. A tuning fork is a good example of a low-damped system. Energy is imparted to the fork by striking it, and once struck, it might continue to vibrate freely for several seconds, depending, of course, on the force with which it was struck. In contrast, in systems that are **high damped**, the vibrations are very brief and there is a steep decrement in the amplitude of vibration over time.

Figure 2–22 displays examples of the vibrations of a "lossless" system (panel A) where the vibrations continue to infinity, a theoretical concept in which no damping exists, and also of low-damped (panel B) and high-damped (panel C) systems. We can see that in a low-damped system, the amplitude diminishes gradually over time. In a high-damped system, the vibrations last for only a brief period of time, and the decrement in amplitude is steep.

The Damping Factor

Regardless of whether we are considering low-damped or high-damped systems, *the ratio of the amplitudes (A) of any two consecutive cycles of vibration is a constant*. For example, in the low-damped system in panel B, $A_1/A_2 = A_2/A_3 = A_3/A_4$, and so forth. We will learn in Chapter 3 that *constant ratios* can be expressed logarithmically. For that reason, the *magnitude of damping* (the **damping factor**), which we will symbolize as d_f, is given by the natural log ($\log_e$, or ln) of the ratio of the amplitudes of any two consecutive cycles:

$$d_f = \ln\left(\frac{A_1}{A_2}\right).$$

Equation 2.13

Figure 2–23 shows examples of vibrations resulting from five systems with different damping factors, d_f. The amplitudes of A_1

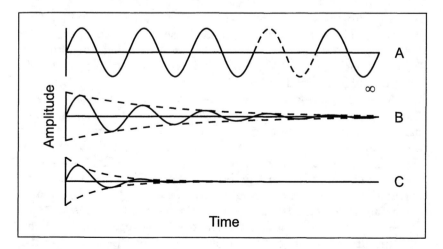

Figure 2–22. Illustrations of **damping** that occurs because of resistance to motion.

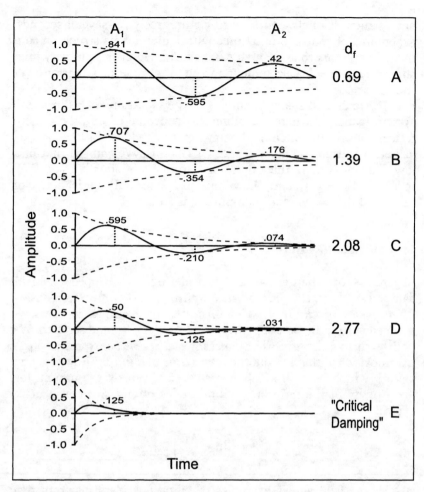

Figure 2–23. Examples of waveforms with different damping factors that range from 0.69, to 2.77, to **critical damping**.

decrease progressively from .841 unit to .5 unit in the first four examples, and the amplitudes of A_2 decrease from .42 to .031 unit. As the amplitude decreases from A_1 to A_2 in each panel, the damping factor increases from 0.69 (a relatively low-damped system) to 2.77 (a relatively high-damped system).

After completing a review of logarithms and antilogarithms in Chapter 3, the interested reader might return to this discussion of damping. It should then be apparent that because we have seen that a constant ratio of 2:1 is preserved between the amplitudes of any two consecutive cycles of the damped system in panel A of Figure 2–23, the damping factor increases linearly in equal (if you carry the calculation to sufficient decimal places) log units of 0.69315 because a constant ratio of 2:1 is preserved and the natural log of 2 is 0.69315.

In a theoretically lossless system, $d_f = 0$, because the ratio of any two amplitudes would equal one, and the log of 1 (regardless of the base) equals 0. The lowest curve in panel E of Figure 2–23 shows what is called **critical damping**. A system that is critically damped is displaced and then returns to equilibrium, but not beyond.

Examples of Damped Systems

We are all familiar with practical examples of damped systems in our daily lives. Shock absorbers on cars, for example, are usually designed to give critical damping (or nearly so) so that the car will not bounce up and down excessively. Of course, as the shock absorbers wear out, they become underdamped, and the car will tend to bounce up and down several times when it hits a bump.

Another example is the level indicator, or needle, on a VU meter of a tape recorder. It too is typically designed to be close to critically damped. If underdamped, the needle would swing back and forth on either side of the "correct value" before finally settling down. On the other hand, if the needle is overdamped, too much time would be required for the needle to reach the correct value and the rapid changes in the level of signals such as speech or music could not be detected. Critical damping represents the boundary between over-damped (nonoscillatory) and underdamped (oscillatory) conditions.

■ ACOUSTIC IMPEDANCE

The tuning fork, pendulum, and simple spring-mass system introduced in Chapter 1 all engage in simple harmonic motion. Moreover, they all engage in what is called **free vibration**, and each system vibrates freely at its own **natural frequency (f_{nat})**.

By **free vibrations** we mean that once energy is imparted to a body that has a low **damping factor**, the body vibrates *freely* for some considerable period of time, and no additional outside force is required to urge the continued vibrations. Thus, once an external force is applied to a system and vibration is initiated, the only forces that are operating are the restoring force of **elasticity** (except for the pendulum, where the restoring force is gravity) and an **inertial force**.

What will be the frequency of vibration? The **natural frequency** of a simple harmonic oscillator depends on the **mass** and the **stiffness** of the system. Specifically, the natural frequency of a system is *directly proportional to the square root of its **stiffness** and inversely proportional to the square root of its **mass***. Thus, if the **natural frequency** of a system were 200 Hz and its stiffness were increased by a factor of 4:1, the **natural frequency** would *increase* by a factor of 2:1 (square root of 4) to a frequency of 400 Hz. If, instead, the mass of that same system were increased by a factor of 4:1, the natural frequency would *decrease* by a factor of 2:1 to a frequency of 100 Hz.

We know, of course, that **free vibrations** will not continue indefinitely. The oscillations will be damped because of **resistance**. There is no such thing as perpetual motion because forces exist that oppose, or **impede**, all motion.

Resistance (R)

All motion is opposed by **resistance (R)**, and resistance contributes to, but is not synonymous with, **acoustic impedance**. We may think of acoustic impedance as *the total opposition to motion*. In other words, there are forces in addition to resistance that help determine the total opposition to motion, which is the **impedance**.

We learned previously that because **friction** opposes, or resists, motion, friction serves to limit velocity of motion. Energy is transformed from **kinetic energy** to **thermal energy** (heat). Importantly, **resistance**, which is measured in units called **ohms**, *is independent of frequency*. Thus, a given magnitude of resistance provides a specified opposition to motion of a system, regardless of the frequency with which that system oscillates. There are, however, additional forces that oppose motion of an elastic system *in a frequency selective way*. Those forces are called **reactance forces** or, simply, **reactances.**

Reactance (X)

When a force is applied to a simple harmonic oscillator, some of the energy associated with the applied force is converted to thermal energy because of resistance. Some of the energy that is applied to a system, however, *is stored in the elastic system as potential energy* **(PE)**. The component of a system that is responsible for storage of energy is called **reactance**.

Reactance opposes motion, but in a way that is very different from the opposition to motion attributable to **resistance**. In the case of resistance, *energy is dissipated*. In the case of reactance, *energy is stored*. Thus, the **impedance** of a system has two components: an *energy-dissipating component* called **resistance** and an *energy-storage component* called **reactance.**

Resistance, the energy-dissipating component of impedance, *is independent of frequency*. Reactance, the energy-storage component of impedance, *is frequency dependent*. We shall see, subsequently, that the total opposition to motion, the **acoustic impedance**, is the complex sum of frequency-independent resistance and frequency-dependent reactance.

Opposition to motion in frequency-selective ways, the reactance, depends on the **mass** and **compliance** of the system. Although a system's **mass** and **compliance** each serve to oppose, or impede, motion, they do so in opposite ways. To explain this, it will be helpful to return to Figure 2–21 and review the phasic relations among displacement, velocity, acceleration, and so forth. The following phasic relations are important for understanding impedance.

1. Opposition to motion due to **resistance,** which is independent of frequency, *is in phase with velocity*.

2. Opposition to motion due to **compliance,** which is frequency dependent, *is in phase with displacement and elasticity,* and *lags resistance by 90°.*

3. Opposition to motion due to **mass,** which also is frequency dependent, *is in phase with acceleration,* and *leads resistance by 90°.*

4. It therefore follows that opposition to motion due to **mass** *is 180° out of phase with* **compliance.**

Reactance has two components. One is **mass reactance (X_m)** and the other is **compliant reactance (X_c).** The two components of reactance, mass reactance and compliant reactance, always act in opposition to one another. When one is storing energy, the other is giving it up.

Mass Reactance (X_m)

The magnitude of **mass reactance (X_m),** which is measured in **ohms,** is given by:

$$X_m = 2\pi f m,$$

Equation 2.14

where **f** is frequency, **m** is the effective mass,

and

2π is a constant.

Recall that $2\pi f$ defines the angular velocity (ω). Therefore it is equally appropriate to say that **mass reactance** is given by the product of angular velocity and mass. *Mass reactance (X_m) is directly proportional to frequency* and is essentially negligible at very low frequencies. For each octave increase (a doubling of frequency or a frequency ratio of 2:1) in frequency ($f_2 = 2f_1$), mass reactance *increases* by a factor of 2:1. Hence, mass reactance contributes to the frequency-dependent nature of impedance.

Compliant Reactance (X_c)

The magnitude of **compliant reactance (X_c),** which also is measured in **ohms,** is given by:

$$X_c = \frac{1}{2\pi f c},$$

Equation 2.15

where **c** is the compliance.

Compliant reactance also can be defined as the reciprocal of the product of compliance and angular velocity, and as we can see in

Equation 2.15, **compliant reactance** *is inversely proportional to frequency.* Thus, compliant reactance also contributes to the frequency-dependent nature of impedance.

Whereas mass reactance is negligible at low frequencies, **compliant reactance** is quite large at low frequencies. For each octave increase in frequency, **compliant reactance** *decreases* by a factor of 2:1.

When $X_m = X_c$, the two opposing reactance forces cancel one another (because they are 180° out of phase), and the only opposition to motion is resistance. When that circumstance exists with a free vibrating, simple harmonic oscillating system, the frequency at which the two opposing forces cancel one another defines the **natural frequency** with which the system will vibrate.

Figure 2–24 shows how the magnitudes of X_m and X_c vary with frequency: $X_m \propto f$ and $X_c \propto 1/f$. For low frequencies, most of the opposition to motion comes from X_c, and the system is described as *compliance dominant.* For high frequencies, most of the opposition to motion comes from X_m, and the system is described as *mass dominant.*

We learned previously that X_m and X_c are 180° out of phase with each other. Therefore, $X_m - X_c$, the net reactance, forms the dashed line in Figure 2–24. The dashed line serves to emphasize the fact that the net reactance $(X_m - X_c)$ is largely attributable to X_c at low frequencies and to X_m at high frequencies.

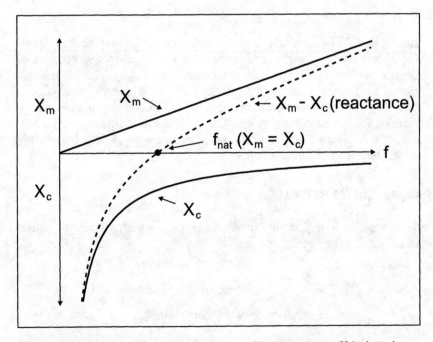

Figure 2–24. Mass reactance (X_m) and **compliant reactance (X_c)** plotted as a function of frequency. The **net reactance (X)** is shown by the curve labeled $X_m - X_c$. The frequency at which $X_m = X_c$ is called the **natural frequency (f_{nat})**.

The dot on the dashed line identifies the frequency where $X_m = X_c$. At that frequency, the net reactance is zero and opposition to motion comes only from **R** (which is not reflected in Figure 2–24). That defines the **natural frequency, f_{nat},** the frequency at which *the system vibrates freely with a maximum amplitude of vibration.*

Impedance (Z)

Resistance causes energy to be dissipated, whereas **mass reactance** and **compliant reactance** cause energy to be stored. Although all three factors serve to oppose motion and the transfer of energy, we cannot add their respective magnitudes algebraically to determine the total opposition (**impedance**) because the three components are not in phase: X_m (**mass reactance**) leads **R** (**resistance**) by 90°; X_c (**compliant reactance**) lags **R** by 90°; and X_m leads X_c by 180°.

Because the three components of impedance are not in phase with one another, they must be treated as vector-like quantities called **phasor quantities**, or just **phasors**, but the mathematics are the same as for vector solution. Consider the phase diagrams in Figure 2–25. In panel A, we show only **mass reactance** (X_m) and **resistance** (**R**). Mass reactance leads resistance by 90°, and the two quantities are drawn at right angles to one another. The resultant **impedance (Z) vector**, which is shown by the dashed line, is determined by use of Pythagoras' theorem, just as we learned to do with velocity (Equation 1.2) in Chapter 1:

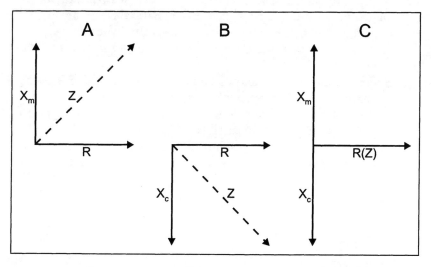

Figure 2–25. Phase diagrams that show the **impedance vectors** that result from **mass reactance** and **resistance** in panel A, **compliant reactance** and **resistance** in panel B, and **mass reactance, compliant reactance**, and **resistance** in panel C.

Equation 2.16

$$Z = \sqrt{R^2 + X_m^2},$$

where **R** is the resistance,

and

X_m is the mass reactance.

In panel B, we show only **compliant reactance** (X_c) and **resistance** (**R**), but of course in this case, compliant reactance lags resistance by 90°. Again, the impedance (**Z**) vector is shown by the dashed line, and the resultant impedance is given by:

Equation 2.17

$$Z = \sqrt{R^2 + X_c^2},$$

where X_c is the compliant reactance.

In panel C, all three components of **impedance** (**R**, X_m, and X_c) are included with the appropriate phasic relations. The impedance vector now is given by:

Equation 2.18

$$Z = \sqrt{R^2 + (X_m - X_c)^2}.$$

Thus, **acoustic impedance** (**Z**), which is expressed in **ohms**, may be defined *as the square root of the sum of the square of the resistance* (**R**) *and the square of the reactance* (**X**). In the case of the specific example that is shown panel C in Figure 2–25, $X_m = X_c$, the two reactance components cancel, and **Z** = **R**. As we learned previously, the frequency at which $X_m = X_c$ defines the **natural frequency** (f_{nat}) of the system. In Chapter 6, we will learn to say that when the $X_m = X_c$ (the two reactance components equal one another), *the system is "in resonance."*

Panel A of Figure 2–26 shows a phase diagram in which $X_m > X_c$. In this case, the contribution of mass reactance to impedance is greater than the contribution of compliant reactance. The opposite relation, $X_c > X_m$ is shown in panel B of Figure 2–26.[4] You should also note that in those two instances, **impedance** is not determined exclusively by **resistance**. The **reactance** components also contribute to the total opposition to motion, the **impedance**. When $X_m = X_c$, impedance (**Z**) is at its minimum.

■ SUMMARY

We have seen that simple harmonic oscillators engage in sinusoidal motion. Once a force is applied to such an oscillator, it engages in free vibration. The waveform has four dimensions of interest: amplitude, frequency (and period), phase, and wavelength. Finally, we have

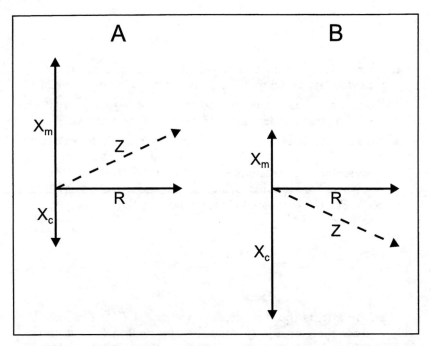

Figure 2–26. Phase diagrams that show the **impedance vectors** that result from all three components of impedance. In panel A, **mass reactance** is dominant, and in panel B, **compliant reactance** is dominant.

learned that free vibrations of a system do not last indefinitely because of opposition to motion from friction. The amplitudes decay over time, and those vibrations are called damped vibrations. The total opposition to motion or energy transfer is called impedance, and impedance has two components, resistance and reactance (mass reactance and compliant reactance).

Chapter 4 will concern the use of **decibels** to express the "magnitude" of a sound wave. To understand the decibel requires knowledge of logs and antilogs. Readers who feel comfortable with those concepts might wish to move directly to Chapter 4. For those who would profit from a review, Chapter 3 contains a detailed description of logs and antilogs.

■ NOTES

1. Those who are familiar with calculus will recognize that particle velocity is the first derivative of particle displacement.

2. Particle acceleration is the first derivative of particle velocity and the second derivative of particle displacement.

3. These equations provide an approximate, but perfectly acceptable, *estimate* of the **rms** sound pressure of sine waves. Precise calculations of the **rms** pressure require knowledge of calculus, which is beyond the scope of this book. For the interested reader, however, the defining equation for **rms** is

$$\text{rms} = \sqrt{\frac{1}{T}\int_0^T x(t)^2\, dt}\,,$$

where **x (t)** is the time-domain waveform, **T** is the period, and the integral sign (∫) indicates summation of an infinite number of instantaneous amplitudes during one period (one cycle) of the wave. For our purposes, and for all practical purposes that most readers will encounter, Equation 2.6 will suffice for calculating the **rms sound pressure** of sine waves.

4. Impedance is a vector-like quantity called a phasor. Solution of Equation 2.18 reveals the *length* of the impedance vectors in Figure 2–26. The impedance vector in each panel of the figure, however, also must reflect the appropriate phase angle, θ. The phase angle of impedance is given by θ = **arctan** [(X$_m$ − X$_c$)/R], which is the same as θ = **tan**$^{-1}$ (X/R). **Tan**$^{-1}$ is the same as **arctan**, and **tan**$^{-1}$ is likely to be the label that you will find on your pocket calculator.

■ FREQUENTLY MISUNDERSTOOD CONCEPTS

1. What is the phasic relation between **particle velocity** and **particle displacement** during simple harmonic motion?

   Particle velocity *leads* **particle displacement** by 90°. Hence, particle velocity is *maximally positive* when the instantaneous phase angle of particle displacement is 0°, and particle velocity is *maximally negative* when the instantaneous phase angle of particle displacement is 180°.

2. Mean square sound pressure = rms^2. Does that mean that **mean square pressure** will always be greater than **rms pressure**?

   No. If rms is less than 1.0, mean square will be less than rms, and if rms equals 1.0, mean square will equal rms. For example, if rms = 0.9, mean square = 0.81 (0.9^2), but if rms = 1.0, means square also = 1.0 (1.0^2). Thus, the numerical value of mean square may be less than, equal to, or greater than rms, depending on the value of rms. Note, however, that the unit of measure for rms (**Pa**) is different from the unit of measure for mean square (**Pa^2**)

3. Sine wave **X** has a frequency of 1000 Hz and a starting phase of 0°. Sine wave **Y** has a frequency of 2000 Hz and a starting phase also of 0°. Describe the relation between the instantaneous phase angles of the two sine waves over the course of one period for sine wave **X**.

   The phasic relation between the two sine waves will vary from moment to moment; they will move in and out of phase. See Figure 2–16. The two waves are *in phase* (0°) when t = 0 ms, **Y** *leads* **X** by 90° when t = .25 ms, **Y** *leads* **X** by 180° when t = .5 ms, and so forth. They are in phase once again when t = 1 ms.

4. How does the magnitude of the elastic restoring force of a spring-mass system change over time when the system is engaged in simple harmonic motion?

   Elasticity is a **restoring force** that *opposes* the force that acts to deform the spring. Hooke's law informed us that the magnitude of the restoring force (**F$_r$**) is directly proportional to the magnitude of the spring's displacement (**x**). The magnitude of the spring's displacement changes sinusoidally over time, and the magnitude of restoring force also varies sinusoidally over time. The sinusoidally changing restoring force is *in phase* with the sinusoidally changing displacement.

Logarithms and Antilogarithms

In Chapter 2 we learned that the magnitude, or amplitude, of a sine wave can be expressed by reference to its sound pressure in newtons per square meter (N/m^2) or pascals (**Pa**). Most of the time, however, the magnitude of the sine wave is described by the **decibel** (**dB**). It is apparent from reading popular literature such as newspapers and magazine articles and, unfortunately, even from reading some professional papers, that the decibel is sometimes used incorrectly and apparently is often misunderstood. We will consider the decibel (actually the decibels) in detail in Chapter 4, but because decibel notation requires a facility with **logarithms** (**logs**) and **antilogarithms** (**antilogs**), those concepts will be reviewed here.

■ THE CONCEPT OF LOGARITHMS AND ANTILOGARITHMS

Some readers might not know the answers to the two antilog problems below:

$$\text{antilog}_2 \ 2 = \underline{\hspace{2cm}} \ ?$$

or

$$\text{antilog}_{10} \ 2 = \underline{\hspace{2cm}} \ ?$$

Almost everyone, however, will know the answers to the next two problems, which might *appear* to be easier to understand and solve:

$$2^2 = \underline{\hspace{2cm}} \ ?$$

and

$$10^2 = \underline{\hspace{2cm}} \ ?$$

Actually, the two sets of problems are equal in difficulty because the second set is identical to the first. If you know that $2^2 = 4$ and that $10^2 = 100$, the *concept* of antilogs will be easily understood. The reason for that assurance lies in the following statement of equivalence:

$$\text{antilog}_2 \ 2 = 2^2 = 4$$

and

$$\text{antilog}_{10} \ 2 = 10^2 = 100.$$

In other words, asking, "$\text{antilog}_{10} \ 2 = \ ?$" is identical to asking, "what is 10 raised to the second power, or what is 10 squared?" The concept of *any* antilog problem is no more difficult than that, and all that remains is to learn some simple steps that make it possible to solve problems that are computationally, but not conceptually, more difficult. For example, it will not be immediately obvious that

$$\text{antilog}_{10} \ 1.7 = 50.12,$$

but asking, "antilog$_{10}$ 1.7 = ?" is identical to asking, "what is 10 raised to the 1.7 power?"

We shall see subsequently that the *concept of logarithms* is as easy to grasp as the concept of antilogs. Before proceeding to some computational details, it will be helpful to review "scales of measurement" briefly.

SCALES OF MEASUREMENT

The word "measurement" describes a process whereby *numerals* are assigned to objects according to specific rules. The word "numerals" was emphasized, because, as we shall see, it is important to distinguish between numerals and numbers. A **numeral** is a **symbol** such as 8, 25, III, A, and so forth. In contrast, a **number** is a **symbol** that bears some fixed relation to other symbols. For example, the numbers 12 and 13 will always sum to the number 25, whereas the numerals 12 and 13 are nothing but names or designators—they cannot be added or manipulated in other mathematical ways. The importance of distinguishing between numerals and numbers should become more clear as we review the various scales of measurement that are available to us.

There are four scales of measurement: **nominal**, **ordinal**, **interval**, and **ratio** (Stevens, 1951).[1] Before any measurement is undertaken, we should be careful to determine which type of scale applies.

Nominal Scale

With the **nominal** scale, we can sort things into different categories by observing that one object is the *same as* or *different from* another. That is the only requirement. For example, we could sort according to two categories of male/female, adult/child, fruit/vegetable, basic/derived quantities, 1s/0s, and so forth, or according to three categories of beef/pork/poultry, or whatever. Within each category, then, we simply count the number of objects that belong: 6 male/14 female, 13 adults/7 children, and so on. This is not a very powerful scale because, basically, the only arithmetic operation that can be performed legitimately on the entries in the categories is to count them.

Ordinal Scale

With the **ordinal** scale, we still can say that two or more things are different, but we also can say that one object has *more or less* of (or the same as) some quantity than another object. Thus, with the familiar letter grades that often are used to describe academic performance, we are accustomed to saying that

$$A > B > C > D > F.$$

With such a scale, we have an implicit ordering of the letters, but *the letters are not numbers and they cannot legitimately be added or subtracted.* We know that A exceeds B, but we do not know by how much A exceeds B. Of equal importance, we have no guarantee that A exceeds B by the same amount that B exceeds C. We often assign *numerals* to represent those letter grades, and from that we generate another ordinal scale,

$$4 > 3 > 2 > 1 > 0.$$

You still cannot perform many arithmetic operations on those numerals, however, even though Offices of Admissions and Records at most colleges and universities do calculate grade point averages (perhaps only athletic departments realize that the GPA is invalid). When the numerals are used on an ordinal scale, you do know that $4 > 3$ and that $3 > 2$, but you do *not* know the amounts by which 4 exceeds 3 or 3 exceeds 2. Furthermore, you do *not* know that 4 exceeds 3 by the same amount that 3 exceeds 2 anymore than you did for the As, Bs, and Cs that the numerals replaced. That is why addition and subtraction of the numerals on the ordinal scale can lead to misleading results.

The problems associated with performing improper mathematics on the numerals of an ordinal scale can be illustrated by a story adapted from Senders (1958). Four men, nicknamed Boomer, Draw, Slice, and Rake, met for the first time at a golf course and wanted to band together to achieve a competitive match. But, who should be paired with whom to achieve the best balance? They decided to settle the question on the driving range. Boomer slammed his drive 280 yards; Draw hooked his to the left, but netted 265 yards; Slice faded his ball to the right, but it still landed 250 yards away from the tee; and then Rake took an awkward swing, topped the ball badly, and watched as it rolled about 50 yards. Thus,

$$\text{Boomer} > \text{Draw} > \text{Slice} > \text{Rake}.$$

The numeral 4 was assigned to Boomer, 3 to Draw, 2 to Slice, and 1 to Rake because

$$4 > 3 > 2 > 1.$$

Because $4 + 1 = 2 + 3$, the men agreed that Boomer and Rake would compete against Draw and Slice in medal play. The outcome was not what they expected. Boomer shot 68, Draw shot 72, Slice managed a respectable 73, and Rake struggled to a 117. Draw and Slice were the obvious winners. How did this happen when the numerical averages showed the two teams to be equal? Boomer, Draw, and Slice were experienced golfers and each had won several local tournaments. With respect to ability, they were closely bunched. Rake, on the other hand had just appeared at the clubhouse after having tended to the sand traps and had never swung a club before. Rake's golfing ability was clearly distant from that of the other three, even though he was only one numeral below the numeral assigned to Slice.

Interval Scale

The **interval** scale, which also is called a **linear** scale, represents a large leap in mathematical power. Order is still preserved, as it was with the ordinal scale, but now *the size of the interval is some constant value.*

The interval is called the **base**. If the numerals 4, 3, 2, 1, and 0 appear on an interval scale, they are *numbers* rather than numerals. Because the base (the size of the interval between adjacent numbers) is a known constant, we know that 4 exceeds 3 by *exactly* the same amount (1) that 3 exceeds 2 (1).

The interval, or linear, scale consists of successive units that are generated by adding (or subtracting) some specified **base** (size of interval) to each successive number along the scale. Consider the examples for different bases that are shown in Table 3–1. In the first series where the base = 1, we add the base of 1 to each successive number to generate a series 1, 2 (1 + 1), 3 (2 + 1), 4 (3 + 1), and so on. Note also that there is no restriction on the starting number in the series. The only difference between the first and second series is that the first series starts with 1 and the second series starts with 0; the base is the same. The third series is formed in an identical way, except that now a base of 2 is added to each successive number in the series: 0, 2 (0 + 2), 4 (2 + 2), 6 (4 + 2), and so on. In the fourth series, another interval scale has been constructed, but in this case a base of 2 is *subtracted* (added negatively) from each successive number: 10, 8 (10 − 2), 6 (8 − 2), 4 (6 − 2), and so forth. In the final series in the table, a base of 10 is added to form the successive numbers.

With each of the five examples in the table, the interval between any two successive units is exactly equal to the interval between any other two successive units, *and the size of that interval is the **base***. Thus, with an interval scale, we can say that one object is different from another (as with the nominal scale), that one object has more or less of some quantity than another (as with the ordinal scale), and

Table 3–1. Examples of interval scales

Base	Scale	Interval Size
1	1, 2, 3, 4, 5, 6, ... , n	1
1	0, 1, 2, 3, 4, 5, ... , n	1
2	0, 2, 4, 6, 8, 10, ... , n	2
2	10, 8, 6, 4, 2, 0, ... , n	2
10	10, 20, 30, 40, 50, ... , n	10

that one object or event is *a certain number of units more or less than another*. With respect to the golfers described earlier, driving distance on the range might have been used to assign *numbers* on an interval scale. In that case it would have been obvious that Boomer and Rake (280 + 50 = 330) would not have been competitive against Draw and Slice (265 + 250 = 515).

Ratio Scale

The final scale is called a **ratio** scale. We shall see in a moment that it also can be called an **exponential**, or **logarithmic**, scale. The ratio scale has the additional requirement that we have an absolute zero point. The principal characteristic of the ratio scale is that we can say that *one unit on the scale is so many times greater (or less) than another*.

One easy way to understand the necessity of an absolute zero for a ratio scale is to consider the fundamental physical quantity of **time**. Calendar time has no absolute zero. The year 1992 A.D. is not twice as late in time as the year 996 A.D. because we do not know when time began. On the other hand, periods of time can be expressed in terms of ratios. Thus, a person who requires only 5 minutes to run a mile can be said to run twice as fast as a person who requires 10 minutes to finish the same distance.

The ratio scale consists of successive units that are generated by multiplying (or dividing) each successive number along the scale by the **base**. Consider the five examples in Table 3–2. In those examples, a base of 1, 2, 1.5, 10, or 0.1 is multiplied by each successive unit along the scale. Thus, in the first series we obtain 1, 1 (1 × 1), 1 (1 × 1), and so forth. In the second series we obtain 1, 2 (1 × 2), 4 (2 × 2), 8 (4 × 2), 16 (8 × 2), and so on. In the fourth series we obtain 1, 10 (1 × 10), 100 (10 × 10), 1,000 (100 × 10), 10,000 (1,000 × 10), and so forth.

In the scales that result with the five different bases in Table 3–2, we see that successive units always are different by some *constant ratio* (1:1, 2:1, 1.5:1, 10:1, and 0.1:1), and *the constant ratio always equals the base*. Thus, when the base = 2: 64/32 = 2; 32/16 = 2; 16/8 = 2; and so on. Similarly, when the base = 10: 10,000/1,000 = 10; 1,000/100 = 10; 100/10 = 10; and 10/1 = 10. The same must be true for the seemingly more unusual base of 1.5, and in fact 5.0625/3.375 = 1.5; 3.375/2.25 = 1.5; and 2.25/1.5 = 1.5. In all cases, the ratio

Table 3–2. Examples of ratio scales

Base	Scale
1	1, 1, 1, 1, 1, ... , 1
2	1, 2, 4, 8, 16, 32, 64, ... , n
1.5	1, 1.5, 2.25, 3.375, 5.0625, ... , n
10	1, 10, 100, 1,000, 10,000, ... , n
0.1	1, .1, .01, .001, .0001, ... , n

between two adjacent numbers in the series is constant and equal to the base.

The **ratio** scale also can be called an **exponential** scale because any such scale of numbers can be represented as a certain **base** that is raised to successively higher and higher **powers**, or **exponents**. For example, if the base = 2, we can describe the series by either of two ways:

$$1, \quad 2, \quad 4, \quad 8, \quad 16, \quad 32, \quad 64$$

$$(or)$$

$$2^0, \quad 2^1, \quad 2^2, \quad 2^3, \quad 2^4, \quad 2^5, \quad 2^6.$$

The general expression that defines the exponential series shown above is:

$$X^n = \#,$$

which means that the base (X) is used n times in multiplication. Thus, in the example above where the base was 2, we used the base some specified number of times (0, 1, 2, 3, 4, 5, or 6) in multiplication, and we generated a scale that consisted of 1, 2, 4, 8, 16, 32, and 64. If the base of 2 is used either 3, 4, or 5 times in multiplication, we obtain the outcome shown in Table 3–3. Thus, 2^3 means that the base of 2 is used 3 (the power) times in multiplication $(2 \times 2 \times 2)$ to yield 8; 2^4 means the base of 2 is used 4 times in multiplication to yield 16 $(2 \times 2 \times 2 \times 2)$; and 2^5 means $2 \times 2 \times 2 \times 2 \times 2 = 32$.

Table 3–4 shows two exponential (ratio) series that are generated with different base numbers: base = 2 and base = 10. Two generaliza-

Table 3–3. Base = 2 raised to powers of 3, 4, and 5

X^n	Operation	Result
2^3	$2 \times 2 \times 2$	8
2^4	$2 \times 2 \times 2 \times 2$	16
2^5	$2 \times 2 \times 2 \times 2 \times 2$	32

Table 3–4. Exponential series for base = 2 and base = 10

Base = 2		Base = 10	
X^n	Result	X^n	Result
2^0	1	10^0	1
2^1	2	10^1	10
2^2	4	10^2	100
2^3	8	10^3	1,000
2^4	16	10^4	10,000
2^5	32	10^5	100,000

tions can be made from the examples in Table 3–4. First, *any base that is raised to the zero power* (X^0) *equals 1*. From the first rule we learn that: $2^0 = 1$; $10^0 = 1$; $3.1416^0 = 1$; and so forth. Second, *any base that is raised to the first power* (X^1) *equals the base*. From the second rule we learn that: $2^1 = 2$; $10^1 = 10$; $3.1416^1 = 3.1416$; and so forth.

■ MORE ON EXPONENTS

We have seen that exponents (or powers) specify how many times a base (X) is used in multiplication or division. When the operation is *multiplication*, the expression is:

Equation 3.1

$$X^n = \#.$$

For example,

$$3^4 = 3 \times 3 \times 3 \times 3 = 81.$$

The exponent (4) indicates that the base (3) is used 4 times in multiplication. When the operation is *division*, the expression is written as:

Equation 3.2

$$X^{-n},$$

$$\text{where } X^{-n} = \frac{1}{X^n}.$$

Thus, $3^{-4} = 1/3^4 = 1/(3 \times 3 \times 3 \times 3) = 1/81 = 0.01234567$.

The two expressions shown as Equations 3.1 and 3.2 will be encountered frequently in decibel notation. There are other defining equations for exponents, although only one of them will appear often:

Equation 3.3

$$X^0 = 1.$$

The importance of remembering the rule given by Equation 3.3 cannot be emphasized too strongly. *Any base (X) raised to the zero power equals 1*. Thus,

$$X^0 = 1,$$

$$1^0 = 1,$$

$$2^0 = 1,$$

$$10^0 = 1, \text{ and}$$

$$\left[\frac{(2.36)}{(a + bx)} \right]^0 = 1.$$

Laws of Exponents

There are three laws that govern the use of exponents, and they will be of tremendous value in helping to solve decibel problems simply.

Law 1 of Exponents

$$X^a \times X^b = X^{a+b}. \qquad \text{LAW 1}$$

According to Law 1, if you wish to determine the product of some *common base* (X) that is raised to two different powers (a and b), you simply raise the base (X) to the sum of the two powers (a + b). For example,

$$2^3 \times 2^2 = 2^{3+2} = 2^5 = 32.$$

It might not seem very useful to use Law 1 to solve such a simple problem, because we certainly know that $2^3 = 8$ and $2^2 = 4$, so it indeed is simpler to just multiply 8×4 to get 32. But, consider the next example.

$$2^{1.5} \times 2^{1.5} = ?$$

It might not be immediately obvious how we proceed to determine the value of $2^{1.5}$, and it also might not be intuitively obvious what it meant by *using the base of 2 one and a half times in multiplication*. The solution is easy, however, if we employ Law 1.

$$2^{1.5} \times 2^{1.5} = 2^{1.5+1.5} = 2^3 = 8.$$

It is important to remember that in order to use Law 1 in solution of exponent problems, *the value of the base (X) must be the same in both terms of the product.* Thus, Law 1 does not apply for a problem such as $X^a \times Y^b$ (e.g., $2^3 \times 10^4$).

Law 2 of Exponents

The second law is undoubtedly the most useful of the three laws in solution of decibel problems:

$$\frac{X^a}{X^b} = X^{a-b}. \qquad \text{LAW 2}$$

According to Law 2, the ratio of some base (X) raised to two different powers is equal to the base (X) raised to the difference between the two powers (a − b). For example,

$$\frac{2^4}{2^2} = 2^{(4-2)} = 2^2 = 4.$$

That problem also is not difficult to solve without use of Law 2 because we know that $2^4 = 16$, and $2^2 = 4$, and 16/4 = 4. Nevertheless, the example does illustrate the simplicity of the law. The next example would be more difficult to solve without Law 2:

$$\frac{2^{17.5}}{2^{15.5}} = 2^{(17.5-15.5)} = 2^2 = 4.$$

As can be seen from Law 2, as long as the same base appears in both the numerator and the denominator of the ratio, you simply subtract the exponents and then raise the base to the difference.

As was mentioned previously, Law 2 will be encountered frequently in decibel problems, and in virtually all instances the base will equal 10. Consider, therefore, four additional examples of Law 2 with the base = 10.

Example 1
$$\frac{10^{-9}}{10^{-12}} = 10^{(-9)-(-12)} = 10^3.$$

Note that in this example you are subtracting one negative number from another negative number. Remember that *minus a minus is a plus*. Thus, the difference between -9 and -12 is $+3$ because it becomes a -9 and a $+12$ (minus a minus is a plus). The solution could have been carried one step further to show that $10^3 = 1,000$, but the additional computational step generally is not necessary. It is perfectly acceptable to show the answer simply as 10^3.

Example 2
$$\frac{10^{-12}}{10^{-9}} = 10^{(-12)-(-9)} = 10^{-3}.$$

Minus a minus is a plus, but in this case that translates to a -12 and a $+9$, which is a -3.

Example 3
$$\frac{10^{-9}}{10^{-16}} = 10^{(-9)-(-16)} = 10^7.$$

You should see that Example 3 is identical in form to Example 1.

Example 4
$$\frac{10^{-9}}{10^{-9}} = 10^{(-9)-(-9)} = 10^0 = 1.$$

The answer of 1 is consistent with Equation 3.3, which defined $X^0 = 1$ (any base raised to the zero power equals one). You should see from Example 4 that this makes sense, because any number (e.g., 10^{-9}) divided by itself (i.e., 10^{-9}) must equal one.

Law 3 of Exponents

The third law of exponents will not be used extensively in decibel problems, but it might be encountered occasionally.

LAW 3
$$(X^a)^b = X^{ab}.$$
For example,
$$(2^2)^3 = 2^{(2\times3)} = 2^6 = 64.$$

■ ANTILOGS AND LOGS

Antilogs

In Table 3–4 we showed two exponential series that were generated with different base numbers, 2 and 10. Those two series are shown again in Table 3–5, but this time the table is organized differently. We can ask either of two questions and then perform either of two arithmetic operations, depending on how the entries in Table 3–5 are arranged. As the table is presently arranged, we are asking the question:

$$X^n = ?$$

For those examples, therefore, we are asking, "what is the value of 2 raised to the 0 power, 2 raised to the 1st power, 2 raised to the 2nd power, and so on?" Stated differently, we are asking, "what is the value of the base (X) raised to the nth power?" That question also is called *determining the* **antilog** *of the number.* Thus, the question can be written in either of two forms, and they are equivalent.

$$X^n = ?$$

is exactly the same as

$$\text{antilog}_X n = ?$$

In other words,

$$X^n = \text{antilog}_X n.$$

Stated differently, "what is the antilog to the base X of n?" is the same as "what is the value of X raised to the nth power?" In the examples below, the same questions are posed both ways.

$$2^3 = 8 \quad and \quad \text{antilog}_2 3 = 8.$$ **Example 1**

$$10^3 = 1{,}000 \quad and \quad \text{antilog}_{10} 3 = 1{,}000.$$ **Example 2**

Table 3–5. Two exponential series of numbers for base = 2 and base = 10

Base = 2		Base = 10	
X^n	Answer	X^n	Answer
$2^0 = ?$	1	$10^0 = ?$	1
$2^1 = ?$	2	$10^1 = ?$	10
$2^2 = ?$	4	$10^2 = ?$	100
$2^3 = ?$	8	$10^3 = ?$	1,000
$2^4 = ?$	16	$10^4 = ?$	10,000

Thus, with a base of 2, we could ask, "2 raised to the third power equals what number?" (Answer = 8), or we could ask, "what is the antilog to the base 2 of 3?" (Answer = 8).

Logs

In Table 3–6 you will see the same two series of numbers that appeared in Table 3–5, but now they are arranged differently to ask a different question. With this new arrangement of the table, *the exponent is not given*, and we are asking, "to what power must some specified base be raised to equal some particular number?" In other words, we are asking:

$$X^? = \#.$$

Table 3–6. Two exponential series for base = 2 and base = 10

Base = 2		Base = 10	
X^n	Answer	X^n	Answer
$2^? = 1$	0	$10^? = 1$	0
$2^? = 2$	1	$10^? = 10$	1
$2^? = 4$	2	$10^? = 100$	2
$2^? = 8$	3	$10^? = 1,000$	3
$2^? = 16$	4	$10^? = 10,000$	4

Consider the following two examples.

Example 1   To what power must the base of 2 be raised to equal 8?
(Answer = 3)

Example 2   To what power must the base of 10 be raised to equal 10,000?
(Answer = 4)

When you solve problems of that kind, you are *taking the **log** of a number*, and the following two expressions are identical to each other.

$$X^? = \#$$

is exactly the same as

$$\log_X \# = ?$$

Thus, the question, "to what power must the base X be raised to equal the number in question?" is equivalent to asking, "what is the log to the base X of the number?" In the examples on the next page, the same questions are posed both ways.

$2^? = 16$ (Answer = 4) *and* $\log_2 16 = ?$ (Answer = 4.)   **Example 1**

$10^? = 1,000$ (Answer = 3) *and* $\log_{10} 1,000 = ?$ (Answer = 3.)   **Example 2**

Bases for Logs and Antilogs

When you attempt to solve either **log** or **antilog** problems, *the base must always be specified.* Thus, log 1,000 = ? is a meaningless question that cannot be solved. How could one possibly know whether you are asking for the power to which 2 must be raised to equal 1,000, the power to which 10 must be raised to equal 1,000, or whatever? *Any number can serve as the base,* but in practice there are three bases that are most common: "2," "10" (which is called the **common**, or **Briggsian**, **log**), and "e" (2.718, which is called the **natural**, or **Naperian**, **log**).

Summary

It is important to note that when you "take the log of a number" (e.g., $\log_{10} 100 = 2$), *you are solving for an exponent.* An exponent is a log, and a log is an exponent. That is why the title to this chapter is "Logarithms and Antilogarithms" rather than "Exponents, Logarithms, and Antilogarithms."

By now you might be able to solve the simple examples of log and antilog problems fairly quickly by inspection. Thus, you undoubtedly know that $\log_{10} 1,000 = 3$ and that $\log_{10} 100 = 2$. You might, for example, have simply counted the number of zeros and accepted that as your answer. That is perfectly acceptable for those particular problems. It must be less obvious, though, that:

$$\log_{10} 121 = 2.08279.$$

Conceptually, the problem $\log_{10} 121 = ?$ is no different from the problem $\log_{10} 100 = ?$. You are asked to answer the questions, "to what power must the base of 10 be raised to equal 121 in one case and to equal 100 in the other?" The concept is the same, but counting zeros will not always provide you with the correct solution. All that remains, then, is to identify a series of computational steps that will enable us to determine the log of any (positive) number.

■ PROCEDURES FOR SOLVING LOG AND ANTILOG PROBLEMS

Components of a Logarithm

A logarithm consists of one or more **integers** (whole numbers) and an endless string of decimal values. Thus,

$$\log_{10} 100 = 2.00000000----$$

and

$$\log_{10} 121 = 2.08278537----.$$

When we take the log of 100, the solution gives us an integer, or whole number, of 2, and the endless string (usually limited to four, and sometimes only to one or two) of decimals that is composed entirely of zeros. When we take the log of 121, the integer also is 2, but in this case the first four values in the string of decimals are 0.0828. Recall, of course, that in the first example we have learned that 10 (the base) must be raised to a power of 2.0000 to equal 100, and in the second example that the base of 10 must be raised to a power of 2.0828 to equal 121.

Because a log is an exponent, we can rephrase both problems to conform to the language that we used previously with exponents. The base of 10 must be used 2.0000 times in multiplication to equal 100, and it must be used 2.0828 times (just a little more than 2.0000 times) in multiplication (a seemingly strange concept) to equal 121.

The **integer** is called the **characteristic** of a log. The decimal values are called the **mantissa** of a log. Thus, in the two examples above, the **characteristic** (integer) was 2 in both cases, but the **mantissa** (decimal values) was 0.0000 when we took the log of 100 and 0.0828 when we took the log of 121.

To find the log of some (positive) number, the pocket calculator is an indispensable aid. The steps to be followed might vary with different brands, but the manual for the calculator should specify the steps. Most generally, to find the log of some number such as, for example, 121, you enter the number 121 and depress the key labeled [**LOG**]. The display, depending on how many decimals your calculator will display, should read "2.08278537," where the integer 2 is the **characteristic** and 0.08278537 is the **mantissa**.

Some might find it useful to solve a few log problems by using a table of logarithms so that you have an opportunity to become more familiar with the concept of logarithms. Therefore, we shall specify the few easy steps with which the log, both the characteristic and the mantissa, can be found for any positive number. Before taking the log of a number, it is convenient to first transform the number from what can be called **conventional notation** to **scientific notation**.

Scientific Notation

In the course of discussing frequency and period in Chapter 2, we encountered examples of both very large and very small numbers such as 890 MHz (890,000,000 Hz) and its reciprocal (0.001123596 μs or 0.00000001123596 s). In Chapter 4, when the concept of sound intensity is introduced, we will encounter numbers such as 0.0000000000000001 watt/cm^2.

It should be obvious that there are at least two problems with this kind of notation, which we will call "conventional notation."

The expression is cumbersome, and it would be quite easy to drop or add a zero or so without noticing it. Expressing the number in scientific notation should minimize those two problems. We will learn that for the example of sound intensity cited above, the number would be written as 1×10^{-16} in scientific notation rather than 0.0000000000000001 in conventional notation.

Let us begin more simply. We know that 100 could be written as 10^2 because $100 = 10 \times 10$. Similarly, 1,000 could be written as 10^3 because $1,000 = 10 \times 10 \times 10$. That being the case, then it should make sense that 2,000 could be written as $2 \times 10 \times 10 \times 10$ or, more simply, as 2×10^3.

When a number such as 2,000 is expressed as 2×10^3, we are using **scientific notation**. With scientific notation, a number is written *as the product* of some "simple number" (e.g., 2), the coefficient, and the base of 10 raised to some power. Hence $2,000 = 2 \times 10^3$, $5,000 = 5 \times 10^3$, and $6,000 = 6 \times 10^3$. What about the number 5,500, which of course is halfway between 5,000 and 6,000? We will see in a moment that it would be written as 5.5×10^3.

The "simple number," which is the first term in the product, is called the **coefficient**, and in scientific notation, the coefficient is always multiplied by the base 10 raised to some power. The coefficient can be any number that is greater than or equal to 1.00, but less than 10 (e.g., 9.99). You could add as many additional decimal values as might be required to achieve the desired precision, but two decimal places will be sufficient for most of the applications that we will encounter.

Conversion From Conventional Notation to Scientific Notation

Table 3–7 contains several examples in which the same number is written conventionally and in equivalent scientific notation. In the first five examples in the table, the conventional numbers are converted to scientific notation by counting the number of places that the decimal point must be moved to the *left* (*successive division by 10*) to yield an integer between 1 and 9. That specifies the *value of the exponent* in scientific notation.

Table 3–7. Comparison of conventional and scientific notation

Conventional Notation	Scientific Notation
10	1.00×10^1
100	1.00×10^2
1,000	1.00×10^3
121	1.21×10^2
800	8.00×10^2
0.1	1.00×10^{-1}
0.0121	1.21×10^{-2}

To transform 10, the decimal point must be moved one place to the left (divided by 10 once) to arrive at an integer between 1 and 9, and the exponent in scientific notation is 1. For 100, the decimal is moved two places to the left (divided by 10 twice) to get the integer, and the exponent is therefore 2. The same is true for the number 121; when the decimal is moved two places to the left, we have a coefficient of 1.21, and thus the exponent is 2.

In the last two examples in the table, the decimal point must be moved to the *right (successive multiplication by ten)* to yield an integer between 1 and 9. That process also provides the value of the exponent, *but in these cases the exponent is negative.* For example, with 0.0121, the decimal point must be moved two places to the right to yield an integer between 1 and 9 (coefficient = 1.21), and therefore the exponent is −2. A few more examples are shown below.

Example 1 $.002 = 2.00 \times 10^{-3}.$

Example 2 $.0002 = 2.00 \times 10^{-4}.$

Example 3 $2002 = 2.00 \times 10^{3}.$

More precisely, 2002 equals 2.002×10^3, but for convenience we are limiting ourselves to two decimal values for the coefficient.

Example 4 $222 = 2.22 \times 10^{2}.$

Solution for Logs

When a number is expressed initially in conventional notation, only three steps are required to take the log of that (positive) number. In stating the steps, we will use the example of $\log_{10} 121 = ?$

Step One: Express the number in scientific notation.

$$121 = 1.21 \times 10^2.$$

Obviously, this step is omitted if the number is expressed in scientific notation form in the problem, that is, $\log_{10} 1.21 \times 10^2$.

Step Two: The exponent in scientific notation is the **characteristic** of the log. Thus,

$$\log_{10} 121 = \log_{10} 1.21 \times 10^2 = 2.?????$$

We now know the characteristic of the log (the integer), but we also need to know the mantissa (the decimal values).

Step Three: If the base is 10, as it will be most of the time, use the Common Log Table in Table 3–8 to find the **mantissa**. Use the three-numbered *multiplier* (the **coefficient**) in the scientific notation expression to find the appropriate row and column in the log table; for this purpose, we ignore the decimal point and view the multiplier simply as three numbers. The first two numbers specify the correct *row* in the table; the third number specifies the correct *column*. The *cell entry* corresponding to that row and column is the **mantissa** of the logarithm. For our example, we locate row 12 and column 1, and the cell entry (the **mantissa** of the logarithm) is .0828. The answer, then, after completing all three steps is:

$$\log_{10} 121 = \log_{10} 1.21 \times 10^2 = 2.0828.$$

By way of brief review, when we say that the log to the base 10 of 121 is 2.0828, that means that we must raise the base of 10 to the 2.0828 power (use the base 2.0828 times in multiplication) to equal 121. We should be able to perform a quick mental check to see if that answer is reasonable. We know without use of a log table that the log of 100 is 2 and that the log of 1,000 is 3. Therefore, the log of 121 (which is larger than 100 and smaller than 1,000) must be a number between 2 and 3, and 2.0828 falls within that range.

That kind of check to determine if an answer is reasonable is generally a good idea. It won't necessarily reveal if the answer that you obtained is precisely correct, but it will tell you if it is approximately correct or at least if it is wildly wrong. For example, suppose you calculated (incorrectly) that the $\log_{10} 163 = 3.2122$. You then think for a moment and realize that the log of 100 is 2 and that the log of 1,000 is 3. Because the number 163 lies between 100 and 1,000, the $\log_{10} 163$ must be 2.????, not 3.????.

Following are additional examples that you might wish to work for yourself before reading the answer.

$$\log_{10} 648 = \log_{10} 6.48 \times 10^2 = 2.8116.$$

$$\log_{10} 707 = \log_{10} 7.07 \times 10^2 = 2.8494.$$

$$\log_{10} 1,000 = \log_{10} 1.00 \times 10^3 = 3.0000.$$

$$\log_{10} 1 = \log_{10} 1.00 \times 10^0 = 0.0000.$$

If $X^0 = 1$ (Equation 3.3), and if an exponent is a log, then it must be the case that the log, to any base, of 1 = 0.

$$\log_{10} 2 = \log_{10} 2.00 \times 10^0 = 0.3010.$$

$$\log_{10} 0.0002 = \log_{10} 2.00 \times 10^{-4} = \overline{4}.3010.$$

Solution of the first five problems above should be accomplished easily if the three steps are followed: (1) Convert the number to scientific notation; (2) the exponent in scientific notation is the characteristic of the log; and (3) the multiplier in scientific notation is used to find the mantissa in the log table.

Table 3–8. Common log table.

N	0	1	2	3	4	5	6	7	8	9
10	0.0000	0.0043	0.0086	0.0128	0.0170	0.0212	0.0253	0.0294	0.0334	0.0374
11	0.0414	0.0453	0.0492	0.0531	0.0569	0.0607	0.0645	0 0682	0.0719	0.0755
12	0.0792	0.0828	0.0864	0.0899	0.0934	0.0969	0.1004	0.1038	0.1072	0.1106
13	0.1139	0.1173	0.1206	0.1239	0.1271	0.1303	0.1335	0.1367	0.1399	0.1430
14	0.1461	0.1492	0.1523	0.1553	0.1584	0.1614	0.1644	0.1673	0.1703	0.1732
15	0.1761	0.1790	0.1818	0.1847	0.1875	0.1903	0.1931	0.1959	0.1987	0.2014
16	0.2041	0.2068	0.2095	0.2122	0.2148	0.2175	0.2201	0.2227	0.2253	0.2279
17	0.2304	0.2330	0.2355	0.2380	0.2405	0.2430	0.2455	0.2480	0.2504	0.2529
18	0.2553	0.2577	0.2601	0.2625	0.2648	0.2672	0.2695	0.2718	0.2742	0.2765
19	0.2788	0.2810	0.2833	0.2856	0.2878	0.2900	0.2923	0.2945	0.2967	0.2989
20	0.3010	0.3032	0.3054	0.3075	0.3096	0.3118	0.3139	0.3160	0.3181	0.3201
21	0.3222	0.3243	0.3263	0.3284	0.3304	0.3324	0.3345	0.3365	0.3385	0.3404
22	0.3424	0.3444	0.3464	0.3483	0.3502	0.3522	0.3541	0.3560	0.3579	0.3598
23	0.3617	0.3636	0.3655	0.3674	0.3692	0.3711	0.3729	0.3747	0.3766	0.3784
24	0.3802	0.3820	0.3838	0.3856	0.3874	0.3892	0.3909	0.3927	0.3945	0.3962
25	0.3979	0.3997	0.4014	0.4031	0.4048	0.4065	0.4082	0.4099	0.4116	0.4133
26	0.4150	0.4166	0.4183	0.4200	0.4216	0.4232	0.4249	0.4265	0.4281	0.4298
27	0.4314	0.4330	0.4346	0.4362	0.4378	0.4393	0.4409	0.4425	0.4440	0.4456
28	0.4472	0.4487	0.4502	0.4518	0.4533	0.4548	0.4564	0.4579	0.4594	0.4609
29	0 4624	0 4639	0.4654	0.4669	0.4683	0.4698	0.4713	0.4728	0.4742	0.4757
30	0.4771	0.4786	0.4800	0.4814	0.4829	0.4843	0.4857	0.4871	0.4886	0.4900
31	0.4914	0.4928	0.4942	0.4955	0.4969	0.4983	0.4997	0.5011	0.5024	0.5038
32	0.5051	0.5065	0.5079	0.5092	0.5105	0.5119	0.5132	0.5145	0.5159	0.5172
33	0.5185	0.5198	0.5211	0.5224	0.5237	0.5250	0.5263	0.5276	0.5289	0.5302
34	0.5315	0.5328	0.5340	0.5353	0.5366	0.5378	0.5391	0.5403	0.5416	0.5428
35	0.5441	0.5453	0.5465	0.5478	0.5490	0.5502	0.5514	0.5527	0.5539	0.5551
36	0.5563	0.5575	0.5587	0.5599	0.5611	0.5623	0.5635	0.5647	0.5658	0.5670
37	0.5682	0.5694	0.5705	0.5717	0.5729	0.5740	0.5752	0.5763	0.5775	0.5786
38	0.5798	0.5809	0.5821	0.5832	0.5843	0.5855	0.5866	0.5877	0.5888	0.5899
39	0.5911	0.5922	0.5933	0.5944	0.5955	0.5966	0.5977	0.5988	0.5999	0.6010
40	0.6021	0.6031	0.6042	0.6053	0.6064	0.6075	0.6085	0.6096	0.6107	0.6117
41	0.6128	0.6138	0.6149	0.6160	0.6170	0.6180	0.6191	0.6201	0.6212	0.6222
42	0.6232	0.6243	0.6253	0.6263	0.6274	0.6284	0.6294	0.6304	0.6314	0.6325
43	0.6335	0.6345	0.6355	0.6365	0.6375	0.6385	0.6395	0.6405	0.6415	0.6425
44	0.6435	0.6444	0.6454	0.6464	0.6474	0.6484	0.6493	0.6503	0.6513	0.6522
45	0.6532	0.6542	0.6551	0.6561	0.6571	0.6580	0.6590	0.6599	0.6609	0.6618
46	0.6628	0.6637	0.6646	0.6656	0.6665	0.6675	0.6684	0.6693	0.6702	0.6712
47	0.6721	0.6730	0.6739	0.6749	0.6758	0.6767	0.6776	0.6785	0.6794	0.6803
48	0.6812	0.6821	0.6830	0.6839	0.6848	0.6857	0.6866	0.6875	0.6884	0.6893
49	0.6902	0.6911	0.6920	0.6928	0.6937	0.6946	0.6955	0.6964	0.6972	0.6981
50	0.6990	0.6998	0.7007	0.7016	0.7024	0.7033	0.7042	0.7050	0.7059	0.7067
51	0.7076	0.7084	0.7093	0.7101	0.7110	0.7118	0.7126	0.7135	0.7143	0.7152
52	0.7160	0.7168	0.7177	0.7185	0.7193	0.7202	0.7210	0.7218	0.7226	0.7235
53	0.7243	0.7251	0.7259	0.7267	0.7275	0.7284	0.7292	0.7300	0.7308	0.7316
54	0.7324	0.7332	0.7340	0.7348	0.7356	0.7364	0.7372	0.7380	0.7388	0.7396
55	0.7404	0.7412	0.7419	0.7427	0.7435	0.7443	0.7451	0.7459	0.7466	0.7474
56	0.7482	0.7490	0.7497	0.7505	0.7513	0.7520	0.7528	0.7536	0.7543	0.7551
57	0.7559	0.7566	0.7574	0.7582	0.7589	0.7597	0.7604	0.7612	0.7619	0.7627
58	0.7634	0.7642	0.7649	0.7657	0.7664	0.7672	0.7679	0.7686	0.7694	0.7701
59	0.7709	0.7716	0.7723	0.7731	0.7738	0.7745	0.7752	0.7760	0.7767	0.7774

Table 3–8. *(continued)*

N	0	1	2	3	4	5	6	7	8	9
60	0.7782	0.7789	0.7796	0.7803	0.7810	0.7818	0.7825	0.7832	0.7839	0.7846
61	0.7853	0.7860	0.7868	0.7875	0.7882	0.7889	0.7896	0.7903	0.7910	0.7917
62	0.7924	0.7931	0.7938	0.7945	0.7952	0.7959	0.7966	0.7973	0.7980	0.7987
63	0.7993	0.8000	0.8007	0.8014	0.8021	0.8028	0.8035	0.8041	0.8048	0.8055
64	0.8062	0.8069	0.8075	0.8082	0.8089	0.8096	0.8102	0.8109	0.8116	0.8122
65	0.8129	0.8136	0.8142	0.8149	0.8156	0.8162	0.8169	0.8176	0.8182	0.8189
66	0.8195	0.8202	0.8209	0.8215	0.8222	0.8228	0.8235	0.8241	0.8248	0.8254
67	0.8261	0.8267	0.8274	0.8280	0.8287	0.8293	0.8299	0.8306	0.8312	0.8319
68	0.8325	0.8331	0.8338	0.8344	0.8351	0.8357	0.8363	0.8370	0.8376	0.8382
69	0.8388	0.8395	0.8401	0.8407	0.8414	0.8420	0.8426	0.8432	0.8439	0.8445
70	0.8451	0.8457	0.8463	0.8470	0.8476	0.8482	0.8488	0.8494	0.8500	0.8506
71	0.8513	0.8519	0.8525	0.8531	0.8537	0.8543	0.8549	0.8555	0.8561	0.8567
72	0.8573	0.8579	0.8585	0.8591	0.8597	0.8603	0.8609	0.8615	0.8621	0.8627
73	0.8633	0.8639	0.8645	0.8651	0.8657	0.8663	0.8669	0.8675	0.8681	0.8686
74	0.8692	0.8698	0.8704	0.8710	0.8716	0.8722	0.8727	0.8733	0.8739	0.8745
75	0.8751	0.8756	0.8762	0.8768	0.8774	0.8779	0.8785	0.8791	0.8797	0.8802
76	0.8808	0.8814	0.8820	0.8825	0.8831	0.8837	0.8842	0.8848	0.8854	0.8859
77	0.8865	0.8871	0.8876	0.8882	0.8887	0.8893	0.8899	0.8904	0.8910	0.8915
78	0.8921	0.8927	0.8932	0.8938	0.8943	0.8949	0.8954	0.8960	0.8965	0.8971
79	0.8976	0.8982	0.8987	0.8993	0.8998	0.9004	0.9009	0.9015	0.9020	0.9025
80	0.9031	0.9036	0.9042	0.9047	0.9053	0.9058	0.9063	0.9069	0.9074	0.9079
81	0.9085	0.9090	0.9096	0.9101	0.9106	0.9112	0.9117	0 9122	0.9128	0.9133
82	0.9138	0.9143	0.9149	0.9154	0.9159	0.9165	0.9170	0.9175	0.9180	0.9186
83	0.9191	0.9196	0.9201	0.9206	0.9212	0.9217	0.9222	0.9227	0.9232	0.9238
84	0.9243	0.9248	0.9253	0.9258	0.9263	0.9269	0.9274	0.9279	0.9284	0.9289
85	0.9294	0.9299	0.9304	0.9309	0.9315	0.9320	0.9325	0.9330	0.9335	0.9340
86	0.9345	0.9350	0.9355	0.9360	0.9365	0.9370	0.9375	0.9380	0.9385	0.9390
87	0.9395	0.9400	0.9405	0.9410	0.9415	0.9420	0.9425	0.9430	0.9435	0.9440
88	0.9445	0.9450	0.9455	0.9460	0.9465	0.9469	0.9474	0.9479	0.9484	0.9489
89	0.9494	0.9499	0.9504	0.9509	0.9513	0.9518	0.9523	0.9528	0.9533	0.9538
90	0.9542	0.9547	0.9552	0.9557	0.9562	0.9566	0.9571	0.9576	0.9581	0.9586
91	0.9590	0.9595	0.9600	0.9605	0.9609	0.9614	0.9619	0.9624	0.9628	0.9633
92	0.9638	0.9643	0.9647	0.9652	0.9657	0.9661	0.9666	0.9671	0.9675	0.9680
93	0.9685	0.9689	0.9694	0.9699	0.9703	0.9708	0.9713	0.9717	0.9722	0.9727
94	0.9731	0.9736	0.9741	0.9745	0.9750	0.9754	0.9759	0.9763	0.9768	0.9773
95	0.9777	0.9782	0.9786	0.9791	0.9795	0.9800	0.9805	0.9809	0.9814	0.9818
96	0.9823	0.9827	0.9832	0.9836	0.9841	0.9845	0.9850	0.9854	0.9859	0.9863
97	0.9868	0.9872	0.9877	0.9881	0.9886	0.9890	0.9894	0.9899	0.9903	0.9908
98	0.9912	0.9917	0.9921	0.9926	0.9930	0.9934	0.9939	0.9943	0.9948	0.9952
99	0.9956	0.9961	0.9965	0.9969	0.9974	0.9978	0.9983	0.9987	0.9991	0.9996

The last example, in which we solved for $\log_{10}$ 0.0002, deserves additional explanation. Notice, that a negative sign is placed *above* the 4 rather than in front of it. That is because the **characteristic** *can be either positive or negative,* but the **mantissa** *can only be positive.* Thus, $\overline{4}.3010$ does not equal -4.3010. When we say "-4.3010," we imply that the number is 4.3010 units *less than zero.* With "$\overline{4}.3010$," however, we have a negative characteristic of 4, but a positive mantissa of .3010. With a very loose analogy, that is like having roughly 30 cents in your pocket (an asset—a positive value) and owing a friend $4.00 (a liability—a negative value). In that case, your net is a deficit of $3.70.

You approach the log problem in the same conceptual manner. Thus, $\overline{4}.3010 = -4.0000 + 0.3010 = -3.6990$. In other words, $\overline{4}.3010$ is really 3.6990 units below zero, not 4.3010 units below zero. Fortunately, when you solve the problem $\log_{10} 0.0002$ with a calculator that has a log function, the answer will automatically show as -3.6990.

Logs with Bases Other Than 10

There might be a few occasions in which you will need to solve a log problem that has a base other than 10, and you might not be able to locate a published log table to help you. There is an equation, however, that will enable you to solve such problems by using a base of 10. Suppose you want to solve the problem $\log_2 8$. Because we have practiced these simple kinds of problems, you probably can see immediately that the answer is 3, which means that the base of 2 must be raised to the 3rd power ($2 \times 2 \times 2$) to equal 8. Now try to get the answer in a different way by use of Equation 3.4.

Equation 3.4
$$\log_Y X = \frac{\log_{10} X}{\log_{10} Y}.$$

Substitute the values from our problem into Equation 3.4.

$$\log_2 8 = \frac{\log_{10} 8}{\log_{10} 2} = \frac{0.9031}{0.3010} = 3.00.$$

The equation tells us that to find the $\log_2 8$, we first find the $\log_{10}$ 8 (0.9031) and divide that answer by the $\log_{10}$ 2 (0.3010). The answer is 3.0 (if you ignore the third and fourth decimal places), which is the answer that we knew by inspection.

Solutions for Antilogs

If your calculator has a log function, it almost certainly has an antilog function. The key normally is not labeled as "antilog," but rather as 10^X. So, to take the antilog of 2.0828, enter that number, activate the antilog function, and the number 121 should appear in the display.

Solution of antilog problems without a calculator is just as easy as solution of log problems. We simply use the same three steps that were described for solving log problems, but in reverse order. Consider the following example.

$$\text{antilog}_{10}\ 2.0828 = ?,$$

which means

$$10^{2.0828} = ?$$

Regardless of the way in which the problem is posed, we are seeking the answer to the question "what is 10 raised to the 2.0828 power?", which as you should recall, means "what is the value of 10 used 2.0828 times in multiplication?"

Step One: The exponent, 2.0828, is a logarithm and it consists of a characteristic (2.) and a mantissa (0.0828). The **mantissa** is 0.0828 and you first locate the cell entry of that value in the log table. The row (12) and column (1) that correspond to the cell entry of 0.0828 yields the *multiplier*, or *coefficient*, in scientific notation. Because the coefficient always is an integer *between 1 and 9* followed by some number of decimal values, row 12 and column 1 tells you that the multiplier is 1.21; that is the only place within those three digits that the decimal can be located to produce an integer between 1 and 9.

Step Two: If an exponent in scientific notation is the **characteristic** of a log, then the characteristic of a log must be the exponent in scientific notation. Thus, the characteristic of 2 tells us to raise the base 10 to the 2nd power (10^2). The answer, in scientific notation, is 1.21×10^2.

Step Three: If you wish to complete the process by expressing the answer in conventional notation, you simply multiply (or divide) the answer obtained in Step Two by 10 by moving the decimal point to the right (for positive exponents) the number of places specified by the exponent or to the left for negative exponents. For most of the problems that will be encountered in this book, the third step will not be executed, and the answer will remain in scientific notation.

$$1.21 \times 10^2 = 121.$$

Because the exponent is 2, the decimal point is moved two places to the right.

To provide an example for the three steps in determining both logs and antilogs, the number 121 was used. From those solutions we can see that:

$$\log_{10} 121 = 2.0828$$

and

$$\text{antilog}_{10}\ 2.0828 = 121.$$

Laws of Logarithms

Earlier we presented three laws of exponents that permit us to accomplish certain computations more easily. There are four laws of logarithms (not all independent), and they will permit us to solve many decibel problems easily. Each of the four laws applies to logarithms with any base, but only a base of 10 will be used in the examples.

Law 1 of Logarithms

LOG LAW 1

$$\log ab = \log a + \log b.$$

The first law tells us that *the log of any product is equal to the sum of the logs of the factors.* Thus,

$$\log_{10} 3 \times 2 = \log_{10} 3 + \log_{10} 2$$
$$= 0.4771 + 0.3010$$
$$= 0.7781.$$

The answer of 0.7781 can be verified by calculating the $\log_{10} 6$. As with some of the earlier examples, we have not saved much time by using Law 1 to solve such a simple problem because it would have been just as simple to multiply 3 by 2 and take the log of 6. Use of Law 1, however, will simplify the solution of more difficult problems.

Actually, we have already applied Law 1 in solution of more difficult log problems without having identified it as such. Look back to Step One in solution of log problems. When the number 121 was converted into scientific notation, we formed the product 1.21×10^2. We can think of that as the log of the product **ab**, in which **a** (the coefficient) = 1.21 and **b** = 10^2. We then found the log of 10^2, which is 2.0000, and that became the **characteristic**. Next, we found the log of 1.21 in the log table, which was 0.0828, and that became the **mantissa**. The log of 1.21×10^2, then, is the sum of the characteristic (2.0000) added to the mantissa (0.0828), which equals 2.0828.

That kind of reasoning is particularly helpful when we express the log of a number less than one as having a negative characteristic and a positive mantissa. The log is the algebraic sum of the negative characteristic and the positive mantissa, which is an application of Law 1 of logarithms. Below are three more examples of the application of Law 1.

$$\log_{10} 10 \times 10 = \log_{10} 10 + \log_{10} 10 = 1 + 1 = 2.$$
$$\log_{10} 20 \times 20 = \log_{10} 20 + \log_{10} 20 = 1.3010 + 1.3010 = 2.6020.$$
$$\log_{10} 648 \quad = \log_{10} 6.48 \times 10^2 \text{ (log of a product)}$$
$$= \log_{10} 10^2 + \log_{10} 6.48$$
$$= 2.0000 + 0.8116$$
$$= 2.8116.$$

Law 2 of Logarithms

$$\log \frac{a}{b} = \log a - \log b.$$

LOG LAW 2

The second law of logarithms states that *the log of some ratio is equal to the difference between the logs of the factors.* Thus,

$$\log_{10} \frac{3}{2} = \log_{10} 3 - \log_{10} 2 = 0.4771 - 0.3010 = 0.1761.$$

The answer, 0.1761, can be verified by calculating the log of 1.5, which corresponds to the ratio of 3/2. It should be apparent that the major advantage to Law 2 is that it allows us to subtract logs rather than perform potentially cumbersome division. It is not imposing to divide 3 by 2, but use of the law will certainly simplify solutions to the two problems below.

$$\log_{10} \frac{1.8}{1.2} = (\log_{10} 1.8) - (\log_{10} 1.2) = 0.2553 - 0.0792 = 0.1761.$$

Example 1

$$\log_{10} \frac{(1 \times 10^0)}{(2 \times 10^{-4})} = (\log_{10} 1 \times 10^0) - (\log_{10} 2 \times 10^{-4})$$

Example 2

$$= 0.0000 - (\overline{4}.3010)$$

$$= 3.6990.$$

Law 3 of Logarithms

$$\log a^b = b \log a$$

LOG LAW 3

The third law of logarithms states that *the log of the number **a** raised to the **b**th power is equal to **b** times the log of **a**.* This law will be particularly helpful in Chapter 4 when we explain the difference in the equations for decibels of intensity and decibels of pressure.

The first example below is a simple problem that will allow you to find the answer with and without use of Law 3. In the second example, you should see how use of the law simplifies computation greatly.

$$\log_{10} 2^2 = 2 \log_{10} 2 = 0.6020.$$

Example 1

The answer of 0.6020 should be easy to verify by calculating the log of 4 (2^2).

$$\log_{10} 2^{1.65} = 1.65 \times \log_{10} 2 = 0.4967.$$

Example 2

Law 4 of Logarithms

$$\log \frac{1}{a} = -\log a.$$

LOG LAW 4

The fourth and final law states that *the log of a reciprocal is equal to minus the log of the number.* Thus,

$$\log_{10} \frac{1}{2} = -\log_{10} 2 = -0.3010.$$

You should be able to see that Law 4 is not an independent law, but rather is a special application of Law 2. Law 2 stated that,

$$\log \frac{a}{b} = \log a - \log b.$$

When we take the log of 1/2, that fits the form of the second law. But, of course, the log of 1 in the numerator is always 0.0000. Therefore, the answer will always be a negative number because you will be subtracting some positive number in the denominator from zero in the numerator. Hence, Law 4 is written simply as **−log a**.

Logs Without Log Tables

You can get an *approximate* answer to many log problems without use of a calculator or log table, and to do so it is necessary to memorize the logs of only four numbers: 1, 2, 3, and 7. This will be particularly useful because it will enable you to check to see if the answer you obtained by following all of the steps and using a log table, or by using your calculator, is *approximately* correct. Consider the numbers between 1 and 10, and because we are only interested in getting an approximate answer, we will only use one or two decimal places in the computations.

1. The log of 1 is 0.0.   **Memorize**
2. The log of 2 is 0.3.   **Memorize**
3. The log of 3 is 0.48.   **Memorize**
4. The log of 4 is ?   Law 1 stated that log ab = log a + log b. Because 4 = 2 × 2, the log of 4 must equal the log of 2 + the log of 2, which already has been memorized, and 0.3 + 0.3 = 0.6.
5. The log of 5 is ?   Law 2 stated that log a/b = log a − log b. Because 5 = 10/2, the log of 5 must equal the log of 10 − the log of 2 = 1.0 − 0.3 = 0.70.
6. The log of 6 is ?   Because 6 = 3 × 2, the log of 6 must equal the log of 3 + the log of 2 = 0.48 + 0.30 = 0.78.
7. The log of 7 is 0.85.   **Memorize**

8. The log of 8 is ?   Because 8 = 4 × 2, the log of 8 must equal the log of 4 + the log of 2 = 0.60 + 0.30 = 0.90. Alternatively, you might see that 8 equals 2^3 (i.e., 2 × 2 × 2). Therefore the log of 8 = 0.30 + 0.30 + 0.30 = 0.90.

9. The log of 9 is ?   log of 3 + log of 3 = 0.96.

10. The log of 10 is ?   With only a little practice you should see that the answer is 1.

It should be helpful to try to use that system to solve the following problems without log tables.

$\log_{10} 20 = ?$ 20 = 10 × 2.   Therefore, the answer is 1.3.

$\log_{10} 30 = ?$ 30 = 10 × 3.   Therefore, the answer is 1.48.

$\log_{10} 100 = ?$ 100 = 10 × 10.   Therefore, the answer is 2.0.

$\log_{10} 300 = ?$ Can you see easily that the answer is 2.48?

A Final Comment About Logarithms

You might have noticed that when you take the log of a series of numbers from a ratio scale, the logs of those numbers are *linearly* spaced. That concept is illustrated below by comparing the two columns of numbers. The first column shows numbers that progressively increase by powers of 10 (1, 10, 100, . . . ,1,000,000). The second column shows that the logs of those numbers are linearly spaced (0, 1, 2, . . . ,6).

Column I	Column II
1	0
10	1
100	2
1,000	3
10,000	4
100,000	5
1,000,000	6

Because logs are linearly spaced, you can convert linear graph paper into logarithmic units by calculating the logs of the numbers you wish to display. That operation enables you to display a large range of numbers in an economical space. Suppose each dot on the next page represents a tick mark on your graph paper, and you wish to display information that ranges from 1 to 1,000,000 units of measurement. Only 60 lines on the graph paper will be required if the resolution that you desire is restricted to one decimal place.

```
|........|........|........|........|........|........|........|
0        1        2        3        4        5        6
1       10      100     1,000   10,000  100,000 1,000,000
```

In Chapter 4 we will introduce the concept of the decibel, and in all decibel computations we will make considerable use of logs and antilogs. The base for all computations involving decibels will be 10.

■ NOTES

1. The discussion of the four scales of measurement is largely a condensed version of the extensive treatment of the topic by S.S. Stevens (1951). Readers who wish to explore this important topic in greater detail are advised to read his chapter in the *Handbook of Experimental Psychology*.

Sound Intensity and Sound Pressure: The Decibel

We learned in Chapter 1 that sound is a form of wave motion in which a pattern of pressure—or a change in density—is propagated through an elastic medium. **Energy** is transferred through the medium and the transfer of energy occurs at some particular rate. *The rate at which sound energy is transferred through the medium* is called the **acoustic power**.

More generally, **power** is defined as the rate at which work is accomplished, or as the rate at which energy is transformed or transferred:

$$\textbf{Power} = \frac{\text{work}}{\text{unit time}} = \frac{\text{energy transformed or transferred}}{\text{unit time}}.$$

For example, **power** refers to the amount of work accomplished by an engine per second, or the amount of electrical energy that is transformed into heat energy per second by an electrical heater.

It is important to realize that **power** and **energy** are not equivalent. Consider the case of a person who is engaged in a physical activity such as shoveling snow. The person might be able to shovel for an hour at a rate of two shovelfuls per minute before the amount of energy stored in the muscles is used up and exhaustion results. If the person is anxious to complete the job more quickly and picks up the pace to four shovelfuls per minute, exhaustion will occur earlier. Thus, our ability to complete such tasks is limited not only by our **energy**, the capacity to do work, but also by the rate at which the energy is expended, the **power**.

The unit of measure of power, including acoustic power, is the **watt (W)**, which was named in honor of James Watt, the developer of the steam engine. If we expend energy at a rate of 1 joule per s (**MKS** system) or 10,000,000 ergs per s (**cgs** system), we have expended *one watt of power*. Therefore,

$$1 \text{ watt} = \frac{1 \text{ joule}}{\sec} = \frac{10,000,000 \text{ ergs}}{\sec} \left(\text{or } \frac{10^7 \text{ ergs}}{\sec} \right).$$

■ ABSOLUTE AND RELATIVE MEASURES OF ACOUSTIC POWER

Absolute Measure of Power

When we say that a particular sound wave has an acoustic power of some number of watts, we refer to the **absolute acoustic power** in the sound wave. In the case of sound waves, we should not expect to encounter large values of power such as 60, 100, or 200 watts, and we certainly will find no acoustic rival to the megawatt electrical power station. Instead, we commonly deal with very small magnitudes of acoustical power such as, for example, 10^{-8} watt or 2.13×10^{-9} watt.

Even though the value of acoustic power is small, the absolute measure of acoustic power in watts refers to *the rate at which energy is consumed or transferred.*

Relative Measure of Power

We frequently speak of **relative acoustic power** rather than absolute power. In this case, *the absolute power in one sound wave is compared with the absolute power in another (reference) sound wave,* and the two absolute sound powers are used to form a ratio. Thus, we might say, for example, that the acoustic power of wave A is 10 times greater than the acoustic power of wave B.

$$A = 10B.$$

We do not know the absolute power in watts of either wave A or wave B, but we do know the relation between the two. If the absolute power of B is 10^{-6} watt, the power of A must be 10^{-5} watt if we are to preserve the ratio of A = 10B. With the example above, if A = 10B, then

$$B = \frac{A}{10}.$$

Thus, if the absolute power of wave A were 6.21×10^{-3} watt, then the power of wave B must be 6.21×10^{-4} watt:

$$B = \frac{(6.21 \times 10^{-3})}{(1 \times 10^1)}$$

$$= 6.21 \times 10^{-4}.$$

That is the only solution in which the 1:10 ratio would be preserved.

Summary

In summary, with relative power we express the **level** of power in a sound wave by forming a ratio of two absolute powers: the ratio of the absolute acoustic power of the sound wave in question (W_x) to the absolute acoustic power of some reference sound wave (W_r).

$$\text{Level} = \frac{W_x}{W_r}.$$

Equation 4.1

Importance of Specifying the Reference Power

Because level of power is simply the ratio of *any* two absolute powers, *the measure of level is generally meaningless unless the value of the reference power is specified.* If we determine that the level of a particular sound wave is 1,000, we know only that its power is 1,000 times greater than the power of some unspecified reference sound wave. It could be that the power of W_x is 10^{-1} relative to (re:) W_r of 10^{-4}. But, of course, a level of 1,000 would apply equally to $W_x = 10^{-13}/W_r = 10^{-16}$. In either case, the ratio of 1,000 is preserved.

A more explicit statement, therefore, would be, "the level of acoustic power is 1,000 re: 10^{-4} watt." When the reference power (W_r) is specified, there should be no ambiguity. *If the reference is not known, the concept of level has little meaning.*

■ SOUND INTENSITY

Imagine that we have what is called an "idealized point source of sound" that operates in a "free, unbounded medium." By an "idealized point source," we mean a very small sphere that is capable of pulsating in and out in a manner similar to the pulsation of the balloon in Figure 2–10. By "free, unbounded medium" we mean that there are no reflecting surfaces or energy-absorbing materials in the medium to affect sound transmission in any way. In such a case, sound energy is transferred uniformly through the medium in all directions.

In essence, *the energy is transferred outward from the point source as an ever-expanding sphere.* To measure the acoustic power in such a wave at some distance from the point source, we would have to integrate over the entire surface of the sphere. Generally we are more interested in *the amount of power that acts on, is dissipated on, or passes through some much smaller area.* The smaller area is the square meter $(\mathbf{m^2})$ in the **MKS** metric system or the square centimeter $(\mathbf{cm^2})$ in the **cgs** metric system. Thus, instead of referring to the *energy per second* (the **acoustic power**), we speak of the *energy per second per square meter,* and that is called the **intensity** of the sound wave.

Intensity is *the amount of energy transmitted per second over an area of one square meter.*

1. If the unit of measure of **acoustic power** is the **watt** (energy per second), and
2. if **intensity** is the amount of energy per second per square meter, then it follows that
3. the unit of measure for **intensity** must be the **watt per square meter (watt/m²).**

Absolute and Relative Measures of Sound Intensity

Sound power was expressed in both absolute and relative terms, and the same is true of sound intensity. If we say that a sound has an intensity of 10^{-8} watt/m², we are referring to the **absolute intensity** of the sound wave. Alternatively, we can speak of the **relative intensity**, or the level of intensity (not to be confused with "intensity level," because the label "intensity level" implies a specific reference intensity that will be introduced later), by reference to the same kind of ratio that was used for power:

$$\text{Level} = \frac{I_x}{I_r}.$$

Equation 4.2

where I_x is the absolute intensity of wave **x**,

and

I_r is the absolute reference intensity, **r**.

Importance of Specifying the Reference Intensity

It is just as important to specify the reference for level of sound intensity as it is to specify the reference for level of sound power. Consider the examples in Table 4–1 in which each of six absolute sound intensities in **watt/m²** is referenced to two different reference intensities: $I_r = 10^{-10}$ watt/m² and $I_r = 10^{-12}$ watt/m².

For each absolute intensity (I_x), the ratio (I_x/I_r) depends on the reference intensity. Thus, for example, the level of intensity in the first example in the table is 10^2 when referenced to 10^{-10} watt/m², but 10^4 when referenced to 10^{-12} watt/m². In a similar vein, it is not acceptable to say that some sound has a level of intensity of 10^{-1} because, for the examples in Table 4–1, that would apply equally to 10^{-13} re: 10^{-12} and to 10^{-11} re: 10^{-10}.

■ THE DECIBEL

When we speak of the level of power or the level of intensity in a sound wave, we often are faced with a rather cumbersome number.

Table 4–1. Ratios $\frac{I_x}{I_r}$ for two different reference intensities

Absolute Intensity in watt/m² I_x	Relative Intensity, $\frac{I_x}{I_r}$, in watt/m²	
	$I_r = 10^{-10}$	$I_r = 10^{-12}$
10^{-8}	10^2	10^4
10^{-9}	10^1	10^3
10^{-10}	10^0	10^2
10^{-11}	10^{-1}	10^1
10^{-12}	10^{-2}	10^0
10^{-13}	10^{-3}	10^{-1}

For example, a conservative estimate of the range of intensities to which the human auditory system can respond is about 10^{12}:1, and the range of acoustic powers of interest in noise measurements is even greater: about 10^{18}:1. Thus, we are faced with a wide range of intensities, and that presents us with awkward numerical notations.

The awkwardness can be minimized, though, by some elementary transformations of the numbers. Look again at Table 4–1. Entries in the second and the third columns are the ratios of the absolute intensities (I_x) to each of the reference intensities (I_r). Each of those entries is the base 10 raised to some power.

The base is redundant from one example to another in the table; it is always 10. Thus, we could just as well eliminate the base and only list the exponents. We also know that *an exponent is a log* (Chapter 3). In other words: $\log_{10} 10^2 = 2$; $\log_{10} 10^0 = 0$; $\log_{10} 10^{-3} = -3$; and so on. The numbers are simplified, therefore, by *calculating the logarithm to the base 10 of the ratio of two intensities.*

$$\log_{10} \frac{I_x}{I_r}.$$

The Bel

For the first example in Table 4–1 where the absolute intensity (I_x) equaled 10^{-8} watt/m^2, we calculated that its level was 10^2 re: 10^{-10} watt/m^2. Now we see that one further transformation, the log of the ratio 10^2 ($\log_{10} 10^2$), yields a value of 2. This unit of measurement of relative intensity is called the **bel** in honor of Alexander Graham Bell, an inventor who patented the first telephone. Thus,

Equation 4.3
$$N \text{ (bels)} = \log_{10} \frac{I_x}{I_r}.$$

where I_x is the absolute intensity of the wave in question in watt/m^2,

I_r is the absolute intensity of a *reference* sound wave in watt/m^2,

and

the **bel** is a unit of level of intensity.

Thus, the relative intensities of the six sounds in Table 4–1 can be described as 2, 1, 0, −1, −2, and −3 bels re: 10^{-10} watt/m^2, and as 4, 3, 2, 1, 0, and −1 bels re: 10^{-12} watt/m^2.

Summary

Before proceeding, it might be helpful to provide a brief review of the transformations that have been accomplished for specifying the intensity of a sound wave. Consider the first example in Table 4–1.

1. The absolute intensity is 10^{-8} watt/m^2.

2. The relative intensity, referenced to 10^{-12} watt/m², is 10,000, which can be expressed more simply as 10^4.

3. The base 10 is redundant because the level of intensity will always be described as the base 10 raised to some power. The expression can be simplified more, therefore, by calculating the log of the ratio. Because an exponent is a log, *the log of 10 raised to some power (exponent) is the exponent.* The level in this example, therefore, is 4 (**bels**).

4. Thus, a sound wave with an absolute intensity (I_x) of 10^{-8} watt/m² has a relative intensity of 4 bels re: 10^{-12} watt/m². Because relative intensity varies with the reference that is chosen for comparison, that same sound has a relative intensity of 2 bels re: 10^{-10} watt/m².

From the Bel to the Decibel

The **bel** as a measure of relative intensity is less cumbersome than the ratio of intensities because the wide-range scale of intensities has been compressed by transformation to a logarithmic scale. Thus, instead of expressing the relative intensity for various sounds as 0.0001, 0.01, 1,000, 100,000, or 1,000,000,000,000, we could say simply that the relative intensities are -4, -2, 3, 5, and 12 bels respectively.

Although the bel might be less cumbersome than a ratio (a level of 10^{12} is expressed simply as 12 bels), the scale has been compressed so much that fractional values often are required to reflect desired accuracy of measurement. For example, a sound intensity of 2×10^{-8} watt/m² has a relative intensity of 4.3 bels re: 10^{-12} watt/m².

$$\text{bels} = \log \frac{(2 \times 10^{-8})}{(1 \times 10^{-12})}$$

$$= \log 2 \times 10^4$$

$$= 4.3.$$

Excessive use of decimals can be minimized if we use **decibels (dB)** rather than bels in the same way that we sometimes use inches rather than feet and centimeters or millimeters rather than meters. A length of 5.5 ft can be expressed as 66 in. because each foot contains 12 in.

The prefix, deci, means 1/10. Therefore, *a **decibel** (**dB**) is 0.1 of a **bel**.* Because 1 dB = 0.1 bel and, conversely, 1 bel = 10 dB, Equation 4.3 for bels can be rewritten for decibels as:

$$N \text{ (dB)} = 10 \log_{10} \frac{I_x}{I_r}.$$

Equation 4.4

Thus, with the preceding example, we can say that the relative intensity is 43 dB rather than 4.3 bels. What, then, is a decibel? To say that "a decibel is one-tenth of a bel" is a true statement, but such a definition is not sufficient unless the mathematical definition of the bel is understood. Instead, the decibel is defined most appropriately by reference to Equation 4.4: *the decibel is ten times the log of an intensity ratio or a power ratio.*[1]

A comment about grammar is in order. The singular forms are **bel**, **decibel**, and **dB**, but the plural forms are **bels**, **decibels** and *dB (not dBs)*.

Intensity Level (dB IL)

The decibel, as with intensity ratios and the bel, is ambiguous unless the reference intensity is specified. How, then, can utter confusion be avoided? First, *no confusion should exist if the reference intensity is specified.* A statement that the relative intensity of a sound is 86 dB re: 10^{-12} watt/m^2 is explicit: we know the relative intensity (86 dB), we know the reference intensity (10^{-12}) to which some absolute intensity has been compared, and we can calculate (with the use of antilogs) that the absolute intensity of the sound is 3.99×10^{-4} watt/m^2.

Second, the potential for confusion has been lessened by adoption of *a conventional reference intensity of 10^{-12} watt/m^2* (**MKS** system).[2] Any intensity can be used as the reference for expressing relative intensity, but *when the reference is 10^{-12} watt/m^2, the result is called **intensity level (dB IL)** rather than just "level of intensity."* Strictly speaking, the label **intensity level** and its abbreviation **dB IL** should only be used when the reference is 10^{-12} watt/m^2. There is, however, still sufficient departure from the convention to warrant one final admonition: *the reference intensity should always be specified when the term **decibel** is used.*

The relation between absolute intensity (I_x) in watt/m^2 and dB IL re: 10^{-12} watt/m^2 is shown in the following illustration.

dB IL		I_x
70	=	10^{-5}
60	=	10^{-6}
50	=	10^{-7}
40	=	10^{-8}
30	=	10^{-9}
20	=	10^{-10}
10	=	10^{-11}
0	=	**10^{-12}**
−10	=	10^{-13}
−20	=	10^{-14}

When $I_x = 10^{-12}$, dB IL = 0 because $I_x = I_r$, the reference intensity. As you move up the scale, I_x increases *multiplicatively* by powers of 10 to the quantities 10^{-11}, 10^{-10}, and so on, to a maximum intensity of 10^{-5} in the illustration. For each tenfold increase in sound intensity, dB IL increases *additively* by 10 dB to a maximum of 70 dB IL when $I_x = 10^{-5}$ watt/m^2. Similarly, if you move down the scale, I_x decreases progressively by powers of 10, and for each power of 10 decrease in sound intensity, dB IL decreases by 10 dB to a minimum of -20 dB IL at a sound intensity of 10^{-14} watt/m^2.

Sample Problems

Two steps should be followed to solve decibel problems for relative intensity (any reference) or **intensity level (dB IL)** (reference = 10^{-12} watt/m^2):

1. *Select the proper equation.* If the problem concerns the **intensity** of a sound wave, use Equation 4.4. Later in this chapter we will refer to the **pressure** of a sound wave, and that will necessitate a slight modification of Equation 4.4.

2. *Form a ratio and solve the problem.*

Problem 1: An increase in intensity by a factor of two (2:1) corresponds to how many decibels?

1. Because we are dealing with **intensity**, use Equation 4.4. The ratio is 2:1, which means that some absolute intensity of unspecified value is twice as large as some unspecified reference intensity. It might be that the intensity of one sound wave (A) is twice as great as the intensity of another sound wave (B). Alternatively, it might be that the intensity of one sound wave (A) at one point in time (t_1) has been doubled at another point in time (t_2). In either case, *the ratio is 2:1.*

2. dB = $10 \log \dfrac{2}{1}$

   = 10×0.3010
   = 3.01.   (which normally is rounded to 3 dB)

3. Because the problem could have involved any absolute intensity and any reference intensity that preserved the ratio of 2:1, we see that *as any sound intensity is doubled (the ratio of absolute intensity to reference intensity = 2:1), the level is increased by 3 dB.* Correspondingly, if intensity were halved (ratio = 1:2), the level is decreased by 3 dB because:

   dB = $10 \log \dfrac{1}{2}$

   = $-10 \log 2$ **(Log Law 4)**
   = -3.

Problem 2: An increase in intensity by a factor of ten corresponds to how many decibels?

1. $dB = 10 \log \dfrac{10}{1}$

   $= 10 \times 1$

   $= 10.$

2. Thus, as intensity increases *multiplicatively* by 10, relative intensity increases *additively* by 10 dB. Similarly, if intensity were decreased by a factor of 10, relative intensity would decrease by 10 dB:

   $dB = 10 \log \dfrac{1}{10}$

   $= -10 \log 10$

   $= -10.$

Problem 3: What is the intensity level re: 10^{-12} watt/m^2 of a sound with an absolute intensity of 10^{-6} watt/m^2?

1. Follow the same steps that were used with the first two problems, but note that the ratio is now different. The intensity was not simply increased (or decreased) from some unknown value by a stated ratio such as 2:1 or 10:1, but rather a specific absolute intensity was compared with a standard reference intensity:

   $dB = 10 \log \dfrac{10^{-6}}{10^{-12}}$

   $= 10 \log 10^6$

   $= 10 \times 6$

   $= 60.$

Problem 4: What is the intensity level re: 10^{-12} watt/m^2 of a sound with an intensity of 2×10^{-6} watt/m^2?

1. There are two approaches that can be taken. First, you can solve the problem in the same way that was used for Problem 3:

   $dB = 10 \log \dfrac{(2 \times 10^{-6})}{(1 \times 10^{-12})}$

   $= 10 \log (2 \times 10^6)$

   $= 63.$

2. A quicker solution is available, however. We learned in Problem 3 that a sound with an absolute intensity of 10^{-6} has an intensity level of 60 dB. The sound in Problem 4 has an intensity of 2×10^{-6}, which is twice as great as an intensity of 1×10^{-6}. We also know from Problem 1 that any time you increase the intensity by 2:1, relative intensity increases by 3 dB. Therefore, if the intensity level of $1 \times 10^{-6} = 60$ dB, the intensity level of 2×10^{-6} must $= 63$ dB. It will almost always be useful to inspect a problem to see if it involves powers of 2 (3 dB) or powers of 10 (10 dB). For example, see if such shortcuts can be used to solve Problem 5.

Problem 5: What is the intensity level re: 10^{-12} watt/m^2 of a sound with an intensity of 4×10^{-5} watt/m^2?

1. We know from Problem 4 that 2×10^{-6} corresponds to 63 dB. In addition, we should see that 10^{-5} is 10 times greater than 10^{-6} (10 dB), and 4 is 2 times greater than 2 (3 dB). Therefore, we should expect the answer to be 13 dB (10 + 3) greater than for Problem 4, which is 76 dB.

2. If we solve the problem step-by-step without taking answers to previous problems into account, we must get the same result:

$$dB = 10 \log \frac{(4 \times 10^{-5})}{10^{-12}}$$
$$= 10 \log (4 \times 10^{7})$$
$$= 10 \times 7.6$$
$$= 76.$$

Problem 6: 3 dB corresponds to what intensity ratio?

1. This is an antilog problem, and the solution requires following the steps suggested in Chapter 3.

2. $3 \text{ dB} = 10 \log X$
   $0.3 = \log X$ (Divide both sides of the equation by 10.)
   $X = 2 \times 10^0$. (Zero is the characteristic of the log and also the exponent in scientific notation; 0.3 is the mantissa of the log and, with the aid of a pocket calculator or a log table, we determine that the multiplier in scientific notation is 2.)

Problem 7: 13 dB corresponds to what intensity ratio?

1. Try to solve the problem initially without paper and pencil. You know that 3 dB corresponds to a ratio of 2:1 and that 10 dB corresponds to a ratio of 10:1. Because 13 dB consists of 3 + 10, the ratio must consist of $2 \times 10 = 20{:}1$.

2. Check the answer above by solving the problem step-by-step.
   $13 \text{ dB} = 10 \log X$
   $1.3 = \log X$
   $X = 2 \times 10^1$ (which is 20:1).

Problem 8: 14 dB corresponds to what intensity ratio?

1. There might not be an obvious combination of 3 dB (2:1) and 10 dB (10:1) that adds to 14 dB, which means that a shortcut that involves powers of 2 and/or powers of 10 does not *seem* to be available. You can, however, use your knowledge of powers of 2 and powers of 10 to at least "bracket your answer." We know that 13 dB corresponds to a ratio of 20:1. We should also know that 16 dB would correspond to a ratio of 40:1 because another 3 dB represents another doubling. Therefore, the answer must lie between 20:1 and 40:1.

2. $14 \text{ dB} = 10 \log X$
   $1.4 = \log X$
   $X = 2.51 \times 10^1$ (and 25.1 lies between 20 and 40).

3. Actually, *a shortcut is available*, even if it is not obvious at first glance. We know that 20 dB corresponds to a ratio of 100:1. Therefore, 17 dB, which is 3 dB less, must correspond to a halving of sound intensity, or a ratio of 50:1. Finally, 14 dB represents another halving of sound intensity, which corresponds to a ratio of 25:1.

Problem 9: An intensity level of 65 dB re: 10^{-12} watt/m^2 corresponds to what intensity?

1. Combinations of 10 dB and 3 dB will not add to 65 (unless you use a long string such as $10 + 10 + 10 + 10 + 10 + 3 + 3 + 3 + 3 + 3 = 65$). In this case it might be less cumbersome to solve the problem step-by-step. We can, however, determine a range within which the answer must lie by use of powers of 10 and 2, and that will enable us to determine if the answer we calculate is reasonable. We should know that 63 dB consists of $10 + 10 + 10 + 10 + 10 + 10 + 3$. Each 10 dB involves a tenfold increase in intensity relative to the reference, which therefore corresponds to 10^{-6} (the reference increased by a factor of 10^6). Similarly, each 3 dB involves a twofold increase in intensity relative to the reference. Thus, 63 dB would correspond to an intensity of 2×10^{-6}, and that is a lower boundary of the bracket. To get an upper boundary add another 3 dB. 66 dB would represent another doubling of intensity, which would be 4×10^{-6}. Because 65 dB lies between 63 and 66, we should expect that the intensity corresponding to 65 dB would lie between 2×10^{-6} and 4×10^{-6}.

2. $65 \text{ dB} = 10 \log \dfrac{I_x}{10^{-12}}$

         $6.5 = \log \dfrac{I_x}{10^{-12}}$

   $3.16 \times 10^6 = \dfrac{I_x}{10^{-12}}$

         $I_x = 3.16 \times 10^6 \times 10^{-12}$
            $= 3.16 \times 10^{-6}.$

■ SOUND PRESSURE

We often wish to refer to the **pressure** associated with a sound wave rather than its acoustic power or intensity. We saw previously (Equation 1.5) that **pressure** is *the amount of force per unit area*. The unit of measure in the **MKS** system is the **N/m^2** (newton per square meter) or **Pa** (pascal), and we learned in Chapter 2 that 1 N/m^2 = 1 Pa. It has now become more common to use the **μN/m^2** (microN/m^2) or the **μPa** (microPa) as the unit of measure, and we will use μPa in most computations involving sound pressure.[3]

If we say that a particular sound has a pressure of 200 μPa (2×10^2 μPa), we refer to the **absolute pressure** of the wave. As with intensity, we also can speak of **relative pressure** in decibels by calculating the log of a pressure ratio. Equation 4.4, however, *cannot be used for decibels of sound pressure*. That equation for decibels of intensity must, therefore, be modified in an appropriate manner. To understand the reasons for the transformation of Equation 4.4, it will be helpful first to reconsider the concepts of sound intensity and sound pressure in relation to **impedance**.

Impedance

We learned in Chapter 2 that the **impedance** of any vibratory system, including a volume of air through which sound is transmitted, is determined by the **resistance**, **mass reactance**, and **compliant reactance** of the system. Moreover, we learned in Chapter 1 that the speed of sound in a medium such as air is determined by properties of the medium, namely, the **elasticity** and the **density**. We might reason, therefore, that **impedance** also would be dependent on the speed of sound in a medium.

The **acoustic impedance** for a plane progressive wave is given by the product of the ambient **density** (ρ_o) in kg/m^3 and the **speed of sound** (**s**).[4] Thus,

$$Z_c = \rho_o s.$$ **Equation 4.5**

The subscript (**c**) is used in the equation because the impedance of the medium with plane progressive waves is called the **characteristic impedance**.

We previously defined intensity as *energy per second per square meter*. Intensity also can be defined as *the ratio of the square of rms pressure to the characteristic impedance*:

$$I = \frac{p_{rms}^2}{\rho_o s},$$ **Equation 4.6**

where **I** is intensity,

p_{rms} is root mean square pressure,

and

the product $\rho_o s$ is the characteristic impedance.

Decibels for Sound Pressure

We can see from Equation 4.6 that intensity is proportional to the square of rms pressure, and conversely, **rms pressure** is proportional to the square root of sound intensity:

$$p \propto \sqrt{I},$$
$$I \propto p^2, \text{ and}$$
$$I = \frac{p^2}{Z_c},$$

where **p** refers to rms sound pressure,

I refers to sound intensity,

and

Z_c is the characteristic impedance.

Thus, if intensity increases by 16:1, pressure increases by only 4:1 (square root of 16); if intensity increases by 10:1, pressure increases by only 3.16 (square root of 10); or if sound intensity is doubled, pressure increases by only 1.414 (square root of 2). It is important to keep in mind that:

1. As sound intensity increases by some factor, rms pressure increases only by the *square root* of that factor; and
2. as rms pressure increases by some factor, sound intensity increases by the *square* of that factor.

The relation between **pressure** and **intensity** is shown in Figure 4–1. The function is linear because the figure is constructed with log-log coordinates. The dashed line reflects what the relation would be like

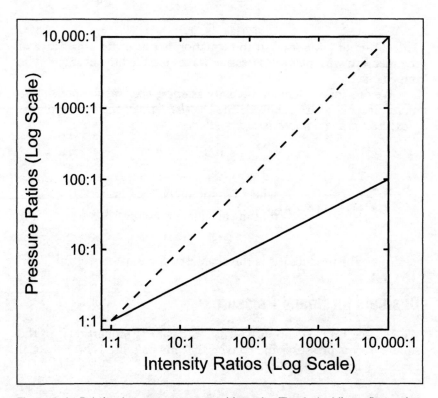

Figure 4–1. Relation between pressure and intensity. The dashed line reflects what the relation would be *if* pressure were proportional to intensity. The solid line reflects the true relation, namely that pressure is proportional to the *square root* of intensity.

if pressure were proportional to intensity. The solid line reflects the true relation, namely that pressure is proportional to the *square root* of intensity.

Equation 4.4 *cannot* be used for decibels of pressure because rms pressure is proportional to the square root of intensity, not to intensity. Equation 4.4 can be modified, however, to be appropriate for measures of pressure from our knowledge of the relation between sound intensity and rms pressure:

$$dB = 10 \log_{10} \frac{I_x}{I_r}. \qquad \text{(Equation 4.4)}$$

Because

$$I = \frac{p^2}{Z_c}$$

$$dB = 10 \log \frac{\left(\frac{p_x^2}{Z_c}\right)}{\left(\frac{p_r^2}{Z_c}\right)} \qquad \text{(by substitution)}$$

$$= 10 \log \frac{p_x^2}{p_r^2} \qquad \text{(canceling } Z_c\text{)}$$

$$= 10 \log \left(\frac{p_x}{p_r}\right)^2$$

$$= 10 \times 2 \log \frac{p_x}{p_r} \qquad \text{(\textbf{Log Law 3}: } \log a^b = b \log a\text{)}$$

$$dB = 20 \log_{10} \frac{p_x}{p_r}. \qquad \text{\textbf{Equation 4.7}}$$

Equation 4.4 should be used to solve problems that involve sound intensity, and Equation 4.7 should be used to solve problems that involve sound pressure. Thus, the decibel now can be defined as *10 times the log of a power or intensity ratio and as 20 times the log of a pressure ratio*. The only difference between the two equations is that a multiplier of 10 is used for intensity problems and a multiplier of 20 is used for pressure problems.

Sound Pressure Level (dB SPL)

Equation 4.7 applies for all instances in which we wish to represent a pressure ratio by decibels, and it is imperative that the reference pressure be specified. We have learned that the standard reference intensity for **dB IL** is 10^{-12} watt/m². The standard reference for **sound pressure** in the **MKS** system is 20 µPa (2×10^1 µPa), which is the pressure created in air by a sound wave with an intensity of 10^{-12} watt/m² under what are called "standard conditions."

"Standard conditions" generally mean a temperature of 20° centigrade and a barometric pressure of 760 mm of mercury. When the reference is 20 µPa, we refer to decibels **sound pressure level (dB SPL)**.[5] This does not mean that 20 µPa is always the reference for sound pressure level. On the contrary, sound pressure level could be (and on occasion has been) referenced to 1 dyne/cm^2 **(cgs)** or to other values. The moral by now should be obvious: *all uses of decibel notation require that the reference be specified*.

In Chapter 1 we emphasized that when an air medium is energized by a vibrating source of sound, *the individual air particles are displaced over a very small distance*. We are now in a position to specify the magnitude of that "small displacement" more precisely to provide some perspective. If the sound wave is a 1000 Hz sinusoid with a sound pressure of 20 µPa (0 dB SPL), the displacement of the air particles is approximately 7.68×10^{-8} m, which is about 1/300 of the diameter of a hydrogen molecule (2.34×10^{-6} m).

Think for a moment about the vastly different magnitudes that we encounter in the study of sound. For the 1000 Hz sine wave, air particles are displaced a nearly infinitesimal distance (7.68×10^{-8} m), whereas the wavelength of that sound wave is about 0.34 m. If we substitute a 100 Hz sine wave at the same sound pressure level, air particle displacement will be unchanged, but now the wavelength will equal about 3.4 m.

The Relation Between Absolute Pressure and Decibels

The relation between absolute pressure (p_x) in µPa and dB SPL re: 20 µPa is shown in the following illustration. When $p_x = 2 \times 10^1$, dB SPL = 0 because $p_x = p_r$.

dB SPL		p_x (absolute pressure)
100	=	2×10^6
80	=	2×10^5
60	=	2×10^4
40	=	2×10^3
20	=	2×10^2
0	=	$\mathbf{2 \times 10^1}$
−20	=	2×10^0
−40	=	2×10^{-1}

µPa

As you move up the scale, p_x increases *multiplicatively* by powers of 10 to the magnitudes $2 \times 10^2, 2 \times 10^3$, and so on, to a maximum pressure of 2×10^6 in the illustration. For each tenfold increase in sound pressure, dB SPL increases *additively* by 20 dB to a maximum of 100 dB SPL when $p_x = 2 \times 10^6$ µPa. Similarly, if you move down the scale, p_x decreases progressively by powers of 10, and for each power of 10 decrease in sound pressure, dB SPL decreases by 20 dB to a minimum of -40 dB SPL in the illustration at a sound pressure of 2×10^{-1} µPa.

Sample Problems

The same two steps that were used to calculate decibels for intensity should be used to calculate decibels for pressure: (1) Select the proper equation, and (2) form a ratio and solve the problem.

Problem 1: An increase in sound pressure by a factor of two (2:1) corresponds to how many decibels?

1. $dB = 20 \log \dfrac{2}{1}$

    $= 20 \times 0.3010$

    $= 6.02$ \qquad (which normally is rounded to 6 dB).

2. We learned previously that as sound intensity increases by a factor of 2:1, the level increases by 3 dB. In contrast, from this problem we see that as sound pressure increases by a factor of 2:1, the *pressure level* increases by *6 dB*. That difference, of course, occurs because with intensity we multiply the log of 2 (0.3) by 10 and with pressure we multiply the log of 2 (0.3) by 20. Correspondingly, if pressure is *halved* (ratio = 1:2), the pressure level *decreases* by 6 dB.

Problem 2: An increase in pressure by a factor of 10 corresponds to how many decibels?

1. $dB = 20 \log \dfrac{10}{1}$

    $= 20 \times 1$

    $= 20.$

2. As pressure increases *multiplicatively* by 10, relative pressure increases *additively* by 20 dB. If the pressure is decreased by a factor of 10 (1:10), the level is decreased by 20 dB.

Problem 3: What is the sound pressure level re: 2×10^1 µPa of a sound with an absolute pressure of 2×10^4 µPa?

$dB = 20 \log \dfrac{(2 \times 10^4)}{(2 \times 10^1)}$

$= 20 \log 10^3$

$= 60.$

Problem 4: What is the sound pressure level re: 2×10^1 µPa of a sound with an absolute pressure of 4×10^4 µPa?

1. First you should note that the pressure in this problem (4×10^4) is exactly twice as great as the pressure in Problem 3 (2×10^4). Because a doubling of pressure corresponds to 6 dB, you should expect that the answer would be 6 dB greater than the answer for Problem 3 $(60 + 6 = 66)$.

2. $\text{dB} = 20 \log \dfrac{(4 \times 10^4)}{(2 \times 10^1)}$

   $= 20 \log (2 \times 10^3)$

   $= 66.$

3. By now, it should not be necessary to use a calculator or log table for this kind of problem, and you might not even need scratch paper. You know that the log of 10^3 is 3 (a log is an exponent), and you should remember that the log of 2 is 0.3. Law 1 of logarithms stated that the log of a product is equal to the sum of the logs of the factors, so the log of 2×10^3 must equal $3 + 0.3$, which multiplied by 20 yields 66.

Problem 5: 26 dB corresponds to what pressure ratio?

1. Before using paper and pencil, see if you can determine the answer by recalling powers of 2 and 10.

2. $26 \text{ dB} = 20 \log X$

   $1.3 = \log X$

   $2 \times 10^1 = X$

   $= 20.$

3. With powers of 2 and 10 in mind, you might have noticed that 26 dB was composed of 20 dB (10:1) and 6 dB (2:1). Because 26 dB consists of $20 + 6$, the ratio must be $10 \times 2 = 20:1$.

Problem 6: A sound pressure level of 65 dB re: 2×10^1 µPa corresponds to what sound pressure?

$$65 \text{ dB} = 20 \log \frac{p_x}{(2 \times 10^1)}$$

$$3.25 = \log \frac{p_x}{(2 \times 10^1)}$$

$$1.78 \times 10^3 = \frac{p_x}{(2 \times 10^1)}$$

$$p_x = 1.78 \times 2 \times 10^3 \times 10^1$$

$$p_x = 3.56 \times 10^4.$$

■ THE RELATION BETWEEN dB IL AND dB SPL

In Table 4–2 we see that an *intensity ratio* of 10:1, for example, corresponds to 10 dB, whereas a *pressure ratio* of 10:1 corresponds to 20 dB. Would you conclude, therefore, that 60 dB IL = 120 dB SPL? *You should not!*

It is true that an intensity ratio of 10:1 corresponds to 10 dB and a pressure ratio of 10:1 corresponds to 20 dB. If, however, the intensi-

Table 4–2. Relation between decibels for intensity and decibels for pressure

Intensity		Pressure	
Ratio	dB	Ratio	dB
$\dfrac{I_x}{I_r}$	$10 \log_{10} \dfrac{I_x}{I_r}$	$\dfrac{p_x}{p_r}$	$20 \log_{10} \dfrac{p_x}{p_r}$
1	0	1.0000	0
10	10	3.1623	10
100	20	10.0000	20
1,000	30	31.6228	30
10,000	40	100.0000	40
100,000	50	316.2278	50
1,000,000	60	1,000.0000	60

ty of a particular sound were increased by a factor of 10:1, the pressure of the same sound wave would be increased only *by the square root of 10:1* (3.1623), and the decibel equivalent would still be 10 (20 log 3.1623 = 10 dB).

Recall that *pressure is proportional to the square root of intensity,* and conversely, *intensity is proportional to the square of pressure.* Other examples of this same relation can be seen in Table 4–2. An intensity ratio of 100:1 corresponds to 20 dB and a pressure ratio of 100:1 corresponds to 40 dB. But, if the intensity of a particular wave were increased by 100:1, the pressure would be increased by only 10:1 and, in either case, the decibel equivalent would be 20 dB.

Thus, we see that 60 dB IL does *not* equal 120 dB SPL. Recall from the derivation of Equation 4.7 that the multiplier of 10 in decibels for intensity was changed to a multiplier of 20 in decibels for pressure. As long as equivalent references are used in the two equations, dB IL = dB SPL, and as we learned previously, 2×10^1 µPa is the pressure equivalent of an intensity of 10^{-12} watt/m^2.

The equivalence of dB IL and dB SPL is illustrated in Figure 4–2, which shows what might be called isodecibel contours. At the left of the figure, intensity in watt/m^2 increases from 10^{-13} at the bottom to 10^{-4} at the top. At the right of the figure, *corresponding* pressure values in µPa increase from 6.32×10^0 to a maximum of 2×10^5.

Thus, we see that as intensity is increased or decreased by a power of 10, pressure changes only by the square root of 10. Each contour is a line that connects a given intensity at the left with a corresponding pressure at the right. The parameter of the figure, then, is decibels, *either dB IL or dB SPL.* They are equivalent.

■ UNITS OF MEASURE FOR PRESSURE

In Chapter 1 we indicated that force is measured in **newtons (MKS)** or **dynes (cgs)**, and therefore that pressure (the amount of force per unit area) is measured in **newtons/m^2 (MKS)** or **dynes/cm^2 (cgs)**. The

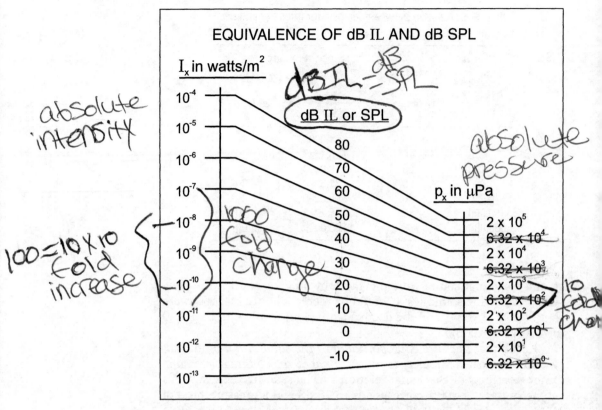

Figure 4–2. Equivalence of dB IL and dB SPL. The reference intensity for dB IL is 10^{-12} watt/m². The pressure created in air by a sound wave that has an intensity of 10^{-12} watt/m² is 20 µPa. Thus, the reference pressure for dB SPL is equivalent to the reference intensity for dB IL, and dB IL *always* equals dB SPL.

popularity of these and other units of measure for pressure has changed over the past several years. It is necessary to compare and understand the relations among the various systems if we are to read all of the scientific literature, not just the literature written in the past few years.

Table 4–3 compares, in approximate order of their appearance in the literature, the dyne/cm² (*and its equivalent, the* **microbar**) with the **N/m²** (*and its equivalent, the* **pascal** [**Pa**]) and with the µN/m² (*and its equivalent, the* **µPa**). The first column of Table 4–3 lists various values of dB SPL ranging from 100 to −6. The second column shows the corresponding *absolute* pressure in **dynes/cm²** or **microbar**. Those two units are equal to each other. The third column shows the equivalent absolute pressures in **N/m²** and **pascals** (**Pa**), which are equal to each other, and the fourth column lists the corresponding absolute pressures in µN/m² and µPa, which also are equivalent to one another.

We can make several observations from the entries in Table 4–3, some of which have been stressed previously.

Table 4–3. Comparisons of various units of measure of pressure

dB SPL	dynes/cm^2 or microbar	N/m^2 or Pa	μN/m^2 or μPa
100	2×10^1	2×10^0	2×10^6
94	10^1	10^0	10^6
80	2×10^0	2×10^{-1}	2×10^5
74	10^0	10^{-1}	10^5
60	2×10^{-1}	2×10^{-2}	2×10^4
54	10^{-1}	10^{-2}	10^4
40	2×10^{-2}	2×10^{-3}	2×10^3
34	10^{-2}	10^{-3}	10^3
20	2×10^{-3}	2×10^{-4}	2×10^2
14	10^{-3}	10^{-4}	10^2
0	2×10^{-4}	2×10^{-5}	2×10^1
−6	10^{-4}	10^{-5}	10^1

1. The **reference pressures** for dB SPL appear in the row for 0 dB SPL, and *the three entries are all equivalent*. Thus, 2×10^{-4} dyne/cm^2 (or microbar) = 2×10^{-5} N/m^2 (or Pa) = 2×10^1 μN/m^2 (or μPa). In a similar vein, all entries of absolute pressure *in any single row are equivalent*. Thus, for the row corresponding to 74 dB SPL, 10^0 dyne/cm^2 (or microbar) = 10^{-1} N/m^2 (or Pa) = 10^5 μN/m^2 (or μPa).

2. Regardless of which unit of measure of sound pressure is selected, any twofold change in pressure corresponds to 6 dB: +6 dB if pressure increases and −6 dB if pressure decreases. For example, 2×10^{-2} Pa = 60 dB SPL; a pressure of 10^{-2} is only half as great as a pressure of 2×10^{-2}, and it corresponds to 54 dB SPL, which is 6 dB less. Similarly, 10^1 μPa = −6 dB SPL, and 2×10^1 μPa, which is twice as great, corresponds to 0 dB SPL, which is 6 dB more.

3. Any tenfold change in sound pressure corresponds to 20 dB: +20 dB if pressure increases and −20 dB if pressure decreases. Thus, 10^{-3} microbar = 14 dB SPL and 10^{-2} microbar (change in pressure by 10:1) corresponds to 34 dB SPL (+ 20 dB).

4. What does 0 dB SPL mean? *It does not mean absence of sound.* It simply means that the pressure in question, p_x, equals the reference pressure, p_r. When $p_x = p_r$, the ratio is 1, the log of 1 = 0, and 20 times 0 equals 0 dB. Of course, the same is true for dB IL or any other decibel. A decibel is 10 (intensity) or 20 (pressure) times the log of a ratio, and 0 dB means that $p_x = p_r$ or that $I_x = I_r$.

5. What do negative decibels mean? It does not matter whether we are dealing with decibels for pressure or decibels for intensity. Negative decibels mean that the value of the reference pressure (p_r) or reference intensity (I_r) *exceeds* the

value of the pressure (p_x) or intensity (I_x) in question, that is, $p_r > p_x$ or $I_r > I_x$. That situation can be seen in the last row of Table 4–3 for all of the units of measure.

■ CONVERSION FROM ONE REFERENCE TO ANOTHER

The values of absolute pressure listed in Table 4–3 opposite 0 dB SPL are the **standard reference pressures** for decibels sound pressure level. There are, however, occasions in which a different reference might be adopted for some reason. In that circumstance, it might be important to compare decibels corresponding to one reference pressure with decibels referenced to a different pressure to determine whether or not they are equivalent.

You are likely to encounter older, but still important, literature in which decibels **sound pressure level** are expressed re: 1 dyne/cm^2 instead of 2×10^{-4} dyne/cm^2 in the **cgs** metric system. Suppose, for example, one author contends that the level of some particular noise is 74 dB SPL re: 2×10^{-4} dyne/cm^2. A second investigator describes the level of the same noise as 0 dB re: 1 dyne/cm^2. Are the results equivalent? We shall see that the answer is "yes," and only a few calculations are necessary to demonstrate the equivalence.

You might encounter a "conversion rule" that says: to convert from a reference pressure of 2×10^{-4} dyne/cm^2 to a reference pressure of 1 dyne/cm^2, *subtract* 74 dB, or, conversely, to convert from 1 dyne/cm^2 to 2×10^{-4} dyne/cm^2, *add* 74 dB. That is a correct rule— if you can remember when to add and when to subtract—but it only applies to those two values. What we need, then, is a system that will permit us to convert between any two reference pressures *expressed in the same metric system* (reference pressures that appear in the same column in Table 4–3). Two alternative approaches can be used.

One choice, albeit cumbersome, is to calculate p_x (an antilog problem) from knowledge of the original reference pressure and then recalculate decibels (a log problem) using the new reference pressure.

1. 74 dB SPL re: 2×10^{-4} dyne/cm^2 = how many dB SPL re: 1 dyne/cm^2? Calculate the pressure, p_x, corresponding to 74 dB re: 2×10^{-4}.

$$74 = 20 \log \frac{p_x}{(2 \times 10^{-4})}$$
$$3.7 = \log \frac{p_x}{(2 \times 10^{-4})}$$
$$5 \times 10^3 = \frac{p_x}{(2 \times 10^{-4})}$$
$$p_x = 10 \times 10^{-1}$$
$$= 1 \times 10^0.$$

2. From that calculation we know that the sound had an absolute pressure (p_x) = 1 dyne/cm^2 (1×10^0). The next step is to recalculate dB SPL using Equation 4.7, but with the new reference pressure, 1 dyne/cm^2, in the denominator.

$$dB = 20 \log \frac{(1 \times 10^0)}{(1 \times 10^0)}$$
$$= 0 \text{ dB SPL.}$$

Consider a second example. 20 dB SPL re: 1 dyne/cm^2 = ? dB SPL re: 2 dynes/cm^2?

1. $20 = 20 \log \dfrac{p_x}{(1 \times 10^0)}$

   $1 = \log \dfrac{p_x}{(1 \times 10^0)}$

   $10^1 = \dfrac{p_x}{(1 \times 10^0)}$

   $p_x = 10^1 \times 1 \times 10^0$
   $= 1 \times 10^1.$

2. $dB = 20 \log \dfrac{(1 \times 10^1)}{(2 \times 10^0)}$

   $= 20 \log (.5 \times 10^1)$
   $= 20 \log (5 \times 10^0)$
   $= 20 \times 0.7$
   $= 14.$

The approach just described required two steps: (1) solve an antilog problem to determine the value of p_x; and (2) solve a log problem to express p_x in decibels re: the new reference. An alternative is to use Equation 4.8, where only one step is necessary.

$$dB_{p_{r(new)}} = dB_{p_{r(orig)}} - 20 \log_{10} \frac{p_{r(new)}}{p_{r(orig)}},$$

Equation 4.8

where $p_{r(orig)}$ = the original reference

and

$p_{r(new)}$ = the new reference.

To illustrate that the two approaches yield identical results, we shall solve the first of the two problems listed above: 74 dB SPL re: 2×10^{-4} dyne/cm^2 = ? dB re: 1 dyne/cm^2:

$$dB = 74 - 20 \log \frac{(1 \times 10^0)}{(2 \times 10^{-4})}$$
$$= 74 - 20 \log (.5 \times 10^4)$$
$$= 0.$$

■ COMBINING SOUND INTENSITIES FROM INDEPENDENT SOURCES

If the intensity of some sound is 10^{-5} watt/m^2, we can calculate with Equation 4.4 that the intensity level is 70 dB IL re: 10^{-12} watt/m^2.

Suppose, then, that two independent sound sources are operating simultaneously and that each produces a sound with an intensity of 10^{-5} watt/m^2. We know that each source has an intensity level of 70 dB, but what is the *total intensity level* from the two sources combined? It is *not* 140 dB. Work through the problem and see why 140 dB is not a reasonable answer. To have an intensity level of 140 dB would require an absolute intensity of 10^2 watt/m^2:

$$140 = 10 \log \frac{I_x}{10^{-12}}$$

$$14 = \log \frac{I_x}{10^{-12}}$$

$$I_x = 10^{14} \times 10^{-12}$$

$$= 10^2.$$

It should be apparent that it is clearly *impossible* to have a total intensity of 10^2 watts/m^2. Each independent source produces a finite amount of energy. If the intensity (**energy/s/m^2**) from each source is an identical 10^{-5} watt/m^2, then the total intensity from the combined sources can only be twice as great, 2×10^{-5} watt/m^2, not 10^2 watts/m^2. If the total **intensity** from the two sources combined is 2×10^{-5} watt/m^2, what is the **intensity level** from the two combined?

$$dB = 10 \log \frac{(2 \times 10^{-5})}{10^{-12}}$$

$$= 73.$$

If the **intensity level** is 73 dB, what is the **sound pressure level** from the combined sources? If the reference pressure is 2×10^1 µPa, dB SPL also equals 73. First, a brief calculation should demonstrate the equivalence. The **intensity** from the combined sources was twice as great as for either source alone. A doubling of intensity corresponds to +3 dB, and we saw that the total of 73 dB was 3 dB greater than the intensity level from only one of the sources. If the intensity were increased by a factor of 2:1, what would have happened to the pressure? It would have increased by the square root of 2 ($p \propto \sqrt{I}$), or 1.414. From Equation 4.7 we see that sound pressure level also would have increased by 3 dB from 70 dB SPL:

$$dB = 20 \log 1.414$$

$$= 3.$$

Second, we learned previously (see Figure 4–2) that dB IL always equals dB SPL *when equivalent reference intensities and pressures are used*. Thus, 70 dB IL (the level for either source alone) equals 70 dB SPL, and if the intensity level increases by only 3 dB, the same must be true for the sound pressure level, which produces a total level of 73 dB SPL.

Unfortunately, the equivalence of dB IL and dB SPL is not always understood. Several years ago a person took a national examination that is required for certification by the American Speech-Language-Hearing Association and encountered the following kind of problem: If two sound sources each produce an identical sound pressure level, by how much will the total sound pressure level of the two combined sources exceed the level for either source alone? By now, you should know that the answer is 3 dB because it is the energies, powers, or intensities that should be added, which requires us to use the "10-log" equation (Equation 4.4). The person wrote a letter-to-the-editor of the journal *Asha* to complain that the examination was unfair because the alternative answers included 3 dB, but not 6 dB, and the writer was certain that 6 dB was the correct choice.

That letter produced some lively (and correct) responses from Mitchell Kramer (1997), who then was a doctoral student at Northwestern University, and from Professors Larry Feth (1977) and the late W. Dixon Ward (1977) that were published in *Asha* (March, 1977). Some comments from those three individuals should serve to emphasize the main point that has been stressed in this section:

> Both sound pressure and power change with a change in energy of an acoustic signal, with power changing as the square of pressure. But, a 3 dB change in pressure is equal, identical, and the very same as a 3 dB change in power or intensity. Of course, a doubling of pressure results in a 6 dB increase (of both pressure and intensity or power) but unless two signals are (1) the same frequency, and (2) added in phase, the intensities add, and a 3 dB increase results. This is equivalent to doubling the sound power, or increasing pressure by a factor of 1.41. But a dB is still a dB. (Kramer, p. 225)

> What students often carry away from the lecture on combining sound sources is the rule of thumb: "Double the intensity means a 3 dB increase; double the sound pressure results in a 6 dB increase." That rule by itself is correct. The errors arise in not understanding how sound pressure waveforms are added and in thinking that there is a difference between intensity level (IL) and sound pressure level (SPL) . . . . It must be kept in mind that sound pressure level (SPL) and intensity level (IL) are always synonymous and further are always numerically equal . . . . When two independent sound sources are combined, one must always add their intensities. Two sound pressure waveforms can only be added if their relative phase is known, and it seldom is. (Feth, pp. 225–226)

> What I suspect happened is that the problem went something like this: "If we put two machines side by side, each of which develops an SPL of 80 dB, what will be the SPL when they are both running?" The question is designed to lead the unwary down the primrose path by using SPL instead of IL, so that he or she is hoodwinked into thinking: "Oh yes, doubling the pressure is a 6-dB increase"—which is correct, but, alas, irrelevant, because the pressure simply does not get doubled in this situation. The correct answer is indeed 83 dB SPL—and, assuming that it is still taking place here on earth, also 83 dB IL. In air at standard temperature and pressure, the zeros on the SPL and IL scales have been chosen to represent the same acoustic conditions, so X dB SPL is also X dB IL . . . . To double the pressure (still under optimum conditions) would require four equal machines. (Ward, p. 226)

It is important to remember that when the total intensity level or sound pressure level from uncorrelated (independent) sound sources is desired, it is *the energies, or powers, or intensities that should be summed, not the pressures.* As Feth stated in his letter cited above, we cannot add the pressures unless the relative phases are known, and they seldom are.

There are two approaches that can be taken to solving problems such as these: one for when the source intensities are equal, and another for when the source intensities are unequal.

Equal Source Intensities

We will consider first the easier situation in which all of the contributing sources are characterized by an identical intensity level or sound pressure level. In that case,

Equation 4.9
$$dB_N = dB_i + 10 \log_{10} N,$$

where i = dB SPL (or dB IL) from one of the equal sources

and

N = the number of sources combined.

We do not have to determine the **intensity** of any of the sources or of the total. We simply want to know the total **intensity level** in dB.

Example 1 Two snowmobiles each produce 94 dB IL. What is the total level from the two combined?

$$dB_N = 94 + 10 \log 2$$
$$= 97.$$

Each source produces some finite amount of intensity that we do not need to calculate. Because there are two such sources, *the two sources combined must produce twice the intensity as either one alone.* If we increase intensity by a factor of 2:1, decibels increase by 3: 94 + 3 = 97. Why does Equation 4.9 "apparently" not contain a ratio? Actually it does. We are asking what happened to the intensity level when we increased from one source to two sources. Thus, the reference is 1 and need not be shown in the denominator.

Example 2 What is the total **sound pressure level** for eight sound sources, each of which produces 92 dB when operating alone?

Even though the level in the problem is expressed in SPL rather than IL, it is the intensities that must be added, not the pressures. Thus, we proceed just as we did with Example 1.

$$dB_N = 92 + 10 \log 8$$
$$= 92 + 9$$
$$= 101.$$

By now you should be able to work this kind of problem by thinking of powers of 2. Eight (8) is 2^3, which means that 8 is the result of the base 2 being used 3 times in multiplication. Each doubling corresponds to 3 dB. Thus, eight sources would produce a sound with an intensity that is 9 dB (3 + 3 + 3) greater than just one of the sources alone.

Unequal Source Intensities

When the contributing sources are not all characterized by equal intensity, Equation 4.9 will not apply, but the problem can still be solved by following three steps: (1) calculate the **intensity** of each source; (2) add the intensities, and the sum becomes the numerator of the ratio; and (3) calculate decibels with Equation 4.4 with a reference of 10^{-12} watt/m^2. The result will be either dB IL or dB SPL because the two are equivalent.

What is the total SPL that results from combining one source that produces 90 dB SPL with a second source that produces 80 dB SPL?   **Example 1**

1. $90 = 10 \log \dfrac{I_x}{10^{-12}}$,   Therefore, $I_{x(1)} = 10^{-3}$,

    and

    $80 = 10 \log \dfrac{I_x}{10^{-12}}$,   Therefore, $I_{x(2)} = 10^{-4}$,

2. $10^{-3} + 10^{-4} = 1.1 \times 10^{-3}$,

3. $dB = 10 \log \dfrac{(1.1 \times 10^{-3})}{10^{-12}}$

    $= 10 \log (1.1 \times 10^9)$

    $= 90.4$.

There are two important observations to make. First, when the levels of two sources differ by 10 dB, the total level is only 0.4 dB greater than the level of the source with the higher intensity. That is true of any two levels that differ by 10 dB: 90 and 80 (90.4), 80 and 70 (80.4), 0 and -10 (0.4), and so on. Second, one must be careful with addition of the intensities in Step 2 because the exponents are different.

$$\begin{aligned} I_{x(1)} &= 1 \times 10^{-3} \\ + I_{x(2)} &= 1 \times 10^{-4} \\ \hline &= \quad ? \end{aligned}$$

Before the two intensities can be added, the exponent for one must be converted to be the same as the other exponent. We will illustrate the process by converting $I_{x(2)}$ to have an exponent of -3 rather than -4. To convert from -4 to -3 we *multiply* by 10. To preserve equivalence, therefore, we must *divide* the other term in the product, the coefficient, by 10: Thus,

$$1 \times 10^{-4} = .1 \times 10^{-3}.$$

Now when we add the two intensities, we obtain:

$$
\begin{array}{r}
1 \times 10^{-3} \\
+ \ .1 \times 10^{-3} \\
\hline
= 1.1 \times 10^{-3}.
\end{array}
$$

If the validity of that series of steps is not obvious, the two intensities are added below in conventional notation rather than scientific notation:

$$
\begin{array}{r}
1 \times 10^{-3} = .001 \\
+ \ 1 \times 10^{-4} = .0001 \\
\hline
= .0011,
\end{array}
$$

and .0011 in conventional notation equals 1.1×10^{-3} in scientific notation.

Example 2   A fan is operating at an unknown level in a noisy environment. You wish to determine the sound pressure level of the fan, but it cannot be removed from its location and the surrounding noise cannot be turned off.

1. Measure the sound pressure level of the combined noise produced by the fan and the surrounding equipment. Suppose this total level is 90 dB SPL.

2. Turn off the fan and measure the level produced by the surrounding equipment. Suppose that this new measurement is 86 dB SPL.

3. From those two measurements we know that the surrounding equipment and the fan together produce a noise of 90 dB SPL and that the surrounding equipment alone produces a noise of 86 dB SPL. The fan, therefore, must be responsible for the difference of 4 dB, but *do not conclude that its level is 4 dB SPL*. Before we solve the problem, try to approximate the answer by using powers of 2. Recall the earlier problem involving the two snowmobiles. We learned that combining two sound sources that have the same intensity produced a 3 dB increase from the level produced by either machine alone. In the present problem, the surrounding noise is 86 dB. Therefore, if the noise from the fan also were 86 dB, the two combined would produce a noise of 89 dB, which is just 1 dB less than the 90 we measured. Therefore, we should expect the true noise level of the fan to be just a little more than 86.

   a. (Intensity of fan *plus* surrounding noise)

   $$90 = 10 \log \frac{I_x}{10^{-12}}, \quad \text{Therefore, } I_x = 10^{-3}.$$

b. (Intensity of surrounding noise *alone*)

$$86 = 10 \log \frac{I_x}{10^{-12}}, \quad \text{Therefore, } I_x = 3.98 \times 10^{-4}.$$

c. (Intensity of fan alone—by subtraction)
$(1 \times 10^{-3}) - (3.98 \times 10^{-4}) = 6.02 \times 10^{-4}.$

d. (Intensity level of fan alone)

$$dB = 10 \log \frac{(6.02 \times 10^{-4})}{10^{-12}}$$

$$= 87.8.$$

Because the preceding computational methods might sometimes be inconvenient, published charts are available to aid with combining decibels. Direct computations are preferable, however, if precise determination of small differences is required.

■ SUMMARY OF DECIBELS FOR SOUND INTENSITY AND SOUND PRESSURE

Earlier in this chapter two steps were suggested for solution of decibel problems. First, select the proper equation. Second, form a ratio and solve the problem. When the problem involves **intensity** or **power**, use Equation 4.4—the so-called "10 log equation." When the problem involves **pressure**, use Equation 4.7—the "20 log equation."

The distinction between power and pressure applies if decibels are used to express the level of some quantity other than sound. For example, if you have three dollars, and someone gives you three more dollars, that represents an increase of 3 dB. In contrast, if a committee comprises three people, and three more members are added, that represents an increase of 6 dB. We might justify use of the 10 log equation in one case, but the 20 log equation in the other, because "money is power," but "people are pressure."

The only confusion that should remain might stem from problems that involve combining sound levels from independent sources. In those instances it is important to keep in mind that unless the relative phases are known, *it is the energies or powers or intensities that should be added, not the pressures*. Thus, it does not matter whether the problem is stated by reference to dB IL or dB SPL. *As long as the references are equivalent, dB IL = dB SPL, and you must always use Equation 4.4—the "10 log equation."*

■ NOTES

1. The proper form for all equations concerning the decibel is "$\log_{10} X$" preceded by a multiplier of either 10 (intensity) or 20 (pressure), where "X" refers to some ratio. Because the **base** for all calculations of decibels is **10**, the base will frequently be omitted for convenience.

2. The equivalent reference intensity in the **cgs** metric system is 10^{-16} watt/cm^2.

3. The unit of measure in the **cgs** metric system is the **dyne/cm^2** or the **microbar**.

4. In many reference texts, the symbol for the speed of sound is **c** rather than **s**. Thus, the equation for characteristic impedance ordinarily is expressed as $Z_c = \rho_o c$. We have elected to use **s** so that we can consistently distinguish between speed (**s**), which is a scalar quantity, and velocity (**c**), which is a vector quantity.

5. The equivalent reference pressure in the **cgs** metric system is **2×10^{-4} dyne/cm^2** or **2×10^{-4} microbar**. See Table 4–3 for a more complete description of equivalent measures of pressure in the two metric systems.

■ FREQUENTLY MISUNDERSTOOD CONCEPTS

1. If intensity level increases by 23 dB, the **intensity** increases by what factor?

200:1. The problem is solved with Equation 4.4:

$$N \text{ (dB)} = 10 \log \frac{I_x}{I_r}$$
$$23 = 10 \log X$$
$$2.3 = \log X$$
$$X = 2 \times 10^2$$
$$= 200.$$

2. An increase in **sound pressure** by a factor of 4:1 corresponds to an increase by how many decibels?

12 dB, not 12 dB IL or 12 dB SPL. The problem is solved with Equation 4.7:

$$N \text{ (dB)} = 20 \log \frac{p_x}{p_r}$$
$$= 20 \log 4$$
$$= 20 \times .6$$
$$= 12 \text{ dB}.$$

It cannot be 12 dB SPL or 12 dB IL because those answers require a reference pressure of 20 µPa (SPL) or 10^{-12} watts/m^2 (IL). We do not know the value of the reference pressure before the pressure was increased. We know only that whatever the value of the pressure originally, it was then increased by a factor of 4:1. Suppose, for example, that the original pressure was 2×10^4 µPa, which corresponds to 60 dB SPL. When the pressure is increased by a factor of 4:1, it becomes 8×10^4 µPa, which corresponds to 72 dB SPL. The increase, however, was by 12 dB, not 12 dB SPL.

3. An increase in sound **pressure** by a factor of 6:1 corresponds to an increase in sound **intensity** by what factor?

   36:1. *Intensity is proportional to the square of **pressure**.* Therefore, if pressure increases by 6:1, intensity increases by a factor of 6^2, or 36:1.

4. If sound **pressure** decreases by one half (1:2), sound **intensity** decreases by how many *decibels*?

   6 dB. Because intensity is proportional to the square of pressure, if pressure decreases by one half (1:2), intensity would decrease by $1/2^2$, or a factor of 1:4. Then, 10 log 1/4 = −6 dB.

5. 90 dB re: 2×10^{-4} microbar (cgs system) corresponds to how many dB re: 1 microbar?

   16 dB. The problem is solved with Equation 4.8:

   $$dB_{P_{r(new)}} = dB_{P_{r(orig)}} - 20 \log_{10} \frac{P_{r(new)}}{P_{r(orig)}}$$

   $$= 90 - 20 \log \frac{(1 \times 10^0)}{(2 \times 10^{-4})}$$

   $$= 90 - 74 = 16.$$

6. Four independent sound sources each produce a sound level of 60 dB SPL. What is the **intensity** (not intensity level) of the four combined?

   4×10^{-6} **watt/m².** The answer is *not* 66 dB SPL (or 66 dB IL) because the question specifically asked for the **intensity**, which is expressed in watt/m², not intensity level, which is expressed in dB. This problem can be solved easily by breaking it into two parts. First, if each source produces a level of 60 dB SPL, what will be the SPL of the four sources combined? Use Equation 4.9:

   $$dB_N = dB_i + 10 \log N$$

   $$= 60 + 10 \log 4$$

   $$= 66 \text{ dB SPL.}$$

Second, use Equation 4.4 to solve for intensity, I_x:

$$dB = 10 \log \frac{I_x}{I_r}$$

$$66 = 10 \log \frac{I_x}{10^{-12}}$$

$$= 4 \times 10^{-6}.$$

7. Four independent sound sources each produce a sound level of 60 dB SPL. What is the **sound pressure** (not sound pressure level) of the four combined?

4 × 10⁴ µPa. The answer is *not* 66 dB SPL, because the question specifically asked for the *pressure*, which is expressed in µPa, not the sound pressure level, which is expressed in dB. We already know the total level for the four sources combined from solving #6: 66 dB SPL. Next, use Equation 4.9 to solve for pressure, p_x:

$$dB = 20 \log \frac{p_x}{p_r}$$

$$66 = 20 \log \frac{p_x}{(2 \times 10^1)}$$

$$= 4 \times 10^4.$$

Complex Waves

All of the sound waves that have been described to this point were of the **sinusoidal** form that appears in panel A of Figure 5–1. Although the sine wave is not the type of vibratory motion that we are likely to experience in our daily lives, it is important to understand it thor-

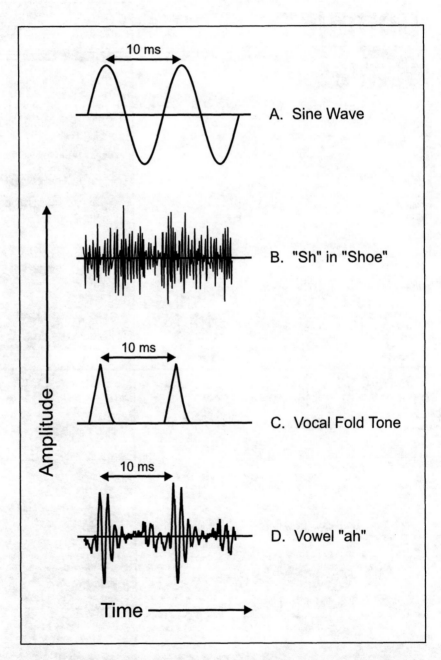

Figure 5–1. Comparison of a sine wave with three complex waves: the "sh" sound from the word "shoe"; the sound wave created by vibratory movement of the vocal folds; and the vowel /a/.

oughly because *the sine wave is the fundamental component of other sound waves that will be encountered.*

The other sound waves shown in Figure 5–1 are much more complex in form than the simple sine wave, and they are, indeed, called **complex waves**. The wave in panel B is similar to the "sh" sound in the word "shoe." Panel C shows one kind of sound wave that results from vibratory motion of the vocal folds during production of a vowel. Finally, panel D shows the same vowel as recorded near the mouth opening rather than deep in the throat just above the vocal folds.

■ FOURIER'S THEOREM

A **complex wave** can be characterized as *any sound wave that is not sinusoidal.* That characterization, though, does not reveal exactly what a complex wave is, but the following theorem should help. The complex waves in Figure 5–1—and all other sound waves that are not sinusoidal—*are composed of a series of simple sinusoids that can differ in amplitude, frequency, and phase.* Thus, when two or more sine waves that differ in amplitude, frequency, or phase are added together, a complex wave is produced.

The degree of complexity of a complex sound wave depends on the number of sine waves that are combined and on the specific dimensional values (amplitude, frequency, and phase) of the sinusoidal components. The theorem was first stated by Joseph Fourier, a French mathematician who lived at the time of Napoleon I; hence, the series of sine waves that are combined to compose a complex periodic wave is called a **Fourier series** in his honor.

Fourier's theorem has two important implications for the study of complex waves. First, because a complex wave consists of some number of sinusoids of different amplitudes, frequencies, and phases, the nature of any complex wave should be easy to comprehend if we understand the concept of simple harmonic motion that is associated with each of the sinusoidal components, and if we recall the relevant dimensions of sine waves: **amplitude, frequency,** and **phase.** Second, we can derive the **Fourier series** by a process called **Fourier analysis**, which means that *a complex waveform can be decomposed, or analyzed, to determine the amplitudes, frequencies, and phases of the sinusoidal components.*

All sound waves can be classified by reference to (1) the presence or absence of **periodicity** in the wave and (2) the degree of complexity of the wave.

■ PERIODIC WAVES

A **periodic wave**, whether sinusoidal or complex, is a wave that *repeats itself at regular intervals over time.* Because the wave repeats itself periodically over time, it is characterized as a **periodic time function.** The sine wave in Figure 5–1 provides an obvious example of periodicity because the characteristics of any one cycle of the wave are duplicated exactly in all other cycles—each cycle in the wave is repeated regularly over time.

Sine waves are not the only forms of wave motion that are periodic. The vocal fold wave (panel C) and the vowel (panel D) in Figure 5–1 appear to be reasonably periodic (they are in fact called **quasiperiodic**) because we can verify that all of the features within one "cycle" of vibration are duplicated *almost exactly* during the next and all other cycles. Thus, there are two kinds of **periodic waves**: sinusoidal and complex. A **sinusoidal wave** *is a wave that results from simple harmonic motion and that comes from a mathematical relation that contains a sine function.* A **complex periodic wave** *is a periodic wave, but it is not sinusoidal.*

Components of a Complex Periodic Wave

According to Fourier's theorem, any complex periodic wave consists of some number of simple sinusoids that are summed, but the sinusoidal components cannot be selected randomly if the resultant sound wave is to be periodic. Instead, they must satisfy a basic mathematical requirement that is called a **harmonic relation**.

The term **harmonic relation** means that *the frequencies of all of the sinusoids that compose the series must be integer (whole number) multiples of the lowest frequency component* in the series. For example, if the lowest frequency sinusoid is 100 Hz, the other sinusoidal components of the complex wave must be selected from the frequencies 200, 300, 400, 500 Hz, and so forth, because other frequency values would not satisfy the requirement of being integer multiples of the lowest frequency. Similarly, if the lowest frequency sinusoid is 110 Hz, the other sinusoidal components must be selected from the frequencies 220, 330, 440, 550 Hz, and so on. We say "must be selected from" because, as we shall see subsequently, all components must be integer multiples of the lowest frequency, but not all integer multiples need be present.

A Harmonic Series

When a harmonic relation exists among frequency components, the series of frequencies is called a **harmonic series**, and all of the sinusoids in the harmonic series are called **harmonics**. The harmonics are numbered consecutively from lowest to highest frequency: 1st harmonic, which also is called the **fundamental frequency (f_0)**, 2nd harmonic, 3rd harmonic, and so on until we reach the nth harmonic, the last component in the series.

In the case of the first example above, the 1st harmonic (also called the f_0) = 100 Hz, the 2nd harmonic = 200 Hz, the 3rd harmonic = 300 Hz, and so on. There also is a special circumstance in which the fundamental frequency (1st harmonic) is missing from the series.

In that case, all of the higher frequencies in the harmonic series are integer multiples of what is called the **repetition rate**.

Figure 5–2 shows the waveform of one example of a complex periodic wave that consists of an infinite number of sinusoidal components. Its periodicity should be apparent, and because it obviously is not sinusoidal, it must be a complex periodic wave. This particular wave is called a **sawtooth wave** because its shape resembles the shape of the teeth of a saw. The sawtooth wave will be of interest to those who become interested in the study of speech acoustics because the waveform of the sawtooth wave resembles the waveform of the sound produced by the vibrating vocal folds.

The period of the fundamental frequency (the 1st harmonic) of the sawtooth wave in Figure 5–2 is 8 ms, which means that f_0, the fundamental frequency, is 125 Hz. All components—the **harmonics**—of the sawtooth wave are *odd and even whole number (integer) multiples of the fundamental frequency*. Thus, if the fundamental frequency is 125 Hz, the harmonic components are: 125 ($f_0 \times 1$), 250 ($f_0 \times 2$), 375 ($f_0 \times 3$), 500 ($f_0 \times 4$), 625 ($f_0 \times 5$) Hz, and so on for an infinity of odd and even integer multiples.

We see in Table 5–1 that the lowest frequency, 125 Hz, is called the fundamental frequency, f_0, and it also is called the 1st harmonic. The other components are labeled the 2nd harmonic, 3rd harmonic, 4th harmonic, and so on.

Partials and Overtones

You occasionally will find that the components in a complex periodic wave are called **partials** or **overtones** instead of **harmonics**. Table 5–1 also shows the relations among these different labels.

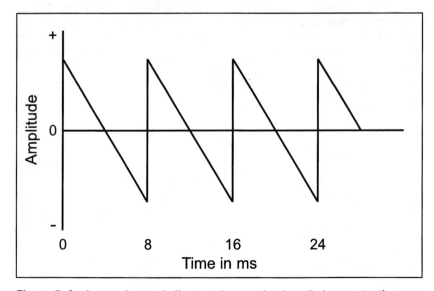

Figure 5–2. A **complex periodic** sound wave that is called a **sawtooth wave** because its shape resembles the teeth of a saw.

Table 5–1. Fundamental frequency, harmonics, partials, and overtones in a complex periodic sound wave

Frequency	Harmonic	Partial	Overtone
125 (f_0)	1	1	
250	2	2	1
375	3	3	2
500	4	4	3
625	5	5	4
750	6	6	5

We can see from the entries in the table that the designations of **harmonic** and **partial** are synonymous *if all components are integer multiples of the fundamental frequency*: the 1st harmonic (also the fundamental) is the 1st partial, the 2nd harmonic is the 2nd partial, and so on. The word, **overtone**, which might, for example, be encountered in musical literature derives from the fact that the complex wave can be described as consisting of a fundamental frequency, or fundamental tone, and a series of other tones whose frequencies lie *over* the fundamental. Thus, the 2nd harmonic is the 1st overtone, the 3rd harmonic is the 2nd overtone, and so on.

Summary

If the complex wave is to be periodic, the sinusoidal components *must be integer multiples of the fundamental frequency*. Thus, if f_0 = 100 Hz, the other components must be selected from 200 Hz, 300 Hz, 400 Hz, and so forth. When that occurs, the partials are harmonics, and the sound wave is exactly periodic. In that circumstance, at the end of one cycle of vibration (10 ms), we will have completed one cycle of the 1st harmonic (100 Hz; T = 10 ms), two cycles of the 2nd harmonic (200 Hz; T = 5 ms), three cycles of the 3rd harmonic (300 Hz; T = 3.33 ms), four cycles of the 4th harmonic (400 Hz; T = 2.5 ms), and so on.

Summation of Sine Waves

As more and more sine waves are added (summed) in the harmonic series, the shape of the resultant complex wave changes. The left side of Figure 5–3 shows four sine waves (S_1, S_2, S_3, and S_4) that have different frequencies and amplitudes, but identical **starting phases** (180°).

The exact frequency of each wave to be summed is unimportant, but an appropriate frequency relation among the four components is maintained; the three higher frequencies must be harmonics of the lowest one—the fundamental frequency. Notice, however, that not all harmonics are present in this example. In fact, we have used only

Shape when sine waves are combined

one cycle

h_1 or S_1
F0

sine wave

complex wave

$C_1 = S_1 + S_2$

h_3 S_2   *3 cycles*

$C_2 = S_1 + S_2 + S_3$

h_5 S_3   *5 cycles*

h_7 S_4   *7 cycles*

$C_3 = S_1 + S_2 + S_3 + S_4$

as go up in frequency, amplitude decreases
—this has to happen for a square wave

Amplitude / Time

all starting phases are the same

$C_n = S_1 + S_2 + \ldots + S_n$

to infinity

Square wave - do not occur naturally, computer generated

Figure 5–3. Summation of sine waves to form complex waves. The sine waves at the left (S_1 through S_4) are added progressively to form the complex waves (C_1 through C_3) at the right. At the bottom, **a square wave** is created by summation of an infinite number of sine waves of *appropriate* **amplitudes, frequencies,** and **starting phases**.

the odd integer multiples so that we have the 1st (f_0), 3rd, 5th, and 7th harmonics. Thus, if the frequency of S_1 were 1000 Hz, the frequencies of the other sinusoids would be 3000, 5000, and 7000 Hz; if the frequency of S_1 were 400 Hz, the frequencies of the other sinusoids would be 1200, 2000, and 2800 Hz.

At the right of Figure 5–3 we show what happens when the sinusoidal components are summed progressively to form three different complex waves (C_1, C_2, and C_3). The complex wave at the top of the figure (C_1) results from $S_1 + S_2$. Wave C_1 is not a sinusoid—it is complex—and it is composed of two sinusoids that differ in amplitude and frequency.

Although the **starting phases** of the two components of C_1 are identical, it should be apparent that the **instantaneous phases** of the two sinusoidal components vary from moment to moment because of their different frequencies. If the two sinusoidal components had any other values of frequency and amplitude, the complex wave that results would be different from the one shown as C_1 because the resultant wave depends upon all of the specific dimensions of the sine waves that compose it.

Wave C_2 looks different from wave C_1 because its shape results from summation of three sinusoids: $S_1 + S_2 + S_3$. Wave C_3 contains all four sinusoidal components. You might notice that the complex waves at the right are becoming more and more "square" in shape as more and more sine waves are added. At the bottom right of Figure 5–3 we show what happens if we combine an infinite number of odd integer multiples ($1\times$, $3\times$, $5\times$, $7\times$, $9\times$, $+ \ldots + n\times$) with appropriate relative amplitudes and starting phases. If, for example, the lowest frequency were 100 Hz, the other components would be 300, 500, 700 Hz, and so on. A complex wave with a perfectly square shape is created by summing an infinity of sinusoids with frequencies that are odd integer multiples of the fundamental frequency and that have appropriate relative amplitudes and identical starting phases.

Figure 5–4 provides another example of summation of sine waves to form a different complex periodic wave. The left side of Figure 5–4 shows three sine waves (S_1, S_2, and S_3) that have different frequencies and amplitudes, but identical **starting phases** ($0°$). S_2 and S_3 are even and odd integer multiples of S_1. Thus, if S_1 were 1000 Hz, the two other components would be 2000 Hz (S_2) and 3000 Hz (S_3).

At the right of Figure 5–4 we see the results of progressive summation of the sinusoidal components to form the complex waves

Figure 5–4. Summation of sine waves to form a different **complex periodic wave**. Because the shape of this complex wave is different from those shown previously, the parameter values for amplitude, frequency, and starting phase of the sinusoidal components must also be different.

$(C_1 = S_1 + S_2;$ and $C_2 = S_1 + S_2 + S_3)$. The two resultant waves, C_1 and C_2, look different from the resultant waves seen in Figure 5–3 because both odd and even harmonics are included rather than just odd integer multiples of f_0.

When an infinity of *odd* harmonics with appropriate relative amplitudes and starting phases is summed, the result is the square wave that was shown in Figure 5–3. When an infinity of *odd and even* harmonics with appropriate relative amplitudes and starting phases is summed, the result is a sawtooth wave such as that shown at the bottom right of Figure 5–4. In fact, with only three components (C_2), and a bit of imagination, you can see that the resultant wave in Figure 5–4 is beginning to assume a sawtooth kind of shape.

In the two examples cited thus far, the **starting phase** was identical for the individual components. Variations in the resultant wave also will occur if we vary the starting phase of the components while holding their amplitudes and frequencies constant, as is illustrated in Figure 5–5.

Figure 5–5. Effects of variations in **starting phase** on the shape of a complex wave that results from summation of sine waves.

The left side of Figure 5–5 shows the sinusoidal components that will be summed to form the complex waves at the right of the figure. The **starting phase** of S_1 is 0° in all four panels. Four different **starting phases** are used for S_2: 0° (panel A); 90° (panel B); 180° (panel C); and 270° (panel D). The four complex waves at the right of Figure 5–5 differ from one another, and the differences are attributable *exclusively* to the differences in the **starting phase** of S_2.

■ APERIODIC WAVES

The principal distinguishing characteristic of complex periodic waves is their regularity over time, or **periodicity**. They repeat themselves indefinitely. The **aperiodic wave** is a second category of waveform, and its name derives from an absence of periodicity. Thus, it is very difficult, and ordinarily impossible, to predict what the wave will look like during one time interval from knowledge of its characteristics during a preceding time interval of equal duration.

The vibratory motion of an aperiodic wave is **random**, and therefore unpredictable, and vibratory motions of this type are called **random time functions**. In acoustics, this is called an **aperiodic sound wave.** The sound wave shown in Figure 5–6 is an aperiodic, or random, wave and you should see that it is virtually impossible (except by chance) to identify any two time intervals of equal duration in which the characteristics of the vibratory motion are identical in all respects.

We encounter aperiodic sound waves daily. Familiar examples are the noises from aircraft, automobiles, or speedboats. Each of those sounds is characterized by random vibratory motion—aperiodicity—but that does not mean that all aperiodic sounds are unpleasant. The water cascading down the side of the mountain produces an aperiodic sound wave, but under the right circumstances it might produce a

Figure 5–6. An **aperiodic** sound wave.

very satisfying sensation. Many of the sounds of speech ("sh" in "she"; "s" in "see"; "f" in "foolish"; "th" in "three"; and so on) are characterized by random vibratory motion, but we usually don't think of such sounds as "noise."

■ WAVEFORM AND SPECTRUM

Waveform

Each picture of periodic (both sinusoidal and complex) and aperiodic waves that has been shown to this point has focused on the **waveform**. By that we mean, we have plotted changes in one variable (pressure, velocity, acceleration, displacement, and so forth) *as a function of time.* The waveform defines, for example, the distribution of instantaneous amplitudes of a sinusoidal or complex wave over time.

Return to the waveforms for the sawtooth wave in Figure 5–2 and the square wave in Figure 5–3. We can identify the **fundamental period** of each wave, and from that we can calculate the **fundamental frequency**. Unless we happen to remember, however, that the square wave consists of all odd harmonics and that the sawtooth wave consists of all odd and even harmonics, we would have no way of knowing what **frequencies** other than the fundamental frequency were present by visual examination of the waveform.

We also cannot determine the **amplitudes** or the **starting phases** of the sinusoidal components by visual inspection of the waveform. We shall see subsequently that both the square wave and the sawtooth wave must satisfy very specific requirements relative to both the amplitudes and starting phases of the components, but the point we wish to emphasize now is that visual inspection of the waveform will not reveal sufficient details about these important dimensions of the sinusoidal components.

Amplitude Spectrum

A graphic alternative to the **waveform** is the **amplitude spectrum in the frequency domain**, or just **amplitude spectrum**. Whereas the waveform shows instantaneous magnitudes such as amplitude as a function of time, the **amplitude spectrum** *shows amplitude (in either absolute or relative values) as a function of **frequency***.

In Figure 5–7, the waveforms of the sawtooth and the square wave are shown at the left and their respective amplitude spectra are shown at the right. The amplitude spectrum is shown by plotting relative amplitude in dB as a function of frequency. The location of each vertical line along the horizontal axis indicates the frequency of that component, and the height of each line is proportional to its relative amplitude. Zero dB represents the amplitude of the component with the greatest energy, and all other amplitudes therefore are shown as

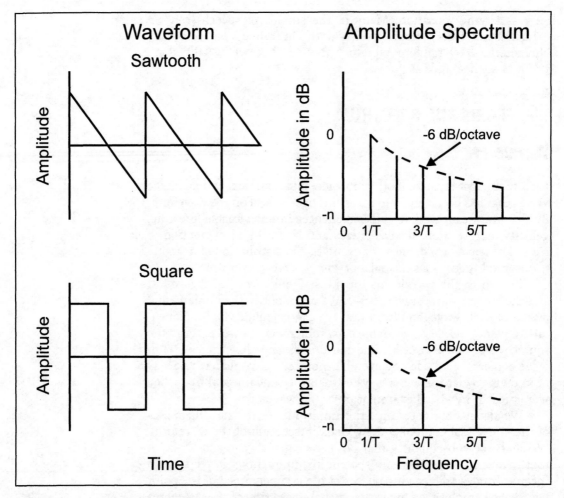

Figure 5–7. A comparison of **waveforms** and **amplitude spectra** for sawtooth and square waves, each of which is a complex periodic wave. Each spectrum is a **line spectrum**.

negative because their amplitudes are shown in dB relative to the amplitude of the fundamental.

The **envelope** of the amplitude spectrum in Figure 5–7 is shown by a dashed line that connects the peaks of each of the vertical lines. We can see that the **square wave** has energy at all *odd harmonics* and the **sawtooth wave** has energy at all *odd and even harmonics*, just as was described previously.

Inspection of amplitude spectra reveals information that, although present in the waveform, was not readily apparent from visual inspection. You might have noticed that when the sinusoidal components in Figure 5–3 were summed to create a square wave, the amplitudes of the components decreased with increasing frequency. That also can be seen in the amplitude spectrum for the square wave in Figure 5–7, and now the relation among the amplitudes of the components can be seen. For the square wave, the **spectral envelope** in the frequency domain *decreases at a rate of 6 dB per octave*, which is the same as saying that the spectral envelope has a slope of -6 dB per octave.

An **octave** refers to *a doubling or halving of frequency* (2f or 1/2f). Thus, 250 Hz is one octave above 125 Hz, 500 Hz is one octave above 250 Hz, and 500 Hz is two octaves above 125 Hz. An octave always refers to *a frequency ratio of 2:1 or 1:2, not to a frequency difference*. Thus, 2000 Hz is one octave above 1000 Hz and 200 Hz is one octave above 100 Hz because, in both cases, a ratio of 2:1 exists. The fact that the frequency difference is 1000 Hz in one case, but 100 Hz in the other, is irrelevant.

The white keys on a piano correspond to the musical notes that are designated "A,B,C,D,E,F,G,A." The lowest note is A_1, which has a frequency of 27.5 Hz. Seven white keys to the right of A_1 is A_2, which has a frequency of 55 Hz. Thus, A_2 is one octave above A_1. At the extreme right of the keyboard is A_8, which has a frequency of 3520 Hz ($27.5 \times 2^7 = 3520$). Thus, A_8 is one octave above A_7, which has a frequency of 1760 Hz, and seven octaves above A_1.

Another example of octave relations can be seen by returning to Table 5–1 where the harmonic components of a complex periodic wave are listed. There we see that the 2nd harmonic is one octave above the 1st harmonic, and conversely, the 1st harmonic is one octave below the 2nd. The 4th harmonic is one octave above the 2nd and two octaves above the 1st, and so forth. In each case, the frequency ratio was either 2:1 or 1:2.

Line Spectra

The amplitude spectra in Figure 5–7 are called **line amplitude spectra**, or just **line spectra**, because the sinusoidal components of the complex periodic waves can be represented by *a set of lines*. The location of a particular line in the frequency domain (horizontal axis) identifies the frequency of that component, and the height of the line along the amplitude scale (vertical axis) identifies the amplitude.

With a line spectrum, *energy is present only at frequencies represented by the vertical lines*. Even though, for example, the spectral envelope is shown by a line that connects the harmonics of the sawtooth wave, *there is no energy at frequencies between two adjacent components*.

Continuous Spectra

The random, or aperiodic, waveform of the noise in Figure 5–6 is shown again in Figure 5–8 along with its amplitude spectrum. The result is called a **continuous amplitude spectrum**, or just **continuous spectrum**, in contrast to the line spectrum shown previously.

A **continuous spectrum** is one in which *energy is present at all frequencies between certain lower and upper frequency limits*. Thus, the complex aperiodic wave does not result from summation

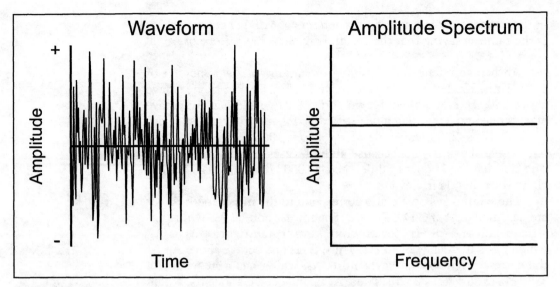

Figure 5–8. Waveform and amplitude spectrum for a complex aperiodic wave. The spectrum is a **continuous spectrum**.

of a harmonic series—integer multiples of the fundamental frequency—but rather there is energy present at all frequencies between some lower and upper limits.

In the case of the noise shown in Figure 5–8, energy is present at all frequencies and the spectral envelope has a slope of 0 dB. In other words, an identical amount of energy is present at all frequencies throughout the range. Equal energy at all frequencies, however, is not a requirement for all aperiodic waveforms, and subsequently we shall describe different types of aperiodic waveforms and their corresponding amplitude spectra.

Phase Spectrum

In addition to the **amplitude spectrum** of a sound wave, we can also describe the **phase spectrum in the frequency domain**, or just the **phase spectrum**. Whereas the amplitude spectrum describes relative amplitude as a function of frequency, the **phase spectrum** defines *the starting phase as a function of frequency*. The combination of the amplitude spectrum and the phase spectrum defines the waveform completely in the frequency domain.

■ EXAMPLES OF COMPLEX SOUND WAVES

Examples of four different complex signals, both periodic and aperiodic, are shown in Figure 5–9 and are compared with the familiar sine

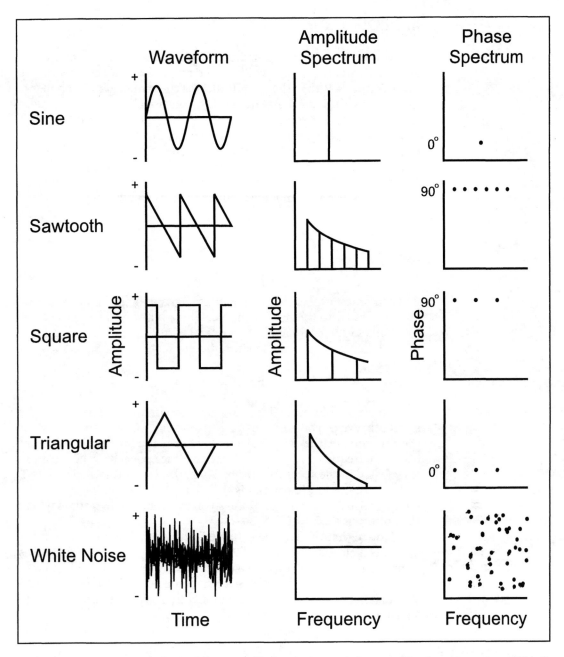

Figure 5–9. A comparison of **waveforms**, **amplitude spectra**, and **phase spectra** for a sine wave, sawtooth wave, square wave, triangular wave, and white noise.

wave at the top of the figure. The panels at the left show the **waveforms**, the middle panels show the **amplitude spectra**, and the panels at the right show the **phase spectra**. The waveform of the sine wave should be thoroughly familiar by now with no further discussion.

Sawtooth Wave

A **sawtooth wave** is a complex periodic wave with energy at all, odd and even, integer multiples of the fundamental frequency. We can see from Figure 5–9 that the amplitudes of the sinusoidal components decrease with increasing frequency. Specifically, the amplitudes decrease as the inverse (the reciprocal) of the harmonic number. Thus, the amplitudes of the harmonics are: h_1 (f_0) = 1/1; h_2 = 1/2; h_3 = 1/3; h_4 = 1/4; ... h_n = 1/n. If the amplitude of h_1 (f_0) = 2 V, the amplitudes of the next three higher harmonics are: h_2 = 1 V (1/2 × 2); h_3 = 0.67 V (1/3 × 2); and h_4 = 0.5 V (1/4 × 2). The relative amplitude, in decibels, for each component frequency is given by:

Equation 5.1
$$dB = 20 \log_{10} \frac{1}{h_i},$$

where h_i is the harmonic number.

By **harmonic number** (h_i) we mean 1st harmonic (h_1), 2nd harmonic (h_2), and so on to the nth harmonic. Thus, **h** always is an integer: 1, 2, 3, and so forth. By application of Law 4 of logarithms (log 1/a = −log a), Equation 5.1 can be simplified to read:

Equation 5.2
$$dB = -20 \log_{10} h_i.$$

The first column of Table 5–2 lists the first nine harmonics of a sawtooth wave. For purposes of illustration, we will arbitrarily set the rms voltage (the electrical analog of acoustic pressure) of the fundamental frequency, f_0, to be 2 V. The voltage of each of the harmonics is listed in the second column. Thus, the 2nd harmonic is 1 V (1/2 × 2 = 1 V), the 3rd harmonic is 0.67 V (1/3 × 2 = 0.67), the 4th harmonic is 0.5 V (1/4 × 2 = 0.5), and so on until the 9th harmonic where the voltage is 0.22 V (1/9 × 2 = 0.22).

Notice that the voltage is halved with each doubling of frequency. Thus, between the 1st and 2nd harmonics, the voltage decreases from 2 V to 1 V. The voltage also is halved between the 2nd and 4th, the 3rd and 6th, and 4th and 8th harmonics. Recall from Chapter 4 that halving of acoustic pressure or electrical voltage corresponds to a change in amplitude of −6 dB:

$$dB = 20 \log_{10} \tfrac{1}{2} = -6 \text{ dB}.$$

Therefore, because each doubling of frequency corresponds to an octave, and for each octave increase the amplitude decreases by 6 dB, we can say that the spectral envelope has a slope of −6 dB per octave.

The third column of Table 5–2 expresses the amplitude of each harmonic in decibels re: the amplitude of the fundamental frequency. Thus, for example, with the aid of Equation 5.2 we can calculate that the level of the 5th harmonic is −14 dB:

$$dB = -20 \log_{10} 5 = -14 \ (-13.98) \text{ dB}.$$

Table 5–2. Amplitudes (in voltage) of sinusoidal components of a **sawtooth** wave in which the amplitude of the fundamental frequency is 2 V

Harmonic Number	rms voltage $\left(\dfrac{1}{h_i}\times 2\right)$	$-20\,\log_{10}\,h_i$
1 (f_0)	$\dfrac{1}{1}\times 2 = 2$	0
2	$\dfrac{1}{2}\times 2 = 1$	−6
3	$\dfrac{1}{3}\times 2 = .67$	−9.5
4	$\dfrac{1}{4}\times 2 = .50$	−12
5	$\dfrac{1}{5}\times 2 = .40$	−14
6	$\dfrac{1}{6}\times 2 = .33$	−15.6
7	$\dfrac{1}{7}\times 2 = .29$	−16.9
8	$\dfrac{1}{8}\times 2 = .25$	−18.1
9	$\dfrac{1}{9}\times 2 = .22$	−19.1

It is important to recognize that the *absolute amplitude* (voltage in this case because the sawtooth wave is an electrical signal) for each harmonic listed in column two of Table 5–2 *depends on the absolute voltage of the fundamental frequency.* You might wish to try a few calculations and confirm that if the voltage of the fundamental of the sawtooth waveform were 1 V rather than 2 V, the voltages of the eight higher harmonics would be: 0.5 V; 0.33 V; 0.25 V; 0.2 V; 0.17 V; 0.14 V; 0.13 V; and 0.11 V.

We have seen with those calculations that the absolute voltage of each of the harmonics in the sawtooth wave depends on the absolute voltage of the fundamental. The relative amplitude, in decibels, for each of the harmonics in a sawtooth wave, however, *is independent of the voltage of the fundamental frequency.* In other words, the level of the 2nd harmonic will always be −6 dB, the level of the 3rd harmonic will always be −9.5 dB, and so on.

If you continue with your computations by calculating $-20 \log_{10} h_i$ (Equation 5.2) for each of the calculations that you just made for the case where $f_0 = 1$ V, you should obtain the same answers for a fundamental frequency of 1 V (subject to rounding error) that appear in the third column of Table 5–2 for a fundamental frequency of 2 V. For example, the relative level of the 5th harmonic still is -14 dB.

What does the amplitude spectrum of a sawtooth wave "look like?" It is a **line spectrum** because energy exists only at discrete frequencies that are integer multiples of the fundamental, or lowest, frequency. The shape of the **spectral envelope**, however, depends on your choice of how to plot the amplitudes as a function of frequency. For example, in panel A of Figure 5–10 the voltage of each harmonic (from column two of Table 5–2) is plotted as a function of harmonic number. The scales for both the y-axis and x-axis are linear, and the resulting spectral envelope is curvilinear.

In panel B of Figure 5–10, the amplitude scale is logarithmic because we have plotted relative amplitudes in decibels re: the amplitude of the fundamental frequency (f_0). In addition, frequency also is

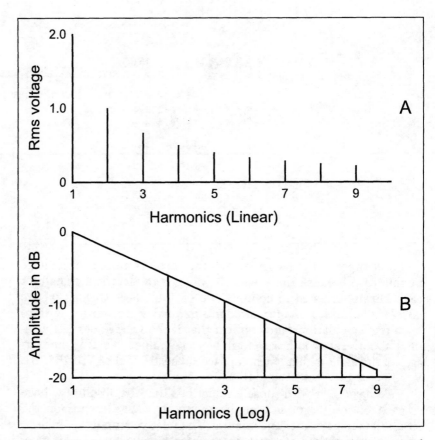

Figure 5–10. Amplitude spectra for a sawtooth wave. In panel A, the measure of amplitude is rms voltage, and the resultant **spectral envelope** is curvilinear. In panel B, the measure of amplitude is decibels, frequency is shown on a logarithmic scale, and the resultant spectral envelope is linear.

plotted on a logarithmic scale. The resulting spectral envelope is now linear. You should see, however, that in either case, panel A or panel B, the spectral envelope has a slope of −6 dB per octave, because for each doubling of frequency, the amplitude decreases by 6 dB.

In summary, a **sawtooth wave** is *a complex periodic wave with energy at odd and even integer multiples of the fundamental frequency with a spectral envelope slope of −6 dB per octave.* In Figure 5–9, each of the sinusoidal components (harmonics) of the sawtooth wave has a starting phase of 90°. The starting phases could just as well be 180°, or 0°, or 270°. It is essential, however, that the starting phases of all frequency components be identical.

Square Wave

A **square wave** also is a complex periodic wave, but it has energy only at *odd integer multiples of the fundamental frequency.* We can see from Figure 5–9 that the amplitudes of the sinusoidal components decrease with increasing frequency, just as they did with the sawtooth wave. Moreover, we shall see that the slope of the spectral envelope of a square wave is identical to the slope of the envelope for a sawtooth wave, because the amplitudes of the frequency components also *decrease as the reciprocal of the harmonic number.*

The first column of Table 5–3 lists five odd harmonics (1, 3, 5, 7, and 9) of a square wave. As with the sawtooth wave, we will arbitrarily set the voltage of the fundamental frequency to be 2 V for pur-

Table 5–3. Amplitudes (in voltage) of sinusoidal components of a **square** wave in which the amplitude of the fundamental frequency is 2 V

Harmonic Number	rms voltage $\left(\dfrac{1}{h_i} \times 2\right)$	$-20 \log_{10} h_i$
1 (f_0)	$\dfrac{1}{1} \times 2 = 2$	0
3	$\dfrac{1}{3} \times 2 = .67$	−9.5
5	$\dfrac{1}{5} \times 2 = .40$	−14
7	$\dfrac{1}{7} \times 2 = .29$	−16.9
9	$\dfrac{1}{9} \times 2 = .22$	−19.1

poses of comparison. We can see that the decrease in voltage for each of the harmonics is identical to the decrease seen for the *same harmonics* in Table 5–2 for the sawtooth wave. For example, the level of the 5th harmonic is −14 dB re: the level of the fundamental frequency for both the square wave and the sawtooth wave.

With the aid of Equation 5.2 you might wish to perform another set of computations with a voltage other than 2 V for the fundamental. Your answers for absolute voltage should differ from those in the second column in Table 5–3, but you should obtain the same answers in decibels that appear in the third column, regardless of the voltage of f_0. Thus, for example, if the voltage of the fundamental frequency is 3 V, the voltage of the 5th harmonic is 0.6 V, but its relative level in decibels is still −14 dB. It therefore is reasonable to conceptualize a square wave as being a sawtooth wave that is devoid of the even harmonics. We should reason, therefore, that the slope of the envelope of the square wave also is −6 dB per octave.

In summary, a **square wave** is defined as *a complex periodic wave with energy at odd integer multiples of the fundamental and a spectral envelope slope of −6 dB per octave*. The amplitude spectrum of a square wave is a **line spectrum**. In the example shown in Figure 5–9, each of the components has a starting phase of 90°, but that is not a requirement. Those who read other introductory reference books or chapters will encounter what, at first glance, might appear to be inconsistencies. Hirsh (1952), for example, shows all components of the square wave to have 0° starting phase, whereas Yost and Nielson (1977) show all starting phases to be 90°.

Figure 5–11 should clarify any confusion. In panel A, starting phases are 0°, and the corresponding waveform begins its first excursion upward (with an infinitely steep slope) from 0°. In panel B, starting phases = 90°, and only half of the first positive-going excursion of the waveform is shown. Regardless of the starting phase that is chosen, we still are faced with the restriction that the starting phase must be identical for each frequency component.

Triangular Wave

The **triangular wave** shown in Figure 5–9 is a complex periodic wave with energy at *odd integer multiples of the fundamental frequency*. Because the exact same statement was made for the square wave, we must look for other explanations to account for the differences in the shapes of the two waveforms.

The first column of Table 5–4 lists the first five harmonics of a triangular wave for which the amplitude of the fundamental frequency has arbitrarily been set at 2 V for easy comparison with our earlier calculations for the sawtooth and square waves. It should be apparent that the amplitudes of the frequency components of the triangular wave decrease at a greater rate than was seen for either the sawtooth wave or the square wave, in which the amplitudes decrease as the reciprocal of the harmonic number.

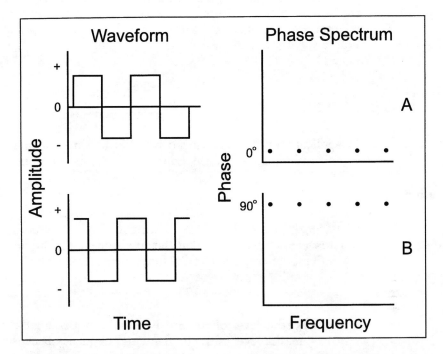

Figure 5–11. A comparison of waveforms and phase spectra for two square waves with different **starting phases**, 0° in panel A and 90° in panel B.

Table 5–4. Amplitudes (in voltage) of sinusoidal components of a **triangular** wave in which the amplitude of the fundamental frequency is 2 V

Harmonic Number	rms voltage $\left(\dfrac{1}{h_i^2} \times 2\right)$	$-40 \log_{10} h_i$
1 (f_0)	$\dfrac{1}{1^2} \times 2 = 2$	0
3	$\dfrac{1}{3^2} \times 2 = .22$	-19.5
5	$\dfrac{1}{5^2} \times 2 = .08$	-29
7	$\dfrac{1}{7^2} \times 2 = .04$	-33.8
9	$\dfrac{1}{9^2} \times 2 = .025$	-38.2

The amplitudes of a triangular wave decrease as the reciprocal of the *square* of the harmonic number (rather than decrease as the reciprocal of the harmonic number itself, as with the sawtooth and square waves), and the relative amplitudes in decibels are given by:

Equation 5.3
$$dB = 20 \log_{10} \frac{1}{h_i^2},$$

where h_i is the harmonic number.

By application of Law 3 of logarithms ($\log a^b = b \log a$) and Law 4 of logarithms ($\log 1/a = -\log a$), Equation 5.3 can be simplified to:

Equation 5.4
$$dB = -40 \log_{10} h_i.$$

Consider, for example, the 3rd harmonic. For a sawtooth wave or square wave, we have seen that the amplitude of the 3rd harmonic is −9.5 dB re: the amplitude of the fundamental frequency because:

$$dB = -20 \log_{10} 3 = -9.5 \text{ dB.}$$

In contrast, the level of the 3rd harmonic of a triangular wave is −19.1 dB re: the level of the fundamental frequency because:

$$dB = -40 \log_{10} 3 = -19.1 \text{ dB.}$$

Thus, the slope of the spectral envelope of a triangular wave is twice as steep, −12 dB per octave, as it is for the sawtooth wave and the square wave.

Therefore, **a triangular wave** is defined as *a complex periodic wave with energy at odd integer multiples of the fundamental and a spectral envelope slope of −12 dB per octave.* The amplitude spectrum of a triangular wave also is a line spectrum because its waveform is periodic. Triangular and square waves are both characterized only by odd harmonics, but the slope of the envelope is −6 dB for the square wave and −12 dB for the triangular wave. For the example shown in Figure 5–9, all frequency components have a starting phase of 0°.

Pulse Train

Panel A of Figure 5–12 shows a **pulse train**, a repetitious series of rectangularly shaped "pulses" of some width or duration (P_d). The repetition occurs at some regular rate. For the example in the figure, the interval between the onset of one pulse and the onset of the next pulse is 10 ms. That defines the **period (T)** of the pulse train.[1] By taking the reciprocal of the period ($1/T$), we calculate the frequency of the pulse train, which for the example in the figure is 100 Hz. This is called the **pulse repetition frequency**.

It should be apparent that the pulse train is a complex periodic waveform, and therefore, there can only be energy at *harmonics* of

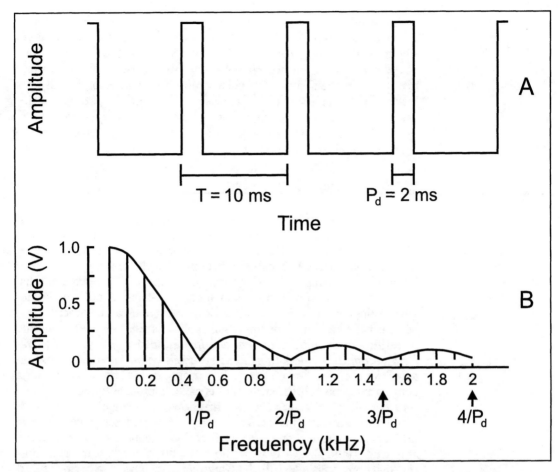

Figure 5–12. Panel A shows a **pulse train** with period = 10 ms and pulse duration (P_d) = 2 ms. Panel B shows the amplitude spectrum corresponding to the waveform in panel A. **Harmonics** are present at integer multiples of the pulse repetition frequency (100 Hz), and nulls are present at integer multiples of the reciprocal of pulse duration.

the pulse repetition frequency: 100 Hz, 200 Hz, 300 Hz, and so on. Panel B of Figure 5–12 shows the amplitude spectrum of the pulse train with frequency plotted on a linear scale. First, note that the component with the greatest amplitude corresponds to 0 Hz, which refers to what is called a *dc* (direct current) component of the signal. Recall from Chapter 2 that direct current means that current is flowing only in a single direction, either positive or negative, in contrast to alternating current that alternates back and forth in positive and negative directions.

Second, notice the irregularly shaped spectral envelope with lobes and valleys in panel B of Figure 5–12. Each valley or "null" occurs at integer multiples of the reciprocal of the pulse duration, P_d. Thus, we should expect to find nulls at frequencies corresponding to $1/P_d$, $2/P_d$, $3/P_d$, and so on. The duration of each pulse in the figure is 2 ms. Therefore, the first null appears at 500 Hz ($1/0.002$ = 500 Hz), the next null appears at 1000 Hz ($2/0.002$ = 1000 Hz), and so on.

The relation among the starting phases of the frequency components is more complicated than the relation observed for the sawtooth, square, and triangular waves. The components within the first lobe below the first null at 500 Hz have a starting phase of 0°, the components within the second lobe between the first and second nulls (500 Hz and 1000 Hz) have a starting phase of 180°, and the pattern continues to alternate in this fashion from lobe to lobe as frequency increases. We shall see subsequently that it is important to emphasize that the amplitude spectrum of a pulse train is a **line spectrum**.

White, or Gaussian, Noise

White, or **Gaussian, nois**e which also was shown in Figure 5–9, is *an aperiodic waveform with equal energy within any frequency band 1 Hz wide* (from $f - 0.5$ Hz to $f + 0.5$ Hz) *and with all phases present in a random array*. It is called **white noise** to be analogous to white light, which is characterized by equal energy in all light wavelengths.

The reason white noise is also called **Gaussian noise** is somewhat more complicated. A random time function can be described by what is called a **cumulative probability distribution**, which reveals *the percentage of the total time that any instantaneous value of the waveform's amplitude is less than some specified value*. Such a distribution for white noise is shown at the left of Figure 5–13. The slope of such a cumulative probability distribution is called a **probability density function**. For white noise, it takes the form shown at the right of Figure 5–13.

Those who have had an elementary course in descriptive statistics undoubtedly will recognize such a function as a **normal curve**, and the amplitudes (and phases) of white noise are distributed normally. A normal distribution is also called a **Gaussian** distribution in honor of Karl Friedrich Gauss, a German mathematician, astronomer, and physicist. Therefore, white noise, which is characterized by a normal probability density function, also can be called **Gaussian noise**.

The amplitude spectrum of white noise is a **continuous spectrum**. You can see in Figure 5–9 that the spectral envelope is a line drawn parallel to the baseline, because white noise has the same amount of energy in every frequency band that is 1 Hz wide regardless of the value of f. We will discuss the slope of the envelope of white noise (and introduce "pink" noise) in more detail in Chapter 6 after the concepts of **pressure spectrum level** and **octave band level** have been presented.

A Single Pulse

Panel A of Figure 5–14 shows the waveform of a **single pulse** that has the same width (duration = 2 ms) as each rectangular pulse in the pulse train that was shown in Figure 5–12. Is the waveform periodic or aperiodic? We must not be deceived by the fact that the shape of the waveform appears to be "regular" instead of random as we saw for white noise; that is irrelevant. The concept of *periodicity* means that an event occurs periodically over time. If there is only a single event (a single pulse), it cannot conceivably occur periodically.

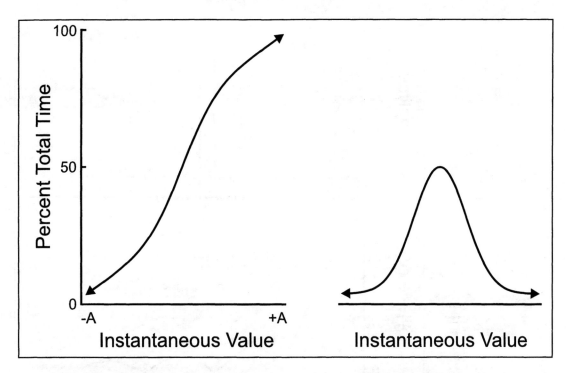

Figure 5–13. At the left is the *cumulative probability distribution* of **white noise**, which shows the percentage of total time that any instantaneous amplitude is less than some specified value. At the right is the *probability density function* for white noise, which is a plot of the slope of the function at the left. Because the probability density function assumes the shape of a normal curve, which also is called a Gaussian curve, **white noise** also is called **Gaussian noise**.

Recall that the period of the pulse train is defined by the interval from the onset of one pulse to the onset of the next successive pulse. From that perspective, the "period" of a single pulse is infinity. If a single pulse is not periodic, we must consider it to be an aperiodic signal, and we therefore should expect that the amplitude spectrum is a **continuous spectrum** rather than a line spectrum.

Look again at the amplitude spectrum of the **pulse train** in Figure 5–12. It is a line spectrum with energy at harmonics of the pulse repetition frequency. For the example in Figure 5–12, the harmonics are spaced at 100 Hz intervals because the period of that pulse train is 10 ms (f = 1/.01 = 100 Hz).

Although it might be difficult to imagine what would happen if the period were increased from 10 ms to infinity, we can, with a few examples, progress in that direction. If the period were increased from 10 ms to 20 ms, the pulse repetition frequency would decrease from 100 Hz to 50 Hz (f = 1/.02 = 50 Hz), and the harmonics would be spaced twice as closely together at intervals of 50 Hz.

Recall from Chapter 1 that each time the period is doubled, frequency is halved. Therefore, for a complex wave, each time the period is doubled, the spacing between harmonics is halved. For example, if we continue to double the period to 40 ms, 80 ms, 160 ms, 320

Figure 5–14. The waveform and spectrum of a **single rectangular pulse**. Nulls appear at integer multiples of the reciprocal of pulse duration, just as they did for a pulse train in Figure 5–12. In this case, however, the spectrum is a **continuous spectrum** in contrast to the line spectrum observed previously for a pulse train because a single pulse *cannot* be periodic.

ms, and so on, the intervals between harmonics in the amplitude spectrum progressively decrease to 25 Hz (f = 1/.04), 12.5 Hz (f = 1/.08), 6.25 Hz (f = 1/.16), 3.125 Hz (f = 1/.32), and so on.

If this process were continued toward infinity, the spacing between harmonics would continue to become smaller and smaller. At infinity, the spacing between harmonics would equal 0, and the result would be a continuous spectrum of the sort shown in panel B of Figure 5–14.

The *shape of the spectral envelope* is the same as was shown previously for the pulse train because the width of the single pulse in Figure 5–14 is the same (2 ms) as the width of each of the pulses in the train of Figure 5–12. Thus, the envelope shows nulls at frequencies that correspond to integer multiples of the reciprocal of the pulse width: $1/P_d$, $2/P_d$, $3/P_d$, and so on.

■ MEASURES OF SOUND PRESSURE FOR COMPLEX WAVES

In Chapter 2 we described several alternative metrics by which the sound pressure of a **sine wave** could be described, and we emphasized that the various equations introduced in Chapter 2 *applied only to the sine wave.* Table 5–5 contains the sine wave equations shown previously, and the modifications to those equations that are required for calculating the rms, mean square, FW$_{avg}$, and peak sound pressure for square waves and for typical aperiodic waveforms.

It is apparent that different equations must be used for different waveforms. This introduces a problem in measurement of sound pressure. Although measurement techniques are beyond the scope of this book, one example can emphasize the importance of knowing the kind of waveform on which a measurement is being performed before the measurement is made. Very often, an acoustical signal is converted (transduced) into an electrical signal and then various measurements are performed. Voltage is an electrical correlate of acoustical sound pressure. Thus, a transduced acoustical sine wave is an electrical waveform with sinusoidally fluctuating voltages over time. Measures of voltage are then performed with the aid of a voltmeter, which registers **rms voltage.**

Rms voltage is analogous to rms sound pressure. But, one type of voltmeter is called an "average-responding meter" and another type is called a "true rms meter." The average-responding meter actually "reads" the peak value of the voltage and then performs a computation to convert the peak reading to an rms reading by dividing the peak value by $\sqrt{2}$. A true rms meter, on the other hand, "reads" the rms directly, thereby avoiding any necessity for conversion.

If the waveform is sinusoidal, you should read the same value with either meter. What happens if an average-responding meter is used to measure the rms voltage of a square wave? Suppose the peak

Table 5–5. Measures of sound pressure for sine, square, and random waveforms. **A** refers to the peak or **maximum amplitude** as defined in Chapter 2

Metrics	Sine Wave	Types of Waveforms Square Wave	Random Wave
rms	$\dfrac{A}{\sqrt{2}}$	A	~ 0.3 A
mean square	$\dfrac{A^2}{2}$	A^2	~ 0.1 A
FW$_{avg}$	$\dfrac{2A}{\pi}$	A	~ .25 A
peak	A	A	A

value is 1 V. We can see from Table 5–5 that the rms value is the same as the peak value, 1 V, for a square wave. The average-responding meter, however, does not "know" that it is responding to a square wave. It will read the peak value of 1, divide the reading by $\sqrt{2}$, and register that the rms voltage is an erroneous 0.707.

The same measurement problem will occur with other complex waveforms. One must either know the appropriate conversions or purchase a more sophisticated and expensive measuring instrument that requires no conversion.

■ SIGNAL-TO-NOISE RATIO IN dB

Without exception, we listen to signals in the presence of some form of background noise. The relation between signal level and noise level is quantified by the **signal-to-noise ratio (S/N)** in dB. A positive S/N ratio means that signal level exceeds noise level, a negative S/N ratio means that noise level exceeds signal level, and an S/N ratio of 0 dB means that signal level and noise level equal one another. Suppose, for example, that a signal with SPL = 70 dB is presented against a background noise with SPL = 66 dB. In that case,

$$dB \ S/N = 70 - 66 = +4 \ dB.$$

If the S/N ratio truly is *a ratio*, why do we solve for decibels by *subtracting* noise level from signal level rather than dividing signal level by noise level? Recall Log Law 2 from Chapter 3, which states that the log of some ratio is equal to the difference between the logs of the factors.

A decibel is (ten times) a log, and therefore we simply subtract the denominator from the numerator rather than divide the numerator by the denominator. If, on the other hand, signal intensity and noise intensity were each expressed in watts/m^2, then division would be the appropriate operation. In the example cited above, the *intensity* of the signal is 10^{-5} watt/m^2 (Equation 4.4) and the *intensity* of the noise is 4×10^{-6} watt/m^2. In that case,

$$dB \ S/N = 10 \ \log \frac{10^{-5}}{(4 \times 10^{-6})}$$
$$= 10 \ \log (0.25 \times 10^1)$$
$$= +4 \ dB.$$

Obviously, it is easier to subtract decibels.

■ NOTES

1. Some authors, for example, Yost and Nielson (1977), use the symbols **P** for **period** and **T** for **pulse duration**. For the sake of consistency, we will continue to use **T** for **period** and we have adopted the symbol $\mathbf{P_d}$ for **pulse duration**.

■ FREQUENTLY MISUNDERSTOOD CONCEPTS

1. If f_0 = 150 Hz for a complex periodic waveform with energy at all integer multiples of f_0, what is the frequency of the third overtone?

   600 Hz. The answer is *not* 450 Hz, which is the frequency of the third harmonic, hence the second overtone. The *third overtone* corresponds to the *fourth harmonic*, which is given by $f_0 \times 4$ = 150 $\times$ 4 = 600 Hz.

2. A complex periodic waveform is composed of two frequencies, each of which has a starting phase of 0°. For one component, f_1 = 100 Hz and the peak amplitude = 2 V. For the second component, f_2 = 200 Hz and the peak amplitude = 1 V. Each component has a starting phase of 0°. After 5 ms, what will be the instantaneous voltage of the resultant wave?

   0 V. The period, **T**, of f_1 = 10 ms, which means that the instantaneous phase angle of f_1 will be 180° at 5 ms; at that moment it will cross the baseline, and the instantaneous voltage will, therefore, be 0 V. The period of f_2 = 5 ms, which means that the instantaneous phase angle of f_2 will be 0° at 5 ms; at that moment it also will cross the baseline, and the instantaneous voltage will, therefore, also be 0 V. Thus, the resultant waveform will cross the baseline at 5 ms, with a resultant instantaneous voltage of 0.

3. A sawtooth wave has a fundamental frequency of 123 Hz and a starting phase of 90°. The amplitude of the 5th harmonic is −14 dB relative to the amplitude of f_0. What is the relative amplitude of the 10th harmonic?

   −20 dB. First, the values of f_0 and starting phase are irrelevant. Second, the slope of the amplitude spectrum of a sawtooth wave is −6 dB/octave. Because the 5th harmonic has a relative amplitude of −14 dB, and the 10th harmonic is one octave above the 5th harmonic regardless of the value of f_0, the relative amplitude of the 10th harmonic must be −20 dB.

Resonance and Filtering

Sound waves, whether sinusoidal or complex, that are produced by vibratory motion often are weak, uninteresting, and perhaps lacking in "richness." Consider, for example, the complex periodic waveform at the left of Figure 6–1 that is produced by the vibrating vocal folds during vowel production. Imagine that a microphone is placed in a location that would permit us to record the sound produced by the motion of the folds in a way that would not be influenced by the supralaryngeal cavities.

The waveform is approximately sawtooth in shape and, perceptually, the result sounds similar to a "buzz."[1] The amplitude spectrum at the right of Figure 6–1 shows that there is a fundamental frequency, f_0, and a series of harmonics that are odd and even integer multiples of the fundamental. An important feature of the vocal fold amplitude spectrum is that the envelope is fairly smooth in the sense that there are no frequency regions with sharp prominences.

Most of the energy is located in the lower frequencies, and the amplitudes of the harmonics diminish in a smooth, regular fashion with increasing frequency. With natural vocal production, those amplitudes decrease at a rate of approximately 12 dB per octave. Recall, of course, from Chapter 5 that if this were a perfect sawtooth, all harmonics would be present and the slope would be −6 dB/octave. If it were a perfect triangular wave, only the odd harmonics would be present, but the slope would be −12 dB/octave.

We would have an extremely limited vowel component of our language system if the sound wave shown in Figure 6–1 was all that was available for human vowel production. Basically, the system would have only three principal parameters that could be varied to produce a set of vowels with which to communicate. We could vary

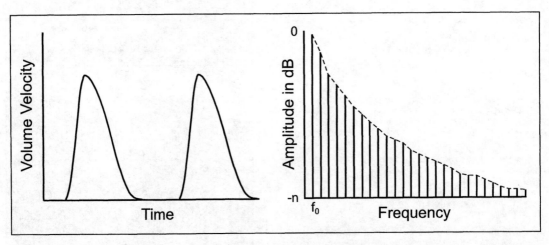

Figure 6–1. The waveform and amplitude spectrum of a sound produced by the vibrating vocal folds. The waveform is approximately sawtooth in shape. The spectrum is a line spectrum with energy at odd and even integer multiples of the fundamental frequency, f_0, and with a spectral envelope slope of approximately −12 dB/octave.

the amplitude to produce a series of tokens that would differ perceptually in loudness, we could vary the fundamental frequency to produce a series of tokens that would differ in perceived pitch, and we could vary the duration. We would not, however, be able to form the series of vowels that actually compose an important part of the phonological system to which we have become accustomed. To compensate for this situation, the sound wave produced by the vocal fold source—and all other sound waves as well—can be "reinforced" or altered by a process called **resonance**, or **filtering**.

The sounds produced by stringed instruments also need to be "enhanced," rather than rely simply on the vibrating strings alone to produce the desired sound waves. This is accomplished by use of what some call a "mechanical amplifier," known as a sounding board. It is more properly called a **resonator**, because it does not truly amplify sound waves, but a resonator such as a sounding board "reinforces" the sound waves emanating from the vibrating strings.

RESONANCE

We will begin by attempting to gain an intuitive understanding of what is meant by the word "resonance," and examine what takes place when a system is "set into resonance." The next step, then, will be to learn *why* resonance occurs.

One easy way to demonstrate the phenomenon of resonance is to strike a tuning fork and hold the vibrating tuning fork in the air medium. The sound wave that results is approximately sinusoidal. It will be characterized by a certain frequency of vibration that is governed by the **mass** and **stiffness** of the fork. As we learned in Chapter 2, the frequency with which a specific fork vibrates is called its **natural frequency**, and that frequency of free vibration of the fork will give rise to the perception of some pitch by listeners. Frequency of vibration will not change as the fork continues to vibrate.

The sound wave will also be characterized by a certain amplitude of vibration that will depend on the force applied to the fork when it is struck, and the amplitude of vibration will give rise to the perception of loudness. We learned previously that the amplitude of vibration will diminish over time because of **resistance**, and the decay of amplitude over time is called **damping**.

Once the loudness of the tone has become noticeably softer, touch the stem of the fork to a wooden table or some other hard surface. That hard surface is also a system that is characterized by **mass** and **stiffness** and therefore it too can be *forced into vibratory motion*. We shall subsequently see that the hard surface does not engage in **free vibration** at its own **natural frequency**. Instead, it is forced to vibrate (initially) by a force imparted to it by the vibrating tuning fork.

When the tuning fork is held against the hard surface, you should observe that the sound immediately becomes louder. It is important to emphasize that, even though the loudness becomes perceptually greater when the fork is held against the hard surface, *no energy is added to the sound wave.* The sound wave that results from touching the stem of the fork to the table does have greater **power** and greater **intensity**, but not greater **energy**.

Power is *the amount of energy per second*, and an increase in power can be realized by either an increase in energy, or *a decrease in time of vibration.* In this case, the greater power that results from touching the vibrating fork to a hard surface is gained at the expense of a shorter time of vibration. The duration of vibration is shorter when the fork is held against the hard surface than if the fork were left to vibrate only in the surrounding air medium.

The Principle of Resonance

The general principle of resonance that is demonstrated by applying the vibrating tuning fork to a hard surface is:

> When a periodically vibrating force is applied to an elastic system, *the elastic system will be forced to vibrate initially at the frequency of the applied force.* The nearer the frequency of the applied force to the **natural frequency** of the elastic system, the greater will be the resulting amplitude of vibration.

A Comparison of Two Elastic Systems

In Figure 6–2 we can examine the amplitude spectra that result from driving two elastic systems that have different characteristics. Instead of assembling a large array of tuning forks that span a wide frequency range, we will generate sine waves of variable frequency with an electronic device called an "audio oscillator," or "sine wave generator."

Sine waves of variable frequency *but constant amplitude* are directed to each of the two different systems represented in the figure. Each system will be forced to vibrate at the frequencies of the applied forces, that is, at the frequencies produced by the sine wave generator. We then can examine, separately for each driving frequency, the amplitudes of vibration *at the outputs of the elastic systems.* Finally, we can plot the results that are shown in Figure 6–2. In that plot, 0 dB corresponds to the amplitude of the frequency that produces the greatest magnitude of vibration.

Let us first consider the example in panel A of Figure 6–2. When the driving frequency is 100 Hz, the elastic system is forced to vibrate with a frequency of 100 Hz, when the driving frequency is 200 Hz, the elastic system vibrates at 200 Hz, and so on. This is an example of **forced vibration** because the elastic system is *forced* to vibrate at the frequency of the applied force. As we move through higher and higher frequencies, the elastic system always vibrates with the frequency of the force applied. In other words, *the process of resonance does not change the frequency of vibration.* This is consistent with

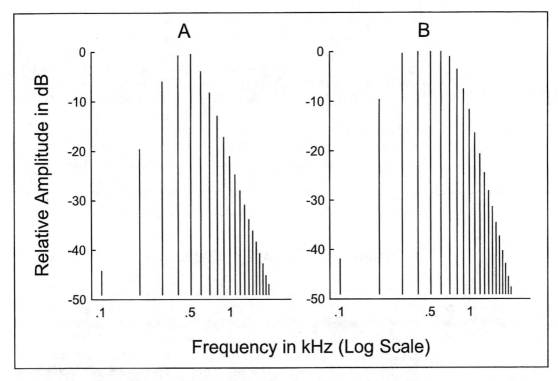

Figure 6–2. An illustration of the **principle of resonance**. Sine waves with different frequencies are applied with equal amplitudes to two resonant systems. The resonant system is forced to vibrate at the frequency of the applied force, and the nearer *the frequency of the applied force* to the **natural**, or **center**, **frequency**, f_c, of the resonant system, the greater will be the amplitude of vibration. As a consequence, the resulting amplitudes of vibration of the resonant system vary as a function of frequency. The system in panel A is a **narrowly tuned** system with a fairly well-defined f_c, whereas the system in panel B is more **broadly tuned**, and maximum amplitude of vibration occurs over a wider range of frequencies.

the first part of the principle of resonance that was stated previously: *When a periodically vibrating force is applied to an elastic system, the elastic system will be forced to vibrate initially at the frequency of the applied force.*

Return now to the lowest driving frequency, 100 Hz, and look at the amplitude of vibration that results at the output of the elastic system. In this example, the resulting amplitude is approximately 45 dB lower than the largest amplitude that is achieved, which occurs at 500 Hz. At 200 Hz, the amplitude of vibration is greater than at 100 Hz, about −20 dB.

As we move to higher and higher frequencies, we see that the amplitude of vibration continues to *increase* until it reaches a maximum, in this case when f = 500 Hz. Then, as the frequency of the applied force continues to increase beyond 500 Hz, the amplitude of vibration *diminishes* in a manner that is symmetric (in log frequency) with the increase that was observed for the lower frequencies.

The driving frequency that produces the greatest amplitude of vibration of the elastic system, 0 dB, corresponds to the **natural fre-**

quency (f_{nat} or f_c) of the elastic system, which is 500 Hz in the case of panel A of the figure. That outcome is in agreement with the second part of the principle of resonance: *The nearer the frequency of the applied force to the **natural frequency** of the elastic system, the greater will be the resulting amplitude of vibration.*

Panel B of Figure 6–2 shows a different outcome when the same driving frequencies are applied to a different elastic system. The second system also is forced to vibrate at the driving frequencies, but the principal difference between the response of this system and the one at the left of the figure is that maximum amplitude (0 dB) is realized for several driving frequencies, not just one. We shall see later that the elastic system in panel A is a more **narrowly tuned** system, and the one in panel B is a more **broadly tuned** system.

A "Shattering" Example of Resonance

Several years ago there was a television commercial sponsored by a maker of one brand of audio tape that showed a drinking glass shatter when the recorded voice of Ella Fitzgerald was reproduced near the glass. The glass, as with any other system that has mass and stiffness, has a **natural frequency**, which also is called a **resonant frequency**.

In accordance with the principle of resonance, the glass was forced to vibrate at the frequency of the applied force (the driving frequency), which in this case was determined by the fundamental frequency, f_0, of Fitzgerald's singing voice. When the fundamental frequency (sometimes referred to as the "fundamental pitch") of her voice reached the resonant, or natural, frequency of the glass, the amplitude of vibration increased until the vibration of the glass became so great that it finally shattered.

■ RESONANCE AND FILTER CURVES

Figure 6–3 shows the same process described for Figure 6–2, but in a slightly different fashion. Frequency of applied force again is shown on the abscissa and amplitude of vibration of the elastic system in dB is shown on the ordinate. In this case, however, there are no tuning forks or other sources of sound. There is, in fact, no sound. Instead, the curve that is shown represents *the relative amplitude of forced vibrations as a function of frequency that would be realized if driving forces were applied to the elastic system.*

From inspection of the curve in Figure 6–3, you can determine the relative amplitude of vibration resulting for any frequency of vibration that is applied to the system as long as all of the driving frequencies are applied with exactly the same force. If the force of application were increased for all of the frequencies, would the curve be displaced upward? *No.* It is true that the amplitude of response would be increased by an identical amount (to some upper limit) for each frequency, but because the ordinate is scaled in *relative amplitude,*

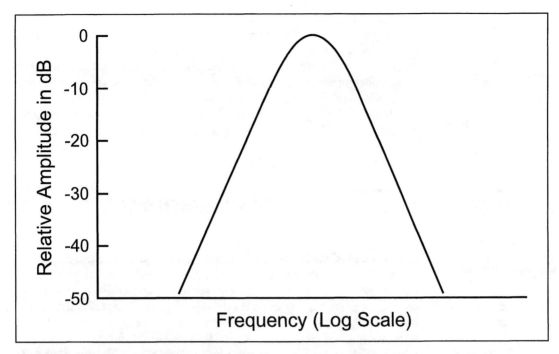

Figure 6–3. A **resonance**, or **filter**, **curve**. The curve shows the relative amplitude of vibration as a function of frequency for a resonator. The curve also can be called a **system transfer function**.

where 0 dB refers to the amplitude of the frequency with the greatest energy, the curve would appear exactly as it does in Figure 6–3.

The curve in Figure 6–3 is called a **resonance curve** because it behaves in a manner consistent with the definition of resonance stated earlier: The system vibrates at the frequency of the applied force, and the amplitude of vibration depends on the proximity of the frequency of the applied force to the natural frequency of the elastic system.

The curve in Figure 6–3 also is called a **filter curve**, which is simply emphasizing a different aspect of the same phenomenon. Look first at the frequency that corresponds to the **natural frequency** of the system—the peak of the curve. The amplitude of vibration is greatest at that point, and therefore corresponds to 0 dB.

As we move upward or downward in frequency from the natural frequency, the system is less responsive, and the corresponding amplitudes of vibration are less than the amplitude at the natural frequency. Thus, we can say that *the system responds differentially, or selectively, as a function of frequency*, and it therefore is called a **frequency-selective system**. Frequencies that are remote from the natural frequency are said to have been filtered.

Summary

When an elastic system is set into resonance, it is forced to vibrate initially at the frequencies of the forces applied to it. The elastic system has mass and stiffness, and those properties determine the **natural frequency**, or **resonant frequency**, of the system. When an elastic system is driven by a frequency that corresponds to its own **natural frequency**, we obtain the greatest amplitude of vibration. Finally, the amplitudes of vibration are less for frequencies that are either lower or higher than the natural frequency.

Why is the amplitude of vibration greatest when the driving frequency equals the natural frequency of the system? To explain this phenomenon, we will review, and expand on, **acoustic impedance**, which was introduced in Chapter 2.

▣ ACOUSTIC IMPEDANCE AND RESONANCE

The **impedance** of a system has two components. One component is an energy-dissipating component called **resistance**. *The magnitude of resistance is independent of frequency.* The second component is an energy-storage component called **reactance**, and unlike resistance, *reactance is frequency dependent.* Recall from Chapter 2 that there are two types of reactance, **mass reactance (X_m)**, which increases with increasing frequency ($X_m \propto f$), and **compliant reactance (X_c)**, which decreases with increasing frequency ($X_c \propto 1/f$). **Impedance (Z)** is the complex sum of its components: R, X_m, and X_c.

Effects of Impedance on a Resonance Curve

Figure 6–4 shows five resonance curves. The characteristics (shapes) of each of the different curves *are determined by the **impedance** of the system being driven.* Importantly, the shape of each curve, and its location in the frequency domain, reflects the relative contribution of the three components of **impedance** to the total opposition to transfer of energy: **resistance**, **mass reactance**, and **compliant reactance**.

If no resistance were present, maximum transfer of energy would occur, and the response of the system would be infinite at the natural frequency. That circumstance is represented by the dashed resonant curve (labeled "Undamped") in the figure with the arrows pointing upward. Consider next resonance curve A with a sharp peak. **Resistance** now is present, which serves to limit the maximum amplitude of vibration relative to the "ideal" or lossless case where there is no dissipation of energy. Curve A is frequency selective and the location of the peak of the curve along the frequency axis corresponds to the **natural frequency** of the system. The greatest amplitude of vibration occurs at the **natural frequency** because that is the frequency at which the least **impedance** is encountered.

At the **natural frequency (f_c)**, $X_m = X_c$, and the impedance, the total opposition to transfer of energy, is determined entirely by the **resistance**. When the driving frequency equals the natural frequency of the system, we say the system has been *set into resonance*. The amplitude of vibration is less for frequencies below f_c, and for those

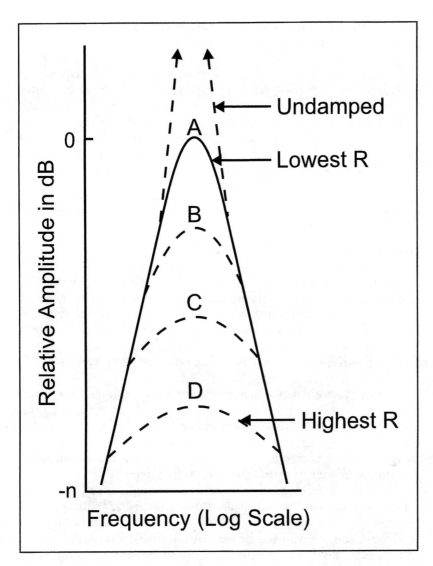

Figure 6–4. A series of resonance curves. The dashed curve labeled "Undamped" reflects the response of a theoretically lossless system with no resistance. From curve A through curve D, resistance increases, which produces two obvious effects on the shape of the curves: (1) the maximum amplitude of response decreases and (2) the system becomes more broadly tuned.

frequencies the system is called **compliance**, or **stiffness, dominant**. By that we mean, the relative contribution of **compliant reactance** to **impedance** is greater than the relative contribution of **mass reactance**. The response of the system also diminishes with increasing frequency above f_c, and for those frequencies the system is called **mass dominant** because the relative contribution of **mass reactance** to impedance is greater than the relative contribution of **compliant reactance**. **Compliance dominance** occurs for lower frequencies because $X_c = 1/2\pi fc$ (Equation 2.15). **Mass dominance** occurs for higher frequencies because $X_m = 2\pi fm$ (Equation 2.14).

Curves B, C, and D in Figure 6–4 show the effects of progressively increasing the **resistance** of a system. The **natural frequency** is unchanged because there has been no change in the **mass reactance** (X_m) or **compliant reactance** (X_c). As **resistance** (which is frequency independent) *increases*, however, more energy is dissipated, damping is increased, and the system becomes more broadly tuned. Stated conversely, as the resistive component of impedance *decreases*, the system becomes less damped and more narrowly tuned.

Admittance

When we have discussed the concept of impedance, we have, in a sense, emphasized the "negative." By that we mean, we have focused on opposition to motion or transfer of energy. Thus, we say that the transfer of energy to an elastic system is **impeded** at frequencies remote from the natural frequency, and *the more remote the **driving frequency** from the **natural frequency** of the system, the greater is the impedance.* The result is a reduction in the response of the system as the driving frequency becomes progressively lower or higher than the natural frequency of the system.

We can just as easily emphasize the inverse, or (musically speaking) "accentuate the positive," by saying, the closer the driving frequency to the natural frequency of the system, the greater will be the transfer of energy to the system. In a sense we are saying that more energy will be accepted by, or *admitted* to, the elastic system when the driving frequency equals the natural frequency.

Admittance is inversely proportional to **impedance** (**Z**) and the appropriate symbol for **admittance** therefore is Z^{-1} (Recall from Equation 3.2 in Chapter 3 that $1/X^n = X^{-n}$). Thus, the ordinate in Figure 6–4 could have been labeled **admittance** (instead of "relative amplitude in dB"). The unit of measure of **impedance** is the **ohm**, whereas the unit of measure of **admittance** is the **mho** (which you might notice is "ohm" spelled backward).

System Tuning

Figure 6–5 shows two resonance curves. The curve in panel A reflects a **narrowly tuned system**, whereas the curve in panel B reflects a **broadly tuned system**. A narrowly tuned system *can be forced to vibrate*, but only with maximum amplitude over *a very narrow range of frequencies*. A tuning fork and the wires or strings of stringed musical instruments are examples of narrowly tuned systems, and they vibrate freely at their own natural frequencies when energized.

We have, for convenience, discussed sources of sound such as the tuning fork or string separately from resonant systems, which might convey *the erroneous impression that a source of sound can-*

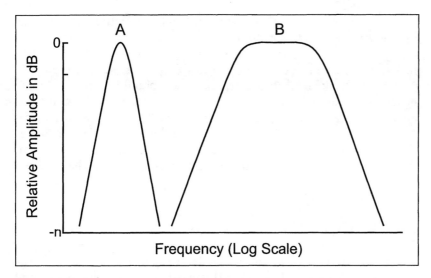

Figure 6–5. Comparison of two resonance systems, one that is narrowly tuned with low damping (panel A) and one that is more broadly tuned with high damping (panel B).

not be set into resonance. Both the source of sound and the resonant system are characterized by **resistance** and **reactance**. Hence, they both are characterized by some amount of impedance. The tuning fork and the string *are indeed resonant systems* as well. Thus, when the string is plucked or the fork is struck, each vibrates freely at its own **natural frequency**, which corresponds to the frequency at which the **mass reactance** equals the **compliant reactance**.

The tuning fork also can be forced to vibrate if it is tightly coupled to another tuning fork, but to transfer energy efficiently from one fork to another requires that the two forks have nearly identical frequency, because the response curve for each reflects very narrow tuning. That is because the impedance increases (and admittance decreases) rapidly as we descend or ascend in frequency from the natural frequency.

In contrast to a narrowly tuned system, a **broadly tuned system**, such as that shown in panel B of Figure 6–5, can be forced to vibrate with maximum amplitude by external forces over a wide range of frequencies. In addition to the table surface we cited previously, other familiar examples of broadly tuned systems include the diaphragms of microphones, earphones, loudspeakers, and our own auditory systems.

Systems that are **narrowly tuned** *always are associated with minimal* **resistance**, which means that such systems have little **damping**. That circumstance allows free vibrations to continue for some considerable amount of time, and narrowly tuned systems, therefore, are efficient *generators of sound.*

On the other hand, systems that are **broadly tuned** *always are associated with higher* **resistance**, which means that they have much higher **damping**. Therefore, the free vibrations that occur after the external force is removed are very brief in duration, and broadly tuned systems are efficient *transducers of sound*, systems that convert energy from one form to another. One example of a transducer is a loudspeaker, which converts electrical voltage to acoustic pressure.

If you think about it for a moment, you should want a transducer such as loudspeaker to be broadly tuned so that it will respond efficiently to a wide range of frequencies with little loss in amplitude. You also should want a transducer to be highly damped so that it does not "ring"—that is, so that the transducer does not continue to vibrate freely for any appreciable amount of time after the external force is removed.

Impedance Matching

When a force is applied to an elastic system, power is transferred from the source (the "driver") to the elastic system (the "load"), and the system is forced to vibrate. We know by now that the maximum amplitude of vibration of the system will be achieved when the frequency of the driving force corresponds to the natural frequency of the system. In that circumstance, **mass reactance (X_m)** equals **compliant reactance (X_c)**, and **resistance (R)** is the only component of impedance. At the natural frequency of the system, therefore, **impedance (Z)** is minimal and, of course, **admittance (Z^{-1})** is maximal.

Transfer of power from the driver to the load is optimal when the impedance of the source equals the impedance of the load (the elastic system). When the strings of a piano are set into vibration, their motion forces the sounding board (a resonator) of the piano to vibrate. As we stated previously, the sounding board *does not amplify the sound produced by the vibrating string*. Instead, it serves to improve the match of the impedance of the driver (the vibrating string) and the surrounding air mass. As a consequence, more sound power is delivered to the air.

The concept of impedance matches or mismatches will be encountered again in Chapter 8 when we discuss sound wave reflection.

■ FREQUENCY-SELECTIVE SYSTEMS: FILTERS

The effects of a frequency-selective system—a filter—on a driving signal that is directed to its input are illustrated in Figure 6–6. Panel A of the figure shows the **amplitude spectrum** of *the input signal*, which is a complex periodic signal *with equal energy in each harmonic* that will be delivered to a filter. Panel B shows the **filter curve** of the **frequency-selective system**. The filter curve depicts the amplitude with which the system will vibrate at each of the harmonics of the complex periodic input signal. The greatest amplitude of response, of course, will be realized at the **natural frequency** of the system where $X_m = X_c$. Frequencies remote from the natural frequency will be **filtered**; their amplitudes will be diminished relative to the amplitude at the natural frequency because of **mass reactance** and **compliant reactance**, each of which varies with frequency. Stated differently, the mismatch of impedances increases as the frequency of the driver departs, upward or downward, from the natural frequency.

The curve in panel B of Figure 6–6 also can be called a **system transfer function**. That simply means that the curve (a resonance, or filter, curve) describes the way in which the sound wave will be altered or transferred (amplitudes changed as a function of frequency) when the input signal is applied to the elastic system.

We emphasize that the filter curve in panel B *is not a sound wave*. It simply shows the way in which the amplitude spectrum of a sound wave will be altered when the sound wave is applied to the elastic system and forces it to vibrate.

Panel C of Figure 6–6 shows the **amplitude spectrum** of *the output signal*, and a comparison of the amplitude spectrum of the output signal in panel C with the amplitude spectrum of the input signal in panel A reveals the consequences of filtering. The amplitudes of the harmonics have been altered. The greatest amplitude in panel C is observed for the 5th harmonic because its frequency matches the **natural frequency** of the filter shown in panel B. The amplitudes of all other harmonics have been attenuated by the filter.

Figure 6–7 is similar to Figure 6–6. In this case, though, the input signal (panel A) is **white noise**. White noise, as you recall, *has equal energy at all frequencies* and the **amplitude spectrum** is a **continuous spectrum**. Thus, all frequencies in the white noise signal are applied

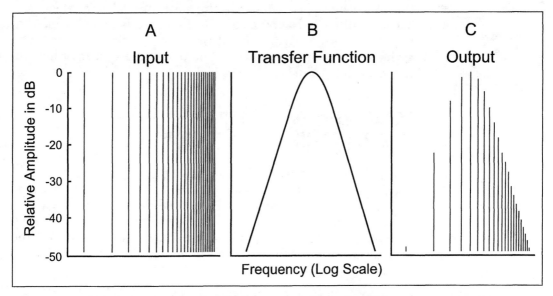

Figure 6–6. The effects of a resonator, or filter, on the amplitude spectrum of sine waves directed to the system. Panel A shows the input signal, panel B shows the transfer function (filter curve), and panel C shows the output signal after filtering. A comparison of the amplitudes of the harmonics in panel C with those in panel A shows the effects of filtering by the transfer function in panel B.

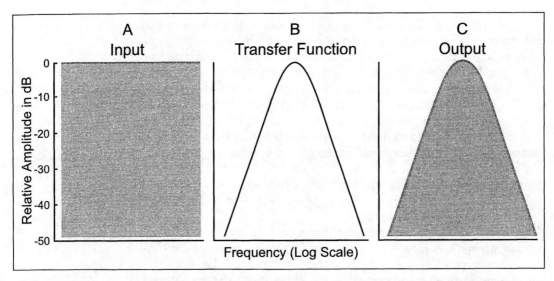

Figure 6–7. This figure is similar to Figure 6–6 except that the input signal (panel A) is white noise. The result (panel C) is called **band-limited white noise** because the output signal was restricted to some smaller band of frequencies due to the transfer function in panel B.

to the filter with equal force. The curve in panel B shows the **system transfer function**, or filter characteristics, and it reveals the way in which the system will respond when the input signal is applied.

Panel C of Figure 6–7 shows the amplitude spectrum of the output signal; the input noise in panel A has been filtered by the frequency-selective device in panel B. The sound wave at the output of the filter (panel C) is no longer white noise. Instead, it is called a **frequency-limited**, or **band-limited, white noise**. It is called a band-limited white noise to signify that it was a white noise signal that was applied to the system, but that the output was restricted, or limited, to some smaller band of frequencies.

▓ PARAMETERS OF A FILTER (SYSTEM TRANSFER FUNCTION)

Figure 6–8 displays two filter curves, or system transfer functions. Filter curves such as those shown in the figure can be described by reference to five parameters: (1) the **natural frequency**, which also is called the **center frequency, f_c**; (2) the **upper cutoff frequency (f_U)**; (3) the **lower cutoff frequency (f_L)**; (4) the **bandwidth (Δf)**; and (5) the **attenuation rate**, which also is called the **rejection rate**.

Natural, or Center, Frequency (f_c)

The **natural frequency**, or **center frequency, f_c**, specifies the frequency that will result in a maximum amplitude of vibration. The center

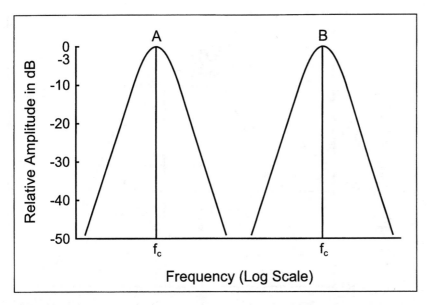

Figure 6–8. Two filter curves with different center frequencies, f_c.

frequency depends on the mass and elastic properties of the system if we are referring to an acoustical system[2] and, as we learned previously, corresponds to the frequency at which $X_m = X_c$.

The two curves in Figure 6–8 have different values of f_c, and f_c is one important parameter that allows us to distinguish one filter from another. It might appear at first glance that the difference in f_c for the two curves is the only distinguishing characteristic between the two curves, but after reading a subsequent section on "band-pass filters" you should return to Figure 6–8 and try to discover another way in which the two curves differ.

Upper Cutoff Frequency (f_U)

A second parameter is called the **upper cutoff frequency, f_U**. We know that frequencies above f_c are attenuated, and we describe this by saying that the higher frequencies are filtered; their amplitudes are attenuated.

At what frequency does the filtering begin? Consider the two examples in Figure 6–9. Both curves (system transfer functions) have exactly the same f_c, but the response of the two systems is different for frequencies above (and below) f_c. Actually, the filtering begins almost immediately above f_c and progresses continuously from there on. A convention has been adopted, however, to describe the "upper limit" of the filter by designating a single frequency as the point above f_c where filtering is said to commence.

By that convention, the **upper cutoff frequency, f_U**, is defined as the **3-dB down point** or as the **half-power point**. More specifically, f_U

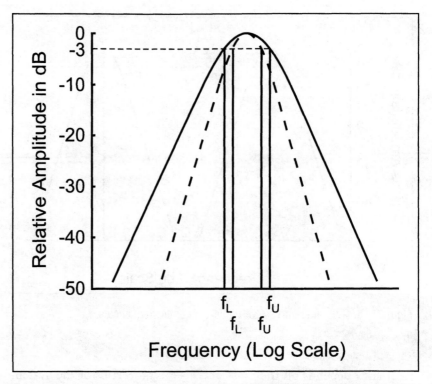

Figure 6–9. Two filter curves with the same center frequency, f_c, but different upper cutoff frequencies, f_U, lower cutoff frequencies, f_L, and bandwidths, Δf.

is that frequency *above* f_c for which the amplitude of response is 3 dB less than the amplitude at maximum, f_c. It is called the **half-power point** because it is that frequency for which the power in the resulting sound wave is one-half the power existing in the wave for f_c. It is called the **3-dB down point** because halving of acoustic power corresponds to -3 dB:

$$10 \log_{10} \frac{1}{2} = -3 \text{ dB}.$$

Thus, f_U for the solid filter curve in Figure 6–9 is *higher* in frequency than f_U for the dashed filter curve.

Lower Cutoff Frequency (f_L)

A third parameter of the filter is the **lower cutoff frequency, f_L.** By convention, f_L is defined as that frequency *below* f_c for which the amplitude of response is 3 dB less than the amplitude of response at maximum, f_c. f_L, like f_U, is also the half-power point because it is that frequency below f_c for which the power in the resulting wave is one half the power existing in the wave for f_c. f_L for the solid filter curve in Figure 6–9 is *lower* in frequency than f_L for the dashed filter curve.

Bandwidth (Δf or BW)

We have seen that the two filter curves in Figure 6–9 have the same f_c, but different upper (f_U) and lower (f_L) cutoff frequencies. It also should be apparent that the two curves in Figure 6–9 differ in another important respect; the solid filter curve *is wider* than the dashed filter curve. The width of a filter is quantified by the fourth parameter, the **bandwidth, Δf.** Δf is defined as the width of the band of frequencies that are "passed" by the filter, and

$$\Delta f = f_U - f_L.$$

Equation 6.1

Thus, bandwidth refers to the width of the band of frequencies between the lower and upper cutoff frequencies, and it defines the range of frequencies over which energy *is passed* by the filter. It can also be called the **passband** of the system to call attention to the band of frequencies that is passed by the filter. The two filter curves in Figure 6–9 have the same f_c, but different upper (f_U) and lower (f_L) cutoff frequencies and different bandwidths (Δf).

Return to Figure 6–4 and examine the resonance curves again. We said previously that as we moved from curve A to curve D, resistance progressively increased and the systems reflected broader tuning. Now we should see that the degree of tuning can be quantified by expressing the bandwidth, Δf. Thus, curve D in Figure 6–4 has a wider bandwidth than curve A.

Attenuation Rate (in dB/Octave)

The fifth parameter describes the *slope* of the skirts of the filter curve. It is referred to variously as: the **attenuation rate**, the rate with which the amplitude of response is attenuated as a function of frequency; the **roll-off rate**, the rate with which the response of the system "rolls off" on either side of f_c; and the **rejection rate**, the rate with which energy for frequencies on either side of f_c is rejected. The terms are synonymous. They all are measures of the slope of the curve on either side of f_c, and the unit of measure is **dB/octave**.

The two curves in Figure 6–10 have the same f_c, but, the attenuation rates for the two filters are different. The response (relative amplitude in dB) at 1000 Hz for filter A is -10 dB re: the response for f_c, and one octave lower (500 Hz), the response for filter A is -20 dB. Thus, the **attenuation rate** over this linear portion of the curve for filter A is 10 dB/octave. For filter B, which has a steeper slope, the response at 1000 Hz is -20 dB, the response at 500 Hz is -35 dB, and the attenuation rate, therefore, is 15 dB/octave. Thus, attenuation rate is a parameter that distinguishes filter A from filter B, and filter B can be described as being "more selective" than filter A. Because it is more selective, that is to say, it is more narrowly tuned, we know that it offers less resistance to the transfer of energy.

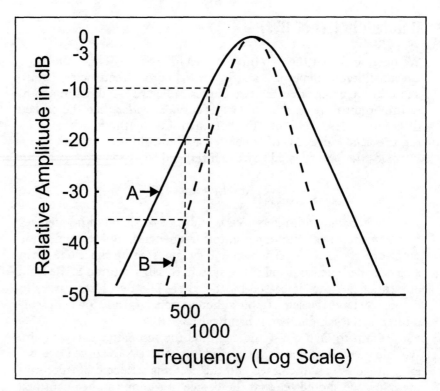

Figure 6–10. Two filter curves with the same center frequency, f_c, but different **attenuation rates**.

■ IDEALIZED VERSUS REALIZED FILTERS

Consider a filter with the following characteristics: f_c = 1000 Hz; f_L = 800 Hz; f_U = 1200 Hz; Δf = 400 Hz; and **attenuation rate** = 24 dB/octave. We would describe such a filter as one that (1) rejects energy below 800 Hz and above 1200 Hz; (2) passes energy in a band 400 Hz wide that is centered on the natural frequency of 1000 Hz; and (3) rejects energy outside the passband (800–1200 Hz) at a rate of 24 dB/octave.

The filter just described can be envisioned as having a rectangular shape, and an **idealized rectangular filter** would take the form of the rectangle in Figure 6–11. *All* energy between 800 (f_L) and 1200 Hz (f_U) is passed by the idealized filter, *all* energy below 800 Hz and above 1200 Hz is rejected, and the filter slopes are infinity. Analog filters that are likely to be encountered will be more of the form shown by the curve in Figure 6–11. Because the slopes in the figure are 24 dB/octave rather than infinity, the analog filter in Figure 6–11 has fallen short of the idealized filter.

When we specify the lower cutoff frequency, the upper cutoff frequency, and the bandwidth of the real filter, we are describing *the real filter* as if it were an **idealized rectangular filter**. Because the slope of the real filter is not infinity, specification of the **attenuation**

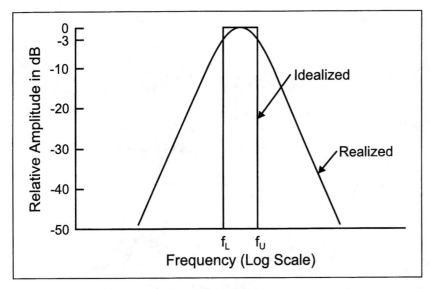

Figure 6–11. A comparison of an analog filter curve with an **idealized rectangular filter** with infinitely steep attenuation rates.

rate provides a measure of the amount by which the real filter *departs* from the idealized filter. Filter B in Figure 6–10 is more like the idealized filter than filter A because it has the steeper slope. If another filter were chosen with an attenuation rate of 72 dB/octave rather than 10 or 15 dB/octave, it would be even more like the idealized filter. Thus, the steeper the attenuation rate, the more the real filter approximates the idealized filter.

■ TYPES OF FILTERS

There are four common types of filters: **low-pass, high-pass, bandpass,** and **band-reject**. We will provide a brief description of each type and also specify the parameters that are necessary to describe each type of filter.

Low-Pass Filter

A **low-pass filter** is one that passes energy *below* some designated upper cutoff frequency (f_U). The two defining parameters are f_U and **attenuation rate**. Figure 6–12 shows four low-pass filters. The two curves in Panel A have the same attenuation rates, but different upper cutoff frequencies. The two curves in panel B have different upper cutoff frequencies and different attenuation rates. In each case, though, energy for frequencies above f_U is rejected.

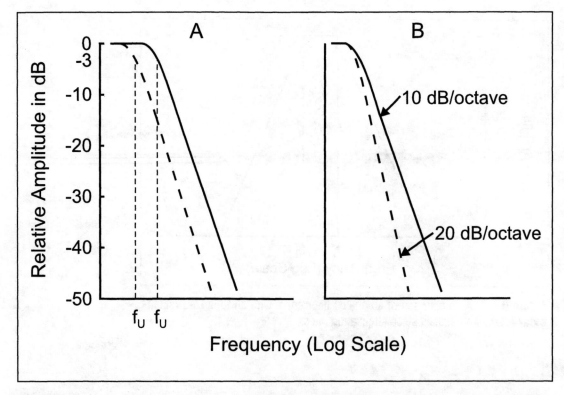

Figure 6–12. Four low-pass filter curves, filters that pass energy *below* some upper cutoff frequency, f_U. The two filter curves in panel A have the same attenuation rates, but different upper cutoff frequencies, f_U. The two filter curves in panel B have different upper cutoff frequencies and different attenuation rates.

High-Pass Filter

A **high-pass filter** is one that passes energy *above* some designated lower cutoff frequency (f_L). The two relevant parameters are f_L and **attenuation rate**. Panels A and B of Figure 6–13 show four high-pass filters that differ in terms of the values of those two parameters. In each case, energy for frequencies below f_L is rejected.

Band-Pass Filter

A **band-pass filter** is one that *passes energy in some specifiable band of frequencies* between a lower cutoff frequency, f_L, and an upper cutoff frequency, f_U. All five parameters are generally relevant: f_L, f_c, f_U, Δf, and **attenuation rate**. Panels A and B of Figure 6–14 show four band-pass filters that are characterized by differences in those five parameters.

A band-pass filter may be thought of as reflecting the combined effects of low-pass and high-pass filtering as is illustrated in Figure 6–15. The low-pass filter (solid line) passes energy below a designated **upper cutoff frequency**, which specifies f_U for the band-pass filter.

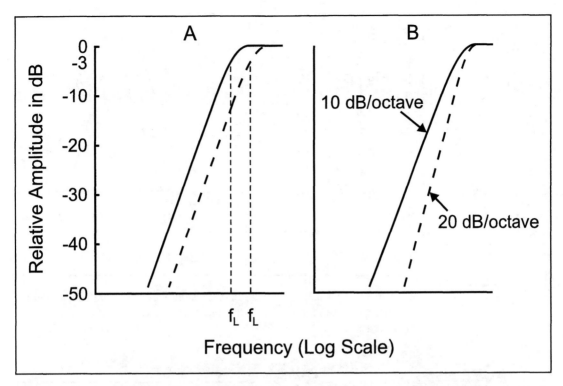

Figure 6–13. Four high-pass filter curves, filters that pass energy above some lower cutoff frequency, f_L. The two filter curves in panel A have the same attenuation rates, but different lower cutoff frequencies, f_L. The two filter curves in panel B have different lower cutoff frequencies and different attenuation rates.

The high-pass filter (dashed line) passes energy above a designated **lower cutoff frequency**, which specifies f_L for the band-pass filter. The bandwidth of the band-pass filter is given by the difference between the upper and lower cutoff frequencies, $f_U - f_L$. Finally, the slope of the low-pass filter curve determines the upper slope of the band-pass filter (the rate of attenuation above f_c), and the slope of the high-pass filter determines the lower slope of the band-pass filter (the rate of attenuation below f_c). Although those two slopes could be different from one another, they are almost always identical.

A word of caution is in order when we say that "a band-pass filter is the combined effect of low-pass and high-pass filtering." That is true *only* if we use what is called a *series, or cascade, system.* By that we mean, a signal is directed to the input of a low-pass filter with an appropriate f_U. Then, the output of the low-pass filter is directed to the input of a high-pass filter with an appropriate f_L. The signal at the output of the second filter will then have been band-passed. The procedure also could be reversed (high-pass followed by low-pass) as long as the output of the first filter is sent to the input of the second filter for additional processing.

For many band-pass filters *the bandwidth, Δf, is independent of the center frequency, f_c.* Thus, Δf and f_c can be manipulated independently of one another. Consider the examples in Figure 6–16.

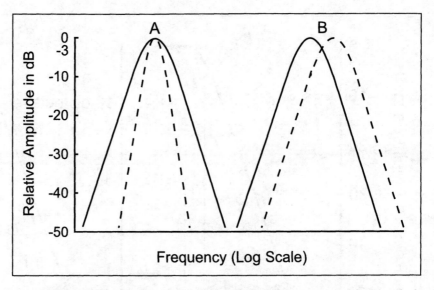

Figure 6–14. Four band-pass filter curves, filters that pass energy in a band of frequencies between f_L and f_U, with different values of f_c, f_L, f_U, Δf, and/or **attenuation rate**.

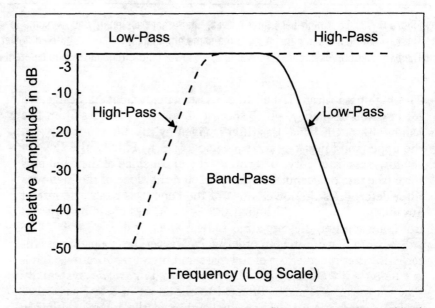

Figure 6–15. An illustration of how a band-pass filter represents the combined effects of a low-pass filter and a high-pass filter connected "in series."

Panel A of Figure 6–16 shows the input signal, white noise, and we label the **amplitude spectrum** of the unfiltered input signal as **X**. Panel B shows the transfer functions of two band-pass filters, one with f_c = 1000 Hz (labeled **Y**) and a second with f_c = 4000 Hz (labeled

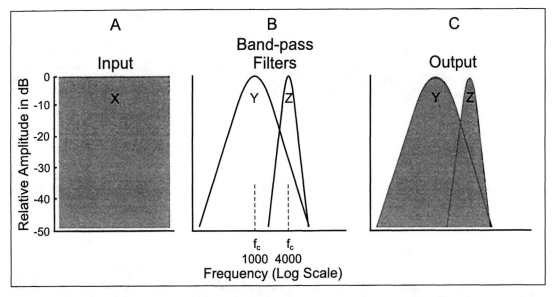

Figure 6–16. A white noise input signal in panel A is filtered by two different band-pass filters in panel B that have identical bandwidths. The different band-limited output noises are shown in panel C. Curve Z at the right in panel B *appears* to have a more narrow bandwidth than curve Y because frequency is plotted on a logarithmic scale, but the bandwidths of the two curves, Y and Z, are identical.

Z). For both filters, Δf = 500 Hz. Filter **Z** *appears* to have a smaller bandwidth than filter **Y**, but that is because frequency is represented on a log scale. On a log scale, the linear distance occupied by 500 Hz (the bandwidth) centered on 4000 Hz is only one-fourth the linear distance occupied by 500 Hz (the bandwidth) centered on 1000 Hz. Thus, because f_c is raised by a factor of 4, filter **Z** has the appearance of being only one-quarter as wide as filter **Y**, but the two bandwidths are, in fact, identical. (Return now to Figure 6–8, as suggested previously, and see if f_c was the only parameter that distinguished one filter curve from the other.) The **amplitude spectra** of the filtered noise are shown in panel C. **Y** represents the amplitude spectrum of the noise as modified by the filter with f_c = 1000 Hz, and **Z** represents the amplitude spectrum of the noise as modified by the filter with f_c = 4000 Hz.

If we were to measure the intensity of the white noise signal *at the input to the filter* (that is, the unfiltered white noise), we observe some level that we will call X_{dB}. At the output of filter **Y** we would observe only a portion of the original spectrum because only a portion of the signal has been passed by the filter; energy at frequencies below f_L and above f_U has been rejected.

The level at the output of this filter, then, can be called some level Y_{dB}, and

$$Y_{dB} < X_{dB},$$

because some of the energy in **X** (the original unfiltered signal) has been filtered. If some of the energy that was present at the *input* of the filter is rejected and therefore is not present at the output of the filter, the output level Y_{dB} must be less than the input level X_{dB}. The signal at the input to the filter has a theoretical bandwidth of infinity because it is white noise, but the output signal has been *band limited* by a filter with a center frequency of 1000 Hz and a bandwidth of 500 Hz.

Consider, now, what happens when f_c is raised from 1000 Hz to 4000 Hz. Even though f_c has been raised by a factor of 4, we have preserved a bandwidth of 500 Hz because *the bandwidth is independent of the center frequency*.

The level at the output of filter Z, Z_{dB}, will be less than the level at the input to the filter, X_{dB}, because, as before, the input signal has been filtered. Thus, $Z_{dB} < X_{dB}$. The critical factor, however, is that:

$$Y_{dB} = Z_{dB}.$$

Why are the output levels from the two different filters identical? The bandwidths of the two filters are identical, and as long as the input signal is white noise, which has equal energy in all frequency bands 1 Hz wide, the output level of the filters will remain constant as f_c is changed to any value *as long as the bandwidth does not change*. Of course, a band-pass filter can be adjusted to have many different values of Δf, and the wider the Δf, the greater will be the energy at the output of the filter. The important characteristic is that Δf *does not vary automatically* with changes in f_c. The two parameters, f_c and Δf, can be adjusted independently of each other.

Constant Percentage Bandwidth Filter

There is one type of band-pass filter, which is called a **constant percentage bandwidth filter**, for which the bandwidth is *not* independent of f_c. The distinguishing feature of a **constant percentage bandwidth filter** is that Δf is always *some constant percentage* of f_c. The concept of a constant percentage bandwidth filter is not unlike the concept of a sales tax. For example, if your state levies a 6% sales tax, that means that the dollar value of tax owed increases as your purchase price increases. If the purchase price is $10, you pay $0.60 of tax. If the purchase price increases by a factor of 4 to $40, your tax also increases by a factor of 4 to $2.40. The purchase price and the sales tax are not independent; the tax is a constant percentage of the purchase price. The same relation exists between Δf and f_c with a constant percentage bandwidth filter. As f_c increases by some factor, Δf increases by the same factor.

Look next at the two filters, Y and Z, in Figure 6–17. As in Figure 6–16, in panel A a white noise signal is directed to the input of the filters, the amplitude spectrum of the unfiltered noise is represented by X, and the level of the noise at the input is some value X_{dB}. For filter Y in panel B, $f_c = 1000$ Hz, and, for this example,

$$\Delta f = 0.707 \, (f_c) = 707 \text{ Hz},$$

which means that the bandwidth has a value that is 70.7% (which would be a very high sales tax) of the value of the center frequency. The level at the output of filter **Y** in panel **C** will be some value Y_{dB}, and as before,

$$Y_{dB} < X_{dB},$$

because the signal has been filtered.

Now, suppose we insert filter **Z** (panel B) with a center frequency of 4000 Hz to replace filter **Y**. Because the filter is a **constant percentage bandwidth filter** with a bandwidth that is always some constant percentage of the center frequency, and because the center frequency of filter **Z** is four times higher than the center frequency of filter **Y**, the bandwidth of filter **Z** is four times greater than the bandwidth of **Y**:

$$\Delta f = 0.707 \ (f_c) = 2828 \text{ Hz.}$$

The bandwidths of filter **Z** and filter **Y** *appear* to be identical in the figure, but again, that is because frequency is represented on a log scale. The bandwidth of filter **Z** is four times greater than the bandwidth of filter **Y**, but on a log scale they occupy the same linear distance.

The level at the output of filter **Z** in panel C, Z_{dB}, will of course be less than the level at the input, X_{dB}, because the signal has been filtered. The important point is that:

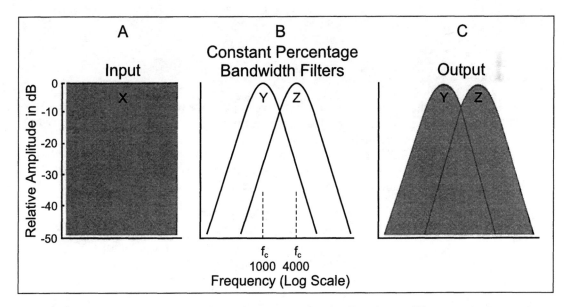

Figure 6–17. This figure is similar to Figure 6–16 except that the filters in panel B are **constant percentage bandwidth** filters in which the bandwidth is a constant percentage of the center frequency. The two curves, Y and Z, in panel B *appear* to have the same bandwidth because frequency is plotted on a logarithmic scale, but the bandwidth of curve Z is four times greater than the bandwidth of curve Y because its center frequency is four times higher.

$$Z_{dB} > Y_{dB},$$

because the bandwidth of **Z** is four times greater than the bandwidth of **Y**. The white noise signal is characterized by equal energy per cycle at the input to the filter, and filter **Z** passes that equal energy per cycle over a frequency range of 2828 Hz, whereas filter **Y** passes that equal energy per cycle over a frequency range of only 707 Hz. Subsequently, we will describe how much greater the level of Z_{dB} is than the level of Y_{dB} *in decibels*, but the impatient reader might wish to try to solve the problem in advance by recalling the discussion on "combining sound intensities from independent sources" in Chapter 4.

Common Constant Percentage Bandwidth Filters. In the preceding example, a percentage of 70.7 was used, but actually any value is acceptable, just as different local and state governmental bodies levy different amounts of sales tax. There are, however, a few common percentages that will be encountered with constant percentage bandwidth filters. One of the most common is called a **1-octave (1/1) filter.**

For a **1-octave filter,**

Equation 6.2 $\Delta f = 0.707\ f_c.$

Thus, the bandwidth (Δf) of a 1-octave filter is always 70.7% of the center frequency (f_c). Why is it called a **1-octave filter**? Recall that an octave is a doubling of frequency ($f_2 = 2f_1$). For a 1-octave filter, *and only for a 1-octave filter,*

Equation 6.3 $f_L = 0.707\ f_c$

and

Equation 6.4 $f_U = 1.414\ f_c.$

Therefore, from Equations 6.3 and 6.4, we can see that the upper cutoff frequency for a 1-octave filter *is 1 octave* (2f) higher than the lower cutoff frequency.

Table 6–1 shows how the parameters of a constant percentage bandwidth filter change with changes in f_c. You should see from the table that as f_c increases by some factor for a 1-octave filter, f_c, f_U, and

Table 6–1. Lower cutoff frequency (f_L), upper cutoff frequency (f_U), and bandwidth (Δf) for various values of the center frequency (f_c) for a 1-octave filter

f_c	f_L	f_U	$\Delta f = f_U - f_L$
100	70.7	141.4	70.7
200	141.4	282.8	141.4
1000	707	1414	707
2000	1414	2828	1414
10,000	7070	14,140	7070

Δf increase by the same factor. For example, if f_c increases by a factor of 2 from 100 Hz to 200 Hz, the values of the other three parameters also increase by a factor of 2.

Figure 6–18 shows the 1-octave filter from Table 6–1 with a center frequency of 1000 Hz. As you look at the filter curve, the center frequency appears to be at the "center" of the passband, and in fact it is located at what is called the "geometric center." That does not mean that the center frequency is the common arithmetic mean of the upper and lower cutoff frequencies. The arithmetic mean of 707 Hz and 1414 Hz is 1060.5 Hz, but we indicate in the table that the center frequency is 1000 Hz, not 1060.5 Hz. For a constant percentage bandwidth filter, the center frequency is *the geometric mean*, not the common arithmetic mean, of the upper and lower cutoff frequencies. Thus,

$$f_c = \sqrt{f_L \times f_U},$$

Equation 6.5

which states that the geometric mean of two numbers is the square root of the product of the two numbers.

There are other common constant percentage bandwidth filters in addition to the 1-octave filter. They include, for example, a **1/2-octave filter**, a **1/3-octave filter**, and a **1/10-octave filter**. Because a constant percentage bandwidth filter can, in principle, be any fractional value

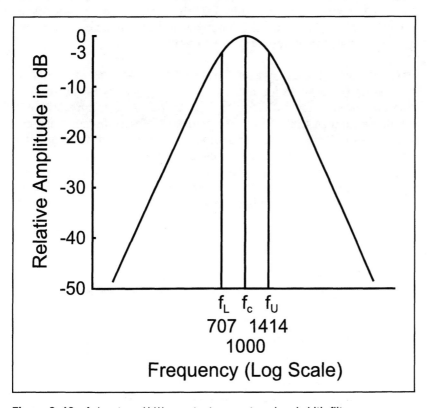

Figure 6–18. A 1-octave (1/1) constant percentage bandwidth filter.

in addition to unity (**1/1**), the general expression is: **1/n-octave filter**. Each is a constant percentage bandwidth filter, and the common defining characteristic in all such filters is that *the bandwidth is always some constant percentage of the center frequency*. The exact constant percentage varies with the value of **n** that specifies the fraction of an octave that characterizes the filter.

Calculation of Parameters of Constant Percentage Bandwidth Filters. The equations for calculating the important parameters of a constant percentage bandwidth filter are:

Equation 6.6

$$f_L = \frac{f_c}{2^{1/2n}} = \text{antilog}_{10} \left(\log_{10} f_c - .3/2n \right);$$

Equation 6.7

$$f_U = 2^{1/n} f_L = \text{antilog}_{10} \left(\log_{10} f_c + .3/2n \right);$$

and

Equation 6.8

$$\Delta f = f_U - f_L.$$

Table 6–2 shows how the lower and upper cutoff frequencies and the bandwidth vary as different fraction-octave filters are employed. Each row in the table represents a different constant percentage bandwidth filter, and, in this example, each of the four filters has the same center frequency, 1000 Hz. For the 1-octave, 1/2-octave, 1/3-octave, and 1/10-octave filters in Table 6–2, the upper cutoff frequency is always 1 octave, 1/2 octave, 1/3 octave, and 1/10 octave, respectively, higher than the lower cutoff frequency.

Preferred Center Frequencies for Constant Percentage Bandwidth Filters. The center frequencies for constant percentage bandwidth filters ordinarily are selected in accordance with national or international standards such as ANSI S1.6-1984, revised 1997 (American National Standards Institute). With that standard, the increment in frequency from one f_c to the next in the series is a constant percentage; hence a geometric, or exponential, series of center frequencies is formed. By that we mean, a ratio scale of frequencies is constructed just as we saw in Table 3–2; successive frequency units differ by a constant ratio

Table 6–2. Parameters of various constant percentage bandwidth filters. The center frequency is a constant 1000 Hz

1/n	f_c	f_L	f_U	Δf	%
1/1	1000	707	1414	707	70.7
1/2	1000	844	1190	346	34.6
1/3	1000	891	1122	231	23.1
1/10	1000	966	1035	69	6.9

(± a small percentage), and that constant ratio is the base for the ratio, or exponential, scale.

Just as we learned from Table 3–2, the lowest, or starting, number (frequency) for the series can, in principle, be any value. The *preferred* reference frequency, however, is 1 Hz. For a 1-octave filter, the constant ratio, or base, is 2. Thus, the **preferred center frequencies** are:

$$1, 2, 4, 8, 16, \ldots, 250, 500, 1000 \text{ Hz}, \ldots,$$

and so on. For 1/3- and 1/10-octave filters, the reference frequency is also 1 Hz, but the base, or constant ratio, is 1.25. For those filters, then, the **preferred center frequencies** are:

$$1, 1.25, 1.6, 2, \ldots, 100, 125, 160, 200 \text{ Hz}, \ldots,$$

and so forth. The base for a 1/2-octave filter is 1.4. One-half octave filters are not used frequently, however, and we will not elaborate further on their center frequencies.

ANSI S1.6 lists all **preferred center frequencies** from 1 Hz to 1 MHz for 1-octave, 1/3-octave, and 1/10-octave filters. For most applications that the student of speech and hearing will likely encounter, however, the preferred frequencies will range from about 100 Hz to 10,000 Hz. Lower or higher values can be determined, however, by moving the decimal place appropriately.

Table 6–3 lists the **preferred center frequencies** from 100 Hz (Band Number 20, where Band Number 1 is 1 Hz) to 10,000 Hz (Band

Table 6–3. Frequency band numbers (**N**) and preferred center frequencies (**f_c**) for nominal 1/3- or 1/10-octave filters and for 1-octave filters (boldface only). Values below band 20 and above band 40 have not been included

N	f_c	N	f_c
20	100		
21	**125**	31	1250
22	160	32	1600
23	200	33	**2000**
24	**250**	34	2500
25	315	35	3150
26	400	36	**4000**
27	**500**	37	5000
28	630	38	6300
29	800	39	**8000**
30	**1000**	40	10,000

Number 40). All values in the table are appropriate for 1/3- and 1/10-octave filters. The frequency values shown in **boldface** are the preferred frequencies for 1-octave filters.

As you can see from the table, the constant ratio for the 1-octave filter is 2 (0.3 log unit). Thus, 250/125 = 2, 500/250 = 2, 1000/500 = 2, and so forth. For both 1/3- and 1/10-octave filters, the base is 1.25 (0.1 log unit). Thus, 125/100 = 1.25, 160/125 = 1.25, 200/160 = 1.25, and so on. Finally, the table reveals that the band numbers for successive octave bands are successive integer multiples of 3, whereas the band numbers for successive 1/3- and 1/10-octave filters are successive integers. Table 6–3 also can be used to identify the preferred frequencies for 1/2-octave filters; in that case, successive integer multiples of 3/2 are used.

Band-Reject Filter

A **band-reject filter**, which also is called a **band-stop,** or **notch, filter**, is one that *rejects, rather than passes, energy for frequencies between the upper and lower cutoff frequencies*. Such filters are usually quite narrow, and all five parameters are useful in helping distinguish among various band-reject filters.

Panels A and B of Figure 6-19 contain two band-reject filter curves that differ in f_c, f_U, and f_L. It should be apparent that the meaning of f_c for a band-reject filter is different from the meaning of f_c for a band-pass filter. Although the two filter curves in Figure 6–19

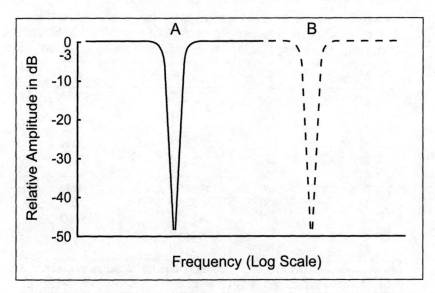

Figure 6–19. A comparison of two band-reject filter curves, filters that reject energy over a band of frequencies.

appear to have the same bandwidth, we shall see subsequently that the two bandwidths are different; the curve in panel B, in fact, has a wider bandwidth than the curve in panel A. Band-reject filters will probably be encountered less frequently than the other three types, but they are important for applications such as measuring distortion.

A **band-reject filter** also represents the combined effects of low-pass and high-pass filtering. In this case, however, the two filters are operated in *parallel*, rather than in *series*. By that we mean, a signal is directed simultaneously (in parallel) to the inputs of each of the two filters, one low-pass and one high-pass. When the outputs of the two filters are summed, the result is a signal that has been band-rejected.

■ SPECIFICATION OF LEVEL AT THE OUTPUT OF FILTERS

We have learned that the sound pressure level of a signal is reduced at the output of a filter (low-pass, high-pass, band-pass, or band-reject) relative to the level of the signal at the input to the filter because the filter *attenuates the energy selectively as a function of frequency*. Energy at some frequencies is passed by the filter, whereas energy at other frequencies is rejected.

We will now describe methods for calculating the actual amount by which signal level is reduced by filtering. Although any sound wave can be filtered, it will be convenient to use **white noise** in most of our examples. White noise, as you recall, is characterized by *equal energy per cycle*. That means simply that energy is present at all frequencies of vibration (to reasonable upper and lower frequency limits), and that the level or intensity *within any frequency band that is 1 Hz wide* (from $f - 0.5$ Hz to $f + 0.5$ Hz) is exactly the same, regardless of the value of f.

The calculations will be much simpler for white noise than for other complex sound waves, but the principles that will be described are applicable for specification of the level of other types of sound waves that are filtered. Before we consider the equations that will be used to accomplish that task, it will be useful to become familiar with a new concept called the **pressure spectrum level, L_{ps}**.

Pressure Spectrum Level

Pressure spectrum level, L_{ps} (commonly called just **spectrum level**), is defined as *the sound pressure level in a frequency band of unit width* (1 Hz), centered at some particular frequency, f. L_{ps} is expressed in decibels, and it refers to the level in any frequency band that is 1 Hz wide, regardless of the frequency upon which that band is centered. For a white noise signal, we could identify an infinity of frequency bands that satisfy that definition, and they need not be integers: for example, $f = 300$ Hz, ± 0.5 Hz; $f = 1300$ Hz, ± 0.5 Hz; $f = 5000$ Hz, ± 0.5 Hz; $f = 425.5$ Hz, ± 0.5 Hz; and so forth.

We stated previously that for a white noise signal, the level or intensity within any frequency band that is 1 Hz wide is exactly the same, regardless of the value of f. That is the same as saying that white noise has a **pressure spectrum level** *slope* of 0 dB; L_{ps} is constant for all values of f.

L_{ps} is given by:

Equation 6.9
$$L_{ps} = SPL_{wb} - 10 \log \frac{\Delta f_{wb}}{\Delta_o f},$$

where L_{ps} is expressed in **dB SPL**,

SPL_{wb} refers to the sound pressure level in some wide-band signal,

Δf_{wb} refers to the bandwidth of the wide-band signal,

and

$\Delta_o f$ is a reference bandwidth equal to unity (1 Hz).

Because the denominator in the ratio in Equation 6.9 is 1, and because the log of 1 = 0, Equation 6.9 for L_{ps} can be simplified to become:

Equation 6.10
$$L_{ps} = SPL_{wb} - 10 \log \Delta f_{wb}.$$

Suppose a white noise signal with a bandwidth of 10,000 Hz has an overall level of 80 dB SPL re: 20 µPa. What is the pressure spectrum level?

$$L_{ps} = 80 - 10 \log 10,000 = 40 \text{ dB SPL}.$$

The reference pressure for pressure spectrum level is the same as the reference pressure used to express the sound pressure level of a sinusoid or of any complex periodic or aperiodic sound wave: 20 µPa (**MKS**) or 2×10^{-4} dyne/cm^2 or microbar (**cgs**). Thus, for the example above, the level of the wide-band (10,000 Hz) signal is 80 dB SPL re: 20 µPa, and the **pressure spectrum level** is 40 dB SPL re: 20 µPa.

To conceptualize pressure spectrum level, simply imagine that the white noise signal is filtered with an **idealized rectangular filter** with a bandwidth of 1 Hz that is centered at any desired frequency (f). The level at the output of the rectangular filter is called the **pressure spectrum level**. For the example above, $L_{ps} = 40$ dB SPL, and, because the wide-band signal is white noise, we will measure that exact same pressure spectrum level of 40 dB SPL for any frequency band that is 1 Hz wide regardless of the value of f.

Suppose we do not know the overall level of a signal, but we are given its bandwidth and **pressure spectrum level**. We can then calculate the overall level of the signal by rearranging Equation 6.10 to read:

Equation 6.11
$$SPL_{wb} = L_{ps} + 10 \log \Delta f_{wb}.$$

For example, suppose the pressure spectrum level of a white noise signal with a bandwidth of 8000 Hz = 45 dB SPL. What is the overall level of the noise?

$$SPL_{wb} = 45 + 10 \log 8000 = 84 \text{ dB SPL}.$$

We have emphasized that with a white noise signal, the level or intensity within any frequency band that is 1 Hz wide (from $f - 0.5$ Hz to $f + 0.5$ Hz) is exactly the same, regardless of the value of f. We can think of each of those frequency bands as being *an independent sound source* and, by definition for white noise, each of those frequency bands, or independent sound sources, has exactly the same level or intensity as any other frequency band.

Recall from Equation 4.9 in Chapter 4 that the total intensity level resulting from combining some number of independent sound sources, each of which has equal intensity, is given by:

$$dB_N = dB_i + 10 \log N,$$

where i refers to the SPL of one of the sources

and

N refers to the number of sources that are combined.

We can now rewrite Equation 4.9 and rename the terms in the equation so that it can be applied to the problem of specifying the level of filtered white noise, which results in Equation 6.11:

$$SPL_{wb} = L_{ps} + 10 \log \Delta f_{wb,}$$

where Δf_{wb} is the bandwidth of the signal

and

L_{ps} is the **pressure spectrum level**.

The bandwidth of the signal (Δf_{wb}) is analogous to "the number of sources being combined" (N), the pressure spectrum level (L_{ps}) is analogous to the "sound pressure level of one of the equal sources" (dB_i), and SPL_{wb} is analogous to "the sound pressure level of the N sources combined." The result, then, is Equation 6.11.

In summary, if we know the bandwidth and overall level of the white noise signal, we can calculate the pressure spectrum level (L_{ps}) with Equation 6.10 by *subtracting* 10 log Δf_{wb} from the overall level. If, on the other hand, we know the bandwidth and the pressure spectrum level, we can calculate the overall level with Equation 6.11 by *adding* 10 log Δf_{wb} to the pressure spectrum level (L_{ps}).

Sample Problems

Problem 1: A white noise signal has a bandwidth of 9000 Hz and an overall level of 72 dB SPL. What is the pressure spectrum level? Use Equation 6.10.

$$L_{ps} = 72 - 10 \log 9000 = 32.5 \text{ dB SPL.}$$

Problem 2: A white noise signal has a bandwidth of 10,000 Hz and an overall level of 34 dB SPL. What is the pressure spectrum level? Use Equation 6.10.

$$L_{ps} = 34 - 10 \log 10,000 = -6 \text{ dB SPL.}$$

What do we mean by saying that the pressure spectrum level in decibels is a *negative* 6 dB? The answer is the same as it was in Chapter 4. Negative decibels simply mean that the sound pressure of the signal of interest *is less than the reference sound pressure*, which for dB SPL is 20 µPa.

Problem 3: A white noise signal has a bandwidth of 7000 Hz and a pressure spectrum level of 51 dB SPL. What is the overall level? Use Equation 6.11.

$$SPL_{wb} = 51 + 10 \log 7000 = 89.5 \text{ dB SPL.}$$

Problem 4: A white noise signal has a bandwidth of 6000 Hz and a pressure spectrum level of -12 dB SPL. What is the overall level? Use Equation 6.11.

$$SPL_{wb} = -12 + 10 \log 6000 = 25.8 \text{ dB SPL.}$$

Specification of Level at the Output of Filters: The More General Case

In the previous section we learned that we can calculate the pressure spectrum level from our knowledge of (1) the bandwidth and (2) the overall level of a signal (Equation 6.10) or, conversely, we can calculate the overall level of a signal from our knowledge of (1) its bandwidth and (2) pressure spectrum level (Equation 6.11). Let us now consider the more general case of how to calculate the level of *any* narrow-band signal (**nb**), not just one that is 1 Hz wide, from our knowledge of the overall level of a wide-band signal (**wb**) and, conversely, how to calculate the level of *any* wide-band signal (**wb**) from our knowledge of the level of a narrow-band signal (**nb**).

In Figure 6–20 we represent a white noise signal with a bandwidth that, because of filtering, becomes progressively more narrow as you move from the top of the figure where the bandwidth is 10,000 Hz to the bottom of the figure where the bandwidth is 1 Hz. It does not matter what type of filter is used (low-pass, high-pass, or band-pass) because our equations only have two parameters: level and bandwidth.

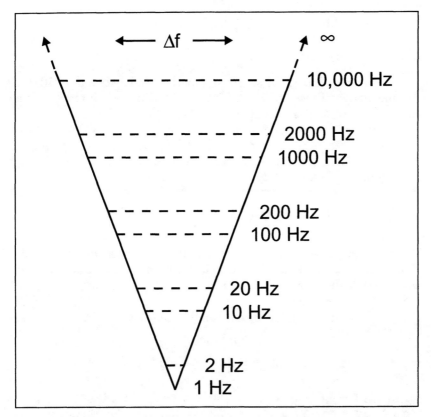

Figure 6–20. Geometric representation of the changing bandwidth of a white noise signal in which the bandwidth becomes progressively more narrow as a consequence of filtering. At the top, the unfiltered bandwidth is infinity. At the bottom, the bandwidth is unity (1 Hz).

With Equation 6.12 we can calculate the level for *any* narrow-band signal (**nb**) from our knowledge of (1) the level of a wide-band signal (**wb**) and (2) the bandwidths of both the wide-band and the narrow-band signal:

$$SPL_{nb} = SPL_{wb} - 10 \log \frac{\Delta f_{wb}}{\Delta f_{nb}}.$$

Equation 6.12

You should see that Equation 6.12 is essentially the same as Equation 6.10 for pressure spectrum level. The only differences are that now the narrow-band signal is not restricted to a bandwidth of 1 Hz and, because of that, the denominator in the ratio can be any value, not just "1."

By rearranging Equation 6.12, we obtain Equation 6.13, which enables us to reverse the process and calculate the level for *any* wide-band signal from our knowledge of (1) the level of the narrow-band signal and (2) the bandwidths of both the wide-band and the narrow-band signals:

Equation 6.13
$$SPL_{wb} = SPL_{nb} - 10 \log \frac{\Delta f_{wb}}{\Delta f_{nb}}.$$

Suppose we have a white noise signal with a bandwidth of 10,000 Hz and an overall level of 90 dB SPL. Next, the noise is filtered with a band-pass filter with f_c = 2000 Hz and Δf = 1000 Hz. What is the level at the output of the filter? You can proceed in one of two ways, but first you should recognize that for this particular problem, the value of f_c is irrelevant because f_c does not appear in Equation 6.12.

By use of Equation 6.12, we compute that:

$$SPL_{1000} = 90 - 10 \log \frac{10,000}{1000} = 80 \text{ dB SPL}.$$

Alternatively, if we first compute the **pressure spectrum level** with Equation 6.10, we can use Equation 6.11 instead of Equation 6.12 and obtain the same answer:

$$L_{ps} = 90 - 10 \log 10,000 = 50 \text{ dB SPL}$$

and then

$$SPL_{wb} = 50 + 10 \log 1000 = 80 \text{ dB SPL}.$$

Sample Problems

The signal is white noise with a bandwidth of 12,000 Hz and an overall level of 95 dB SPL.

Problem 1: What is the level at the output of a band-pass filter with Δf = 1200 Hz? With Equation 6.12, we determine that:

$$SPL_{1200} = 95 - 10 \log \frac{12,000}{1200} = 85 \text{ dB SPL}.$$

Although it is perfectly appropriate to use Equation 6.12, when there are a series of problems to solve, it might be more convenient to first calculate the **pressure spectrum level** with Equation 6.10 and then use Equation 6.11 for the rest of the problems. That approach enables us to avoid the necessity of repeated division. For example,

$$L_{ps} = 95 - 10 \log 12,000 = 54.2 \text{ dB SPL}$$

and then

$$SPL_{1200} = 54.2 + 10 \log 1200 = 85 \text{ dB SPL}.$$

Either approach should produce the same answer, but using pressure spectrum level saves the step of computing the ratio that is required when using Equation 6.12. It also is advantageous to have alternative approaches to solving a problem because it provides you with an independent check on the correctness of your solution.

Problem 2: What is the level at the output of a 1-octave filter with f_c = 2000 Hz? Note that Δf was not given and, therefore, must be calculated by use of Equation 6.2.

$$\Delta f = 0.707 \times 2000 = 1414 \text{ Hz}$$

and then

$$SPL_{1414} = 54.2 + 10 \log 1414 = 85.7 \text{ dB SPL,}$$

or

$$SPL_{1414} = 95 - 10 \log \frac{12,000}{1414} = 85.7 \text{ dB SPL.}$$

Because 85.7 dB SPL is the level at the output of a 1-octave filter, it is referred to as an **octave-band level**. This problem provides a good illustration of why it might be easier to solve some of these problems by first computing the **pressure spectrum level** because, in this instance, is saves us from dividing 12,000 by 1,414.

Problem 3: What is the level at the output of a low-pass filter with f_U = 1200 Hz? Note that Δf was not given. You should know, however, that for a low-pass filter, $\Delta f = f_U$. Therefore,

$$SPL_{1200} = 54.2 + 10 \log 1200 = 85 \text{ dB SPL,}$$

or

$$SPL_{1200} = 95 - 10 \log \frac{12,000}{1200} = 85 \text{ dB SPL.}$$

Problem 4: What is the level at the output of a high-pass filter with f_L = 1200 Hz? As with problem 3, Δf was not given. Unlike problem 3 with a low-pass filter, the value of f_L for a high-pass filter does not equal the bandwidth. The white noise signal that we are dealing with has an upper limit of 12,000 Hz. If that signal is high-pass filtered with a lower cutoff frequency of 1200 Hz, that means that energy below 1200 is attenuated, and all that remains is the energy between the cutoff frequency of 1200 Hz and the upper limit of the unfiltered noise, 12,000 Hz. Thus, to find the bandwidth of the filtered noise, we subtract f_L from the bandwidth of the unfiltered noise ($\Delta f = \Delta f_{unfiltered} - f_L = 10,800$ Hz). Therefore,

$$SPL_{10,800} = 54.2 + 10 \log 10,800 = 94.5 \text{ dB SPL,}$$

or

$$SPL_{10,800} = 95 - 10 \log \frac{12,000}{10,800} = 94.5 \text{ dB SPL.}$$

Problem 5: Suppose we were to remove exactly half of the energy in the white noise ($\Delta f = 12{,}000$ Hz) by some filter. It does not matter what type of filter is used as long as the result is a bandwidth of 6000 Hz. For example, we might use a low-pass filter with $f_U = 6000$ Hz, a high-pass filter with $f_L = 6000$ Hz, or a band-pass filter with $\Delta f = 6000$ centered on some frequency of our choosing. For each of those examples, the resulting bandwidth is the same, 6000 Hz. By how much will signal level be decreased at the output of the filter relative to signal level at the input? The answer must be the same as it was in Chapter 4. If the bandwidth is narrowed to one-half of its original value, the energy or power or intensity of the signal is halved, and if the intensity is reduced to one-half of its original value, the **level of intensity** will decrease by 3 dB because:

$$\text{dB} = 10 \log \frac{1}{2} = -3 \text{ dB}.$$

Thus, signal level will be decreased by 3 dB from 95 dB SPL to 92 dB SPL. We can confirm that answer by using the procedures described for the first four problems.

$$\text{SPL}_{6000} = 54.2 + 10 \log 6000 = 92 \text{ dB SPL},$$

or

$$\text{SPL}_{6000} = 95 - 10 \log \frac{12{,}000}{6000} = 92 \text{ dB SPL}.$$

Does the Type of Filter Affect the Pressure Spectrum Level?

As long as our concern is restricted to **white noise**, the type of filter (low-pass, high-pass, or band-pass) or the bandwidth of the filter, does not affect the **pressure spectrum level**. To illustrate this, suppose we have a white-noise signal with a level of 92 dB SPL and a bandwidth of 20,000 Hz. The **pressure spectrum level** (Equation 6.10) is 49 dB SPL:

$$L_{ps} = 92 - 10 \log 20{,}000 = 49 \text{ dB SPL}.$$

Next, suppose the noise is directed to the input of a **1-octave filter** (a **constant percentage bandwidth filter**) with $f_c = 1000$ Hz. What will be the **pressure spectrum level** at the output of the 1-octave filter?

$$\Delta f = 0.707 \times 1000 = 707 \text{ Hz}$$

and then

$$\text{SPL}_{707} = 92 - 10 \log \frac{20{,}000}{707} = 77.5 \text{ dB SPL}.$$

Finally, calculate L_{ps} from your knowledge of the level of the signal at the output of the 1-octave filter. The answer must be the same as computed above from knowledge of the bandwidth and level of the unfiltered signal, 49 dB SPL:

$$L_{ps} = 77.5 - 10 \log 707 = 49 \text{ dB SPL.}$$

The answer of 49 dB SPL is identical to what we calculated before the 1-octave filter was inserted, and that is as it must be. **Pressure spectrum level** is *the sound pressure level in any band 1 Hz wide*. It does not matter which of the infinite number of frequency bands of the noise we had in mind when we calculated the spectrum level. After all, they each had exactly the same amount of energy— hence the same sound pressure level—which for a unit bandwidth is called the **pressure spectrum level**.

In summary, the **pressure spectrum level** of white noise is the **pressure spectrum level**, and neither the type of filter nor the location of the filter along the frequency axis will alter that basic fact.

■ ANOTHER LOOK AT SELECTED TYPES OF NOISE

We will return to a consideration of a **white noise** signal and expand on what was learned in Chapter 5.

White Noise

We know that **white noise** has energy present at all frequencies (to reasonable upper and lower frequency limits) and that the level, or intensity, within any frequency band that is 1 Hz wide from $f - 0.5$ Hz to $f + 0.5$ Hz is exactly the same, regardless of the value of f. Figure 6–21 shows the amplitude spectrum of such a noise.

In panel A of the figure, the ordinate is **pressure spectrum level** in dB SPL and the abscissa is frequency (log scale). For this example, $L_{ps} = 45$ dB SPL. As stated previously, because L_{ps} is a constant, the **envelope** of the amplitude spectrum is a straight line parallel to the horizontal axis. We must emphasize, however, that such a slope only occurs for white noise if the unit of measure on the ordinate is pressure spectrum level. Thus, we can say that **white noise** has a **pressure spectrum level slope** of 0 dB/octave, which is another way of saying that the pressure spectrum level for white noise does not change as a function of frequency.

Next, let us direct that same white noise to the input of a **1-octave filter** and calculate the **octave-band levels** at the output of the filter for each of several center frequencies, f_c (e.g., 100, 200, 400, 800, 1000, 2000, 4000 Hz, and so on). The results are shown in panel B of Figure 6–21. The ordinate now is **octave-band level** in dB SPL. We use **octave-band level** in this case because we are plotting *the level in a frequency band that is exactly one octave wide* ($f_U = 2f_L$).

When $f_c = 100$ Hz, the octave-band level is 63.5 dB SPL because:

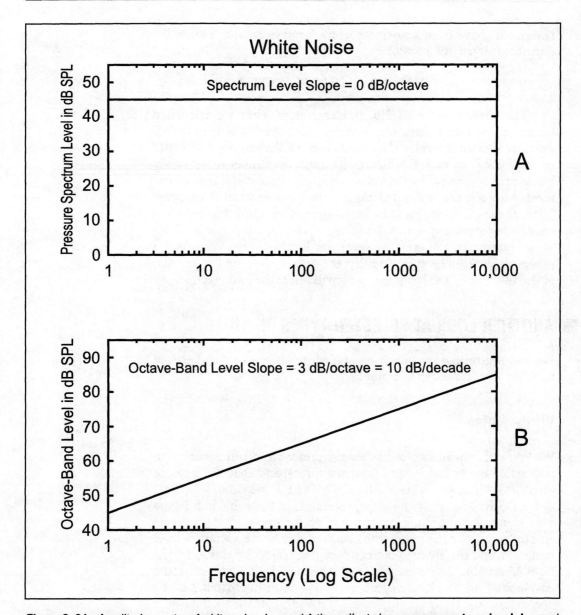

Figure 6–21. Amplitude spectra of white noise. In panel A the ordinate is **pressure spectrum level, L_{ps},** and the envelope has a spectrum level slope of 0 dB/octave. In panel B, for the same signal, the ordinate is **octave-band level,** and the envelope has an octave-band level slope of +3 dB/octave or +10 dB/decade.

$$\Delta f = 70.7 \text{ Hz.}$$

Then,

$$L_{ps} = 45 \text{ dB SPL} \qquad \text{(With Equation 6.10)}$$

and

$$\textbf{octave-band level} = 45 + 10 \log 70.7 = 63.5 \text{ dB SPL.}$$
$$\text{(With Equation 6.11)}$$

With each subsequent increase of f_c by a factor of 2:1, the bandwidth also increases by 2:1, twice as much energy is passed by the filter, and the level at the output increases successively by 3 dB. Thus, the level is 66.5 for f_c = 200 Hz, 69.5 for f_c = 400 Hz, and so on. Correspondingly, with each increase of f_c by a factor of 10:1, the bandwidth increases by 10:1, ten times as much energy is passed by the filter, and the level at the output increases successively by 10 dB. Thus, if the octave-band level for f_c = 100 Hz is 63.5 dB SPL, the octave-band level for f_c = 1000 Hz is 73.5 dB SPL.

We observed in panel A of Figure 6–21 that white noise has a **pressure spectrum level slope** of 0 dB/octave. It is equally appropriate to say that white noise has an **octave-band level slope** of +3 dB/octave or +10 dB/decade (decade = 10:1) because the octave-band level increases by 3 dB with each doubling of f_c (and of bandwidth) and increases by 10 dB with each tenfold increase of f_c (and of bandwidth).

Now, look carefully at panel B of Figure 6–21. We have stated that the **pressure spectrum level** (the sound pressure level in a frequency band 1 Hz wide) is 45 dB SPL for the white noise in the figure. Also observe the values for octave-band level as a function of frequency: 1000 Hz = 73.5 dB; 100 Hz = 63.5 dB; 10 Hz = 53.5 dB; and *1 Hz = 43.5 dB*. If the **pressure spectrum level** *really is the* **pressure spectrum level**, how can it be that L_{ps} = 45 dB, but according to the octave-band level calculations, the level is 43.5 dB when f_c = 1 Hz? There is no discrepancy. The pressure spectrum level is 45 dB SPL just as we calculated, and the octave-band level is 43.5 dB SPL when the filter has a center frequency of 1 Hz. But, if f_c = 1 Hz, Δf = 0.707 Hz , and thus the octave-band level is less than the spectrum level, and specifically the octave-band level is:

$$\text{SPL}_{0.707} = 45 + 10 \log .707 = 43.5 \text{ dB SPL.}$$

We have learned that white noise has a **pressure spectrum level** slope of 0 dB/octave and an **octave-band level** slope of +3 dB/octave or +10 dB/decade. Suppose the white noise in Figure 6–21 had been filtered with a 1/3-octave filter with the same center frequencies used for the 1-octave filter (100, 200, 400, 800, 1000, 2000, 4000 Hz, and so on). The level at the output is called the **1/3 octave-band level**. Can you state the **1/3 octave-band level** slope for white noise? It would be the same as the octave-band level slope: +3 dB/octave or +10 dB/decade. If we were to plot the 1/3 octave-band level as a function of frequency, the result would be a line parallel to the octave-band level function in Figure 6–21, but all 1/3 octave-band levels would be 4.9 dB less than the 1 octave-band levels. Why −4.9 dB? Recall from Table 6–2 that Δf for a 1-octave filter is given by the product of f_c and 0.707, whereas Δf for a 1/3-octave filter is given by the product of f_c and 0.231. Thus,

$$\text{dB} = 10 \log \frac{.231}{.707}$$

$$= -4.9.$$

Therefore, the 1/3 octave-band levels would be 58.6 for f_c = 100 Hz, 61.6 for f_c = 200 Hz, 64.6 for f_c = 400 Hz, 68.6 for f_c = 1000 Hz, and so on. From those calculations, we should see that the **1/3 octave-band level** slope of white noise also is +3 dB/octave and +10 dB/decade.

What if we were to use a 1/10-octave filter with the same values of f_c? The slope would still be +3 dB/octave and +10 dB/decade, but the **1/10 octave-band levels** would be 10.1 dB less than the octave-band levels. $\Delta f = f_c \times 0.069$, and

$$dB = 10 \log \frac{.069}{.707}$$

$$= -10.1.$$

In practice, we ordinarily do not use center frequencies with the values of 100, 200, 400, 800 Hz, and so on for a 1/3-octave filter. The preferred center frequencies are listed in Table 6–3.

Regardless of which constant percentage bandwidth filter we use to analyze white noise, will we achieve sufficient accuracy by making only one measurement for each value of f_c? *Almost certainly, no.* Recall from Figure 5–13 that the probability density function for white noise assumes the shape of a normal curve; the amplitudes (and phases) are distributed normally. Thus, the value obtained from a single measurement has some finite probability of being less than or greater than the mean instantaneous value. Because of the time-varying nature of the instantaneous values, accuracy will be improved by computing the mean of several hundred, or even several thousand, measurements for each center frequency. If the number of measurements is sufficiently large, the mean for each value of f_c should closely *approximate* the values that we computed, which are the *true values*. With the automated measuring equipment that is available, that task is not as daunting as it might seem.

Pink Noise

Consider next the noise shown in Figure 6–22, which is called **pink noise**. In panel A the ordinate again is **pressure spectrum level** and the abscissa is frequency (log scale). It should be obvious from examination of the spectral envelope that this noise has very different characteristics from those for white noise shown in Figure 6–21. In this case, we see in panel A that pink noise has a **pressure spectrum level slope** of −3 dB/octave and, from panel B, that pink noise has an **octave-band level slope** of 0 dB/octave. In other words, the output level from the 1-octave filter for this noise is the same regardless of where in the spectrum the filter is centered.

If f_c = 1000 Hz (Δf = 707 Hz) and the level at the output is, for example, 45 dB SPL, then, when f_c is doubled, the bandwidth is doubled to become 1414 Hz, but the output level, by definition, remains the same. If the bandwidth is doubled, energy is passed at twice as many frequencies. If energy is passed at twice as many frequencies,

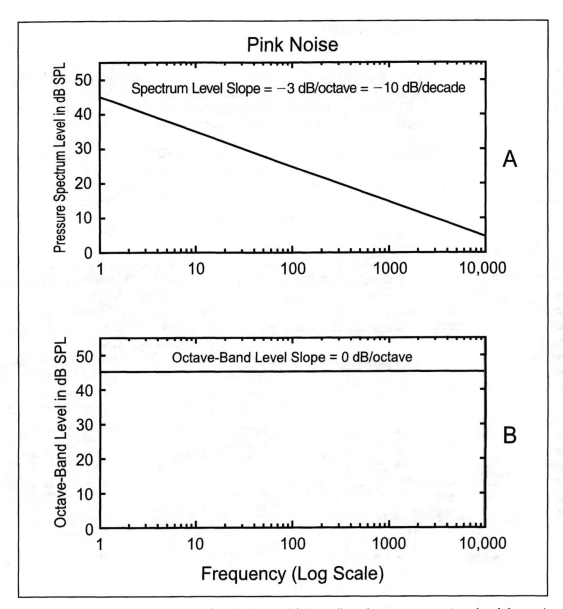

Figure 6–22. Amplitude spectra of pink noise. In panel A the ordinate is **pressure spectrum level, L$_{ps}$,** and the envelope has a spectrum level slope of −3 dB/octave or −10 dB/decade. In panel B, for the same signal, the ordinate is **octave-band level**, and the envelope has an octave-band level slope of 0 dB/octave.

but the octave-band level remains the same, we must conclude that the energy level per unit bandwidth decreases as frequency increases. That is what accounts for a negative **pressure spectrum level slope** of −3 dB/octave or −10 dB/decade.

We can legitimately construct a large array of "acoustic colors" such as red, magenta, and so forth by simply manipulating the pressure spectrum level slopes of the acoustic noises in accordance with standards that have been adopted.

Other Signals

Suppose we wish to determine the **amplitude spectrum** of speech spoken by a single talker. In this case, *we must perform measurements* on the signal, followed by calculations, rather than just calculations, as we did with white and pink noises. The measurement process is complicated by the fact that not only does speech intensity vary over time, but it also varies among speech sounds (phonemes). Moreover, for any given sound (for example, the vowel "ee" in the word "see") the amplitude spectrum is not linear over frequency as it was for white and pink noise.

To compensate for those circumstances, we might proceed as follows. First, we record a passage of a minute or so in duration, and we should make certain that the content of the passage includes all of the phonemes in the language in approximate proportion to the frequency of occurrence of those phonemes in spoken language. Second, we should choose a 1/3-octave filter instead of a 1-octave filter because its bandwidth is only 1/3 as wide. The more narrow filter will increase the accuracy of computation of L_{ps} for each value of f_c. Third, as with measurements of white noise, we *must* make several hundred, or several thousand, measurements for each value of f_c before we compute the mean 1/3 octave-band level and then compute L_{ps}.

Figure 6–23 shows the outcome of measurements made on a recording of a single talker (male) reading a passage of nearly 1 minute in dura-

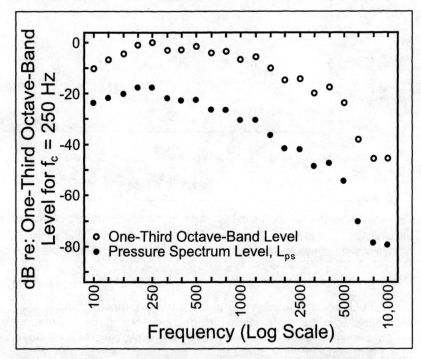

Figure 6–23. Outcome of measurements made on a 1-minute recording of a single (male) talker. The open circles represent the *measured* **1/3 octave-band levels**, and the filled circles represent the **pressure spectrum levels, L_{ps},** that were *calculated* from the 1/3 octave-band levels.

tion. The center frequencies, **f$_c$,** correspond to the **preferred frequencies** listed in Table 6–3 for a 1/3-octave filter.

The open circles represent the *measured* **1/3 octave-band levels,** and the filled circles represent the **pressure spectrum levels, L$_{ps}$,** that were *calculated* from the *measured* 1/3 octave-band levels. The two curves diverge with increasing frequency from 13.6 dB at 100 Hz where $\Delta f = 23.1$ Hz to 33.6 dB at 10,000 Hz where $\Delta f = 2310$ Hz.

■ NOTES

1. The ordinate in Figure 6–1 is labeled "volume velocity," which refers to the particle velocity of air molecules flowing through an area of one cubic meter per second (m^3/s) in the **MKS** system.

2. In an electrical system, inductive reactance and capacitive reactance are the relevant determinants of the natural frequency. Inductive reactance is the electrical equivalent of mass reactance, and capacitive reactance is the electrical equivalent of compliant reactance. In a volume system, such as the vocal tract—the cavity that extends from the vibrating vocal folds at the lower end to the mouth opening at the upper end—the natural frequency will depend on the length of the tube, whether the tube is open at both ends or open at only one end and closed at the other, and on the extent and location of constrictions in the vocal tract.

■ FREQUENTLY MISUNDERSTOOD CONCEPTS

1. A white noise signal has a bandwidth of 5000 Hz and a sound pressure level of 80 dB re: 20 µPa. If you were to insert a high-pass filter with f$_L$ = 4000 Hz, what would be the SPL re: 20 µPa at the output of the filter?

   73 dB. First, calculate the pressure spectrum level of the unfiltered noise with Equation 6.10:

   $$L_{ps} = SPL_{wb} - 10 \log \Delta f_{wb}$$
   $$= 80 - 10 \log (5 \times 10^3)$$
   $$= 80 - 37$$
   $$= 43 \text{ dB SPL.}$$

   Next, calculate the level for the high-pass filtered noise with Equation 6.11, but the equation requires that you know the bandwidth of the high-pass filtered signal. Energy below 4000 Hz was attenuated by the high-pass filter. Therefore, we have energy from 4000 Hz to the upper limiting frequency of the signal before it was filtered, 5000 Hz. Hence, $\Delta f = 1000$ Hz.

$$SPL_{wb} = L_{ps} + 10 \log \Delta f_{wb}$$

$$= 43 + 10 \log 10^3$$

$$= 73 \text{ dB SPL.}$$

Alternatively, the problem could be solved in one step with Equation 6.12:

$$SPL_{nb} = SPL_{wb} - 10 \log \frac{\Delta f_{wb}}{\Delta f_{nb}}$$

$$= 80 - 10 \log \frac{5 \times 10^3}{10^3}$$

$$= 80 - 7$$

$$= 73 \text{ dB SPL.}$$

2. For the same white noise signal (Δf = 5000 Hz; SPL = 80 dB), what is the pressure spectrum level of the noise at the output of a 1/3-octave filter with f_c = 1750 Hz?

   43 dB SPL. Do not make unnecessary calculations. If the answer is not obvious, review **Does the Type of Filter Affect the Pressure Spectrum Level?** As long as the signal is white noise, the pressure spectrum level is unaffected by the type of filter or its bandwidth; **pressure spectrum level** is *the sound pressure level in any band 1 Hz wide*.

3. Suppose the bandwidth of the noise in the two problems listed above were increased from 5000 Hz to 10,000 Hz. What would be the overall SPL of the noise before it is filtered?

   83 dB SPL. The bandwidth is increased by a factor of two (2:1) from 5000 Hz to 10,000 Hz, and white noise has equal energy in every frequency band 1 Hz wide (from $\mathbf{f}$ − 0.5 Hz to $\mathbf{f}$ + 0.5 Hz) with all phases present in random array. If the bandwidth increases by 2:1, the intensity of the signal will increase by the same factor, 2:1. We learned in Chapter 4 that an increase in intensity by a factor of 2:1 corresponds to 3 dB. Therefore 80 dB + 3 dB = 83 dB. Alternatively, we could solve the problem with Equation 6.13:

$$SPL_{wb} = SPL_{nb} + 10 \log \frac{\Delta f_{wb}}{\Delta f_{nb}}$$

$$= 80 + 10 \log \frac{10^4}{5 \times 10^3}$$

$$= 80 + 3$$

$$= 83 \text{ dB SPL.}$$

4. With the bandwidth of the noise now set at 10,000 Hz instead of the original 5000 Hz, what is the pressure spectrum level?

43 dB SPL. L_{ps} is unchanged for reasons explained in answer to #2 above. By way of proof:

$$L_{ps} = SPL_{wb} - 10 \log \Delta f_{wb}$$
$$= 83 - 10 \log 10^4$$
$$= 43 \text{ dB SPL.}$$

5. One band of filtered white noise with $\Delta f = 100$ Hz and SPL = 90 dB is combined with a second band of filtered white noise with $\Delta f = 4000$ Hz and SPL = 90 dB. What is the total SPL of the two noises combined?

93 dB SPL. The fact that the two noises have different bandwidths is irrelevant. The *intensity* of each band is 10^{-3} watt/m^2 (Equation 4.4 from Chapter 4). The intensity of the two combined noises, therefore, will be 2×10^{-3} watt/m^2. Thus,

$$dB = 10 \log \frac{2 \times 10^{-3}}{10^{-12}}$$

$$= 93 \text{ dB SPL.}$$

Alternatively, the problem can be solved with Equation 4.9 from Chapter 4:

$$dB_N = dB_i + 10 \log N$$
$$= 90 + 10 \log 2$$
$$= 93 \text{ dB SPL.}$$

6. White noise is directed to the input of a 1/3-octave filter with $f_c = 1000$ Hz. The level of the noise at the *output* of the filter is 61 dB SPL. If f_c is then raised to 4000 Hz, what is the SPL at the output of the filter?

67 dB SPL. A 1/3-octave filter is *a constant percentage bandwidth filter*. Thus, when f_c increases by some factor, 4:1 in this case, Δf increases by the same factor, 4:1. If the bandwidth increases by 4:1, the intensity also will increase by 4:1, and as we learned in Chapter 4, an increase in intensity by a factor of 4 corresponds to 6 dB:

$$dB = 10 \log \frac{I_x}{I_r}$$
$$= 10 \log 4$$
$$= 6 \text{ dB.}$$

The level of the noise therefore increases by 6 dB from 61 to 67 dB SPL. Note that it was not necessary to complicate solution of the problem by actually calculating the bandwidths for the two center frequencies of the 1/3-octave filter; we simply understand that if f_c increases by some factor, Δf increases by the same factor. By way of proof, however, we learned from Table 6–2 that the bandwidth of a 1/3-octave filter is given by the product of f_c and 0.231. Thus, with f_c = 1000 Hz, Δf = 231 Hz (0.231 × 1000). Correspondingly, if f_c is increased by a factor of four to 4000 Hz, Δf = 924 Hz (0.231 × 4000), which is four times greater than 231 Hz.

Distortion

Suppose a sound wave is delivered to some system, an amplifier for example, and we then compare the waveform at the output of the amplifier with the waveform at the input. If the system reproduces the shape of the waveform faithfully, the signal is said to be *undistorted*. **Distortion**, on the other hand, means that the shape of the waveform has been altered in some way. Three types of distortion will be described: **frequency distortion, transient distortion**, and **amplitude distortion**.

■ FREQUENCY DISTORTION

Amplitude Response of a System

Panel A of Figure 7–1 illustrates a method for evaluating a system (e.g., a tape recorder, amplifier, loudspeaker, etc.) to determine its **amplitude response**, which sometimes is called the **frequency response** of the system. Sinusoidal signals from a signal generator are directed to the input of the system. Frequency of the sine waves is varied over the frequency range of interest, and *the amplitude of the sine waves at the input must be kept constant*.

With the aid of an appropriate measuring device, we then measure the amplitudes of each of the sine waves at *the output of the system*. When the *output amplitudes* are plotted as a function of frequency, we have defined the **amplitude response** of the system. If the system reproduces all frequencies with the same amplitude, the output amplitude spectrum would appear as is shown in panel B of Figure 7–1.

A more realistic output amplitude spectrum is shown in panel C of Figure 7–1. Energy in the low frequency and high frequency regions has been attenuated because *the system did not reproduce all frequencies with the same relative amplitude*. In Chapter 6 we said that the input signal has been filtered, and now we say that *if filtering has occurred*, the signal has undergone **frequency distortion**. A more severe example of **frequency distortion** is shown in panel D of Figure 7–1. One familiar example of frequency distortion is the telephone, which has an amplitude response (frequency response) that extends from approximately 300 Hz to 3000 Hz.

System Transfer Function

The three curves in Figure 7–1 also describe what is called the **system transfer function**. Thus, the **system transfer function**, or **amplitude response**, reveals the extent to which a signal can be expected to undergo frequency distortion. For example, if you examine the specifications for a moderately priced audio tape recorder, you might see that the recorder has an amplitude response (the specifications probably will refer instead to "frequency response") such as that shown by the curve in panel C of Figure 7–1. The system has a relatively flat passband that extends from approximately 100 Hz to 10,000 Hz. Energy for frequencies that lie outside the passband, below 100 Hz and above 10,000 Hz, is attenuated.

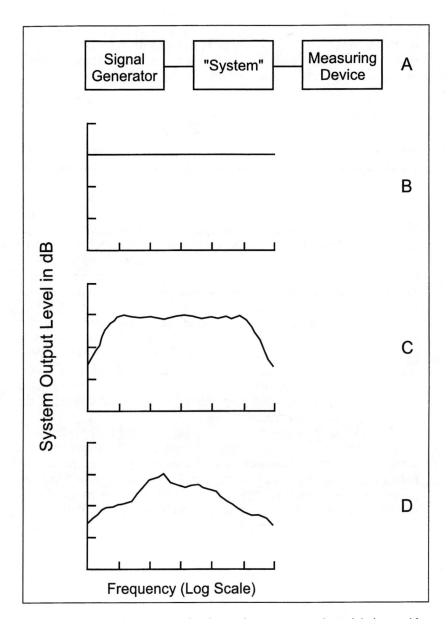

Figure 7–1. Panel A represents the electronic components that might be used for evaluation of a "system." Sinusoidal signals *of constant amplitude and varying frequency* are directed to some device, the "system," and the amplitudes of the various sine waves are then measured at the output of the device. Panels B, C, and D show three examples of amplitude response (frequency response) that might be measured for different systems. The response in panel B shows the absence of frequency distortion (a hypothetical construct), whereas the responses in C and D show different magnitudes of **frequency distortion** because the systems could not reproduce all frequencies with equal amplitudes.

The amplitude response of a system is described more completely by also specifying just how flat the response is *within the passband*. For example, even if the width of the passband is the same for two different systems, one that is flat ±0.5 dB is preferable to one that is flat ±5 dB because the system with the flatter response within the passband has experienced less frequency distortion.

Linear Systems

Systems that produce frequency distortion are **linear systems**. A linear system is one in which only the amplitudes (and phases) of the signal are altered by the system. Panel A of Figure 7–2 shows *an input-output function* for a **linear system**. Output amplitude on the ordinate is plotted as a function of input amplitude on the abscissa, and because the system is linear, *the input-output function is a straight line*. With a linear system, as the amplitude of the input is increased (from left to right in the figure), we achieve a *proportional* increase in output amplitude (from bottom to top in the figure). If, for example, the input amplitude is increased by 3 dB, the output amplitude also is increased by 3 dB.

We should not infer that the level of the output signal *equals* the level of the input signal. It could, but it need not. Output level could equal input level, but it also could be greater than the input level (amplification) or less than the input level (attenuation). That is why we emphasize that changes in input level produce *proportional* changes in output level, and proportional changes occur because the input-output function is *linear*.

In panel B of Figure 7–2 we see that with a linear system, the characteristics of a sine wave at the input of the system (pointing upward) are preserved at the output of the system (pointing toward the right); the shape of the waveform is unaltered. In summary, the **amplitude response** of a linear system describes the way in which signals that are directed to the input will evidence **frequency distortion** in the signal observed at the output.

■ TRANSIENT DISTORTION

When sine waves were introduced from a strictly theoretical perspective in Chapter 2, it was convenient to treat their durations as infinite. Under that circumstance the amplitude spectrum of any sine wave would be a line spectrum. Because duration of sine waves is finite, however, the amplitude spectrum is not a line spectrum.

Effects of Sine Wave Duration on the Amplitude Spectrum

Figure 7–3 shows the effects of sine wave duration on the amplitude spectrum. In panel A, the duration of the sine wave is infinite. It is a

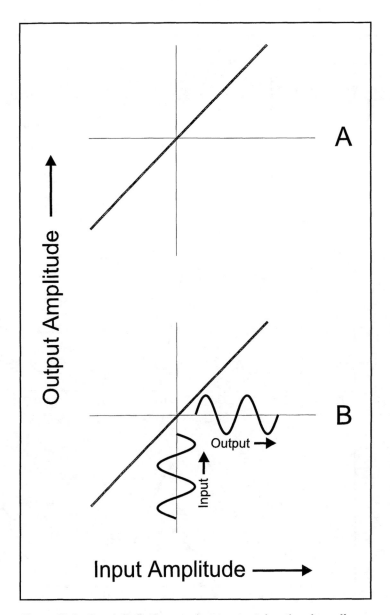

Figure 7–2. Panel A displays an input-output function for a **linear system**, a system for which the amplitude at the output is *proportional* to the amplitude at the input. Panel B shows that the characteristics of the waveform at the input to a **linear system** are faithfully preserved at the output of the system.

periodic signal, and its amplitude spectrum, therefore, is a line spectrum with a single line that corresponds to the frequency of the sine wave, 1000 Hz. In panel B, we can see what happens to the spectrum when the duration is shortened to 100 ms and becomes what is called a **tone burst**, or sinusoidal pulse. Energy is spread to other frequencies, both above and below the frequency of the sine wave. The tone

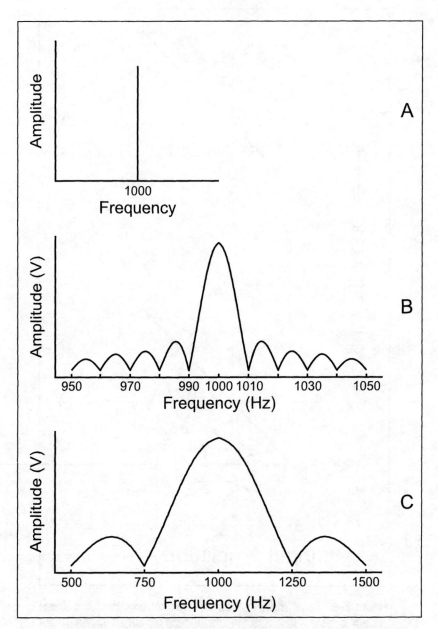

Figure 7–3. Effects of signal duration on the amplitude spectrum of a sinusoid. In panel A, duration is infinite and the amplitude spectrum is a line spectrum with energy at a single frequency. In panel B, duration is 100 ms, and energy is spread to other frequencies to produce a continuous spectrum. In panel C, duration is shortened to 4 ms, which also produces a continuous spectrum. The nulls in panels B and C occur at different frequencies because their locations in the frequency domain are given by integer multiples of the reciprocal of duration. Adapted from *Signals and systems for speech and hearing* (pp. 188–189) by S. Rosen and P. Howell, 1991, Academic Press Inc., San Diego. CA. Copyright 1991 by Academic Press Limited. Reprinted with permission.

burst is aperiodic, not periodic, and the amplitude spectrum is a **continuous spectrum**. We also can see lobes and nulls in the spectrum with a pattern that is similar, but not identical, to the pattern seen in Chapter 5 for a single rectangular pulse. The nulls occur at *integer multiples of the reciprocal of the duration*, in this case at 10-Hz intervals (1/.1 = ±10 Hz; 2/.1 = ±20 Hz; etc.). Unlike the amplitude spectrum for the single rectangular pulse, nulls occur on either side (above and below) of the frequency of the sine wave (1000 Hz).

In panel C of Figure 7–3 we see what happens as duration of the sine wave decreases further, from 100 to 4 ms. In both panels B and C, the nulls appear at the appropriate frequency locations. Thus, for example, when duration = 100 ms, the first nulls are at ±10 Hz (1/.1 = 10 Hz), whereas when duration is shortened to 4 ms, the first nulls increase in frequency to ±250 Hz (1/.004 = 250 Hz). It should be apparent that *the width of each band of energy or lobe* (between adjacent nulls) *is inversely proportional to duration*. Shortening the duration from 100 ms to 4 ms is a factor of 1:25, and the consequence is to widen each band of energy by a factor of 25:1 (from 10 Hz at 100 ms to 250 Hz at 4 ms).

Effects of Rise/Decay, or Rise/Fall, Time on the Amplitude Spectrum

When a sine wave (or other signal) of fairly long duration, say a second or two, is turned on, its maximum amplitude is not allowed to be attained instantly. Instead, the amplitude is made to rise over time from zero to some maximum or steady-state value, as is shown in panel A of Figure 7–4, and then remains steady-state for a duration of our choosing. Similarly, when the tone burst is turned off, the amplitude does not instantly drop to zero; it decays over time from maximum to zero. The dashed curve in panel A of the figure defines the **amplitude envelope** (in the time domain) of the waveform.

Because the signal must be turned on and off, or gated, an amplitude spectrum is created that is more complex than that of a theoretical sine wave, and that outcome is shown in panel B of Figure 7–4. Energy is spread to other frequencies, and the amplitude spectrum is a **continuous spectrum** rather than a line spectrum.

Initiating and terminating a signal produces *transients*, which are sometimes called "on-transients" when the signal is turned on and the amplitude is rising, and "off-transients" when the signal is turned off and the amplitude is decaying. The process of creating *transients* is called **transient distortion**.

The amount of transient distortion varies as a function of the time required for the amplitude to rise from zero toward maximum or to decay from maximum toward zero. The longer the duration over which the signal is rising or decaying, the **rise-decay time**, the narrower the frequency band over which energy is spread in both directions from the frequency of the driving signal. Thus, slowly rising and slowly decaying signals are characterized by less transient dis-

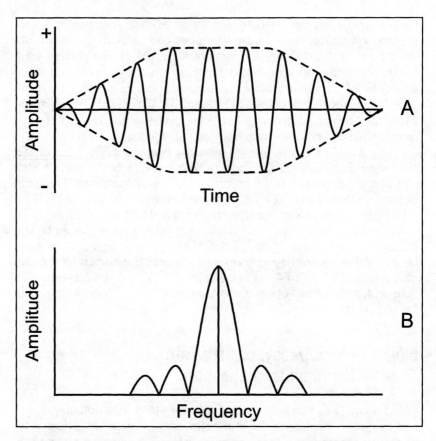

Figure 7–4. Transient distortion. Effects of rise-decay time of the waveform (panel A) on the amplitude spectrum (panel B) of a sine wave. The result is a continuous spectrum and reflects what is called **transient distortion.**

tortion than signals for which the amplitude rises and decays very quickly.

If the rise or decay is very short, an audible "clicking" sound will be heard. Audiologists test a person's hearing by use of an instrument called an *audiometer*, which is a device that generates sine waves at various frequencies with variable sound pressure levels. By manipulating those two variables, the audiologist can determine the lowest sound pressure levels at which an individual can just detect sine waves of various frequencies. But, the sine waves must be turned on and off, and we want to be certain that we determine how well the person hears the sine waves, not the audible clicks that are produced by switching the signal on and off too rapidly.

To ensure that transient distortion is minimized, the *American National Standards Institute* (ANSI) has adopted standards for manufacturers to meet by specifying minimum "rise times" and "decay times" for audiometers. The 1989 standard for rise-decay times (ANSI S3.6-1989), for example, specifies that the time required for the signal amplitude to rise from −20 dB (1%) to −1 dB (79.4%) re: maximum amplitude and to decay from −1 dB to −20 dB shall not be *less* than 20 ms.

■ AMPLITUDE DISTORTION

All systems can be described by an *input-output function* such as the one shown previously in Figure 7–2 *for a linear system.*

Nonlinear Systems

Figure 7–5 compares the input-output function for a linear system in panel A with the input-output function for a **nonlinear** system in panel B. Output amplitude on the ordinate is plotted as a function of input amplitude on the abscissa. We see in panel C that as the input amplitude to *a linear system* is increased, we achieve a *proportional* increase in output amplitude, and the characteristics of a sine wave at the input (pointing upward) are preserved at the output of the system (pointing toward the right). That circumstance, shown previously in Figure 7–2, is shown again in panel C of Figure 7–5.

The same result happens for a **nonlinear system** *if the instantaneous amplitudes of the input signal do not exceed the limits of linearity of the input-output function of the nonlinear system.* Thus, in panel D, if we confine our attention initially to that portion of the function that is *linear* (a straight line), we should observe that as the amplitude of the input signal is increased, we again achieve a *proportional* increase in output amplitude. Furthermore, the characteristics of the input waveform are preserved in the output waveform, just as they were in panel C for a linear system. The characteristics of the input sine wave are preserved faithfully because none of the instantaneous amplitudes exceeds the limits of linearity.

Notice, though, that as we continue to increase the input amplitude from left to right in panel B of Figure 7–5, a point is reached where the input-output function becomes *nonlinear*, and in that region changes in input amplitude *do not produce proportional changes in output amplitude.* Thus, when we operate on the *nonlinear portion* of the function, a 3-dB increase in input amplitude will result in *less* than a 3-dB increase in output amplitude. At the extreme, further increases of the input level produce no increase (or even a decrease) in output amplitude. When input level is increased so much that we are operating on the nonlinear portion of the input-output function, we are said to be "overdriving" or "overloading" the system.

The effects of overdriving a **nonlinear system** on a sinusoidal waveform are shown in Figure 7–6. In panel A, a large-amplitude sine wave is directed to the input of the system (pointing upward). Although many of the *instantaneous amplitudes* of the input sine wave lie within the linear portion of the input-output function, those instantaneous amplitudes of the input signal that are *at or near the*

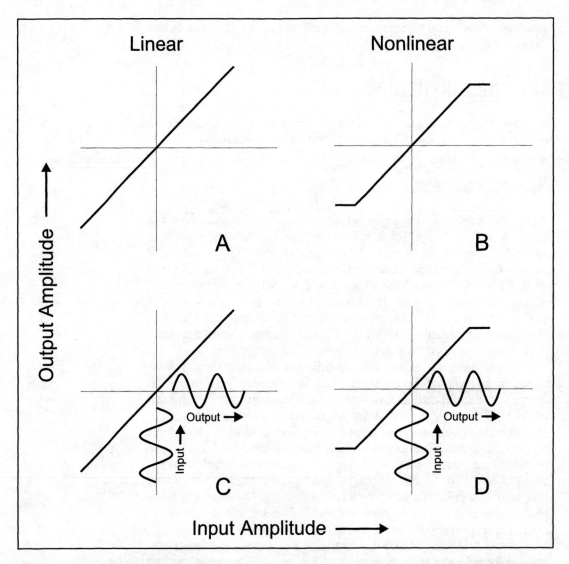

Figure 7–5. Amplitude distortion. Panel A shows an input-output function for the **linear system** that was shown previously in Figure 7–2. Panel B shows an input-output function for a **nonlinear system**. Output amplitude is *proportional* to input amplitude only over the linear portion of the function for the **nonlinear system**. Panel C compares the sinusoidal waveforms at the input and output of the **linear system** in panel A. Panel D compares the sinusoidal waveforms at the input and output of a **nonlinear system**. The waveform characteristics are faithfully preserved at the output of the nonlinear system *because the instantaneous amplitudes of the input signal do not exceed the limits of linearity of the input-output function in panel B.*

maximum amplitude lie on the nonlinear portion of the function. For those amplitudes, *the output amplitude is not proportional to the input amplitude.* Instead, those instantaneous amplitudes are reduced at the output, and the shape of the output waveform (pointing toward the right) has been altered relative to its sinusoidal shape at the input.

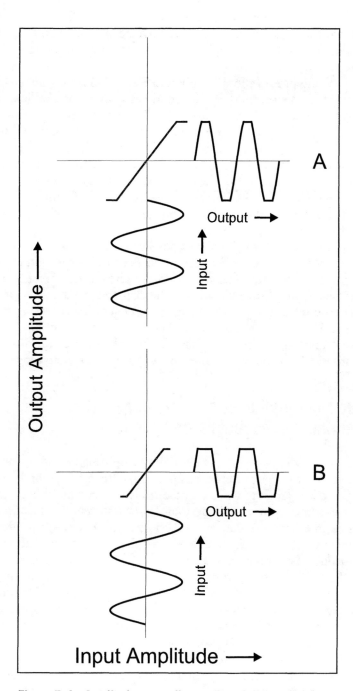

Figure 7–6. Amplitude, or **nonlinear**, **distortion**. In panel A, the instantaneous amplitudes at the input to a **nonlinear system** *do* exceed the limits of linearity of the input-output function. The result is that output amplitude is *not* proportional to input amplitude and the signal is **peak clipped**. Panel B displays more severe peak clipping.

The shape of the output waveform has been altered by virtue of the fact that the peaks of the sine wave have been "clipped off," and this process is called **peak clipping**. More severe peak clipping is shown in panel B of Figure 7–6.

Peak clipping of the sort shown in Figure 7–6 is not the only form of amplitude distortion that can occur. For example, peak clipping can be symmetrical as it is in Figure 7–6. With symmetrical clipping, both the positive and negative peaks of the waveform are clipped, which leaves only the center portions of the waveform unaffected. Peak clipping also can be asymmetrical in which, for example, the positive peaks are clipped and both the center portions and the negative peaks are preserved faithfully. Furthermore, the signal can undergo **center clipping** in which the center portions of the wave are eliminated and only the peaks are preserved.

The waveform of the signal has been altered, and therefore we know that the signal has been distorted. Because the *amplitude* of the waveform is the parameter that has been altered, this form of distortion is called **amplitude distortion**. The distortion to the waveform occurs because the system was overdriven. That is to say, we were operating on the *nonlinear portion* of the input-output function, and this form of distortion, therefore, also can be called **nonlinear distortion**. **Amplitude distortion** and **nonlinear distortion** are synonymous.

Effects of Amplitude, or Nonlinear, Distortion on the Amplitude Spectrum

If the sinusoidal waveform is altered by amplitude, or nonlinear, distortion, what happens to the *amplitude spectrum*? The input signals in Figure 7–6 are sine waves. The output waveforms in both panels A and B of the figure remain periodic, *but they are not sinusoidal*. We learned in Chapter 5 that any waveform that is not sinusoidal is *a complex waveform*. Thus, a sine wave that undergoes **nonlinear**, or **amplitude**, **distortion** becomes *a complex periodic waveform*.

We should expect, from what we learned in Chapter 5, that the complex periodic waveform at the output of a nonlinear system will have energy at **harmonics** of the fundamental frequency, which is the frequency of the driving sine wave at the input. That occurs when a sine wave undergoes **amplitude**, or **nonlinear, distortion**. Therefore, this form of distortion *for a sine wave* also can be called **harmonic distortion** because the output signal contains energy at **harmonics** of the fundamental driving signal.

Figure 7–7 shows the amplitude spectrum of a sine wave that has undergone harmonic distortion. The fundamental frequency (.1 kHz) of the complex periodic wave is the same as the frequency of the input sine wave, but we see that there also is energy at **harmonics** of the fundamental, and the amplitudes of five such harmonics $(A_1 - A_5)$ are shown in the figure; **distortion products** have been created.

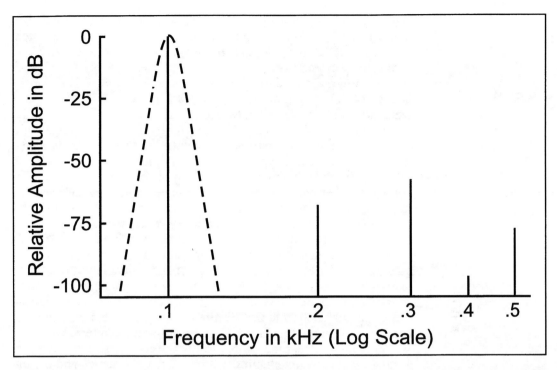

Figure 7–7. The **amplitude spectrum** of a sinusoidal waveform that has undergone **amplitude**, or **nonlinear**, **distortion**. As a consequence of operating on the nonlinear portion of the input-output function, the output signal contains energy at **harmonics** of the fundamental driving signal at the input. The dashed curve illustrates the filter curve of a 1/3-octave filter centered on the fundamental frequency of the distorted signal to aid in measuring its voltage independent of the voltages of the higher harmonics.

Percentage Harmonic Distortion

The magnitude of harmonic distortion usually is expressed in *percentage*. If we return to our mythical purchase of an audio tape recorder, the specifications might say, for example, that you should expect not in excess of 1% harmonic distortion. It might not be intuitively obvious, however, what "1% harmonic distortion" means. To gain a better understanding of that concept, we will attempt a "logical, or intuitive, derivation" of an equation rather than a mathematical one.

Look again at the amplitude spectrum of the signal that has undergone harmonic distortion in Figure 7–7. Suppose we are dealing with a sine wave produced by a sine wave generator and directed to some electronic device, such as an amplifier. In this case, our unit of measure of amplitude is *voltage* rather than sound pressure. With the aid of an instrument called a wave analyzer, we measure the voltage (amplitude) of each of the harmonics in the output signal. A wave analyzer is an electronic instrument that is a combination of a voltmeter (an instrument that measures electrical voltage) and a narrowly tuned band-pass filter with a variable f_c. Thus, one can "tune" the filter (i.e., adjust the center frequency to a desired value) and then measure "only" the voltage of the signal that is passed by the filter.

Suppose, for example, that the wave analyzer contains a 1/3-octave filter centered on the fundamental frequency of the signal, such as that shown by the dashed filter function in Figure 7–7. If the frequency of the input sine wave is 100 Hz, we set f_c of the wave analyzer to 100 Hz. The bandwidth of the filter will be 23.1 Hz (Equations 6.6, 6.7, and 6.8). Thus, virtually all of the voltage registered by the voltmeter will be the voltage of only the fundamental frequency of 100 Hz because voltages associated with the higher harmonics will be well above the passband of the analyzing filter. The voltage of the fundamental frequency is recorded and the measurement process is then repeated several times, each time with the filter tuned to a different center frequency to isolate each of the harmonics of interest: 200 Hz; 300 Hz; 400 Hz; and 500 Hz.

The input signal contains energy only at the fundamental frequency. We shall refer to the voltage of the fundamental (V_1) as reflecting the *desired energy* in the signal. The output signal, of course, contains energy at the desired frequency and it contains *undesired energy* at higher harmonics (limited to four higher harmonics for convenience) of the fundamental; those voltages are referred to as V_2, V_3, V_4, and V_5. The total energy in the output signal is equal to the sum of the *desired energy* in the fundamental frequency and the *undesired energy* that is contained in the other four harmonics of the fundamental frequency. We can conceive of **harmonic distortion** as *the proportion of total energy that is undesired energy*, which if multiplied by 100, would be expressed as **percentage harmonic distortion**. Thus, by reference to the voltages of the fundamental and the higher harmonics in the output signal, we find that:

$$\text{Percentage Harmonic Distortion} = \frac{f(V_2, V_3, V_4, V_5)}{f(V_1, V_2, V_3, V_4, V_5)} \times 100,$$

where f is some undefined function,

and **V** refers to the voltage of some particular harmonic, V_1 through V_5.

Recall from Chapter 4 that we do not ordinarily sum acoustic pressures because we seldom know their relative phases, and the same restriction must apply to their electrical analogs, voltages. We can, however, sum the energies or powers or intensities, which is why the "equation" above does not contain a "+" and therefore is unusable in its present form. We also learned in Chapter 4 that energy, power, or intensity is proportional to the square of pressure ($W \propto p^2$), and electrical energy or power, therefore, also is proportional to the square of voltage ($W \propto V^2$). If we square each of the voltages in the numerator and denominator, we can sum them and compute the ratio. Thus, the equation can be rewritten as:

$$\text{Percentage Harmonic Distortion} = \frac{f'(V_2^2 + V_3^2 + V_4^2 + V_5^2)}{f'(V_1^2 + V_2^2 + V_3^2 + V_4^2 + V_5^2)} \times 100.$$

Finally, we can convert our measures back from "voltage squared" to "voltage" by taking the square root of the ratio of the sum of the squared voltages, and we then arrive at Equation 7.1 for harmonic distortion, which is written more generally to accommodate **n** harmonics.

$$\text{Percentage Harmonic Distortion} = \sqrt{\frac{V_2^2 + V_3^2 + ... + V_n^2}{V_1^2 + V_2^2 + ... + V_n^2}} \times 100.$$ **Equation 7.1**

Approximate Percentage Harmonic Distortion

Because most of the total energy in the denominator comes from only the fundamental frequency, percentage harmonic distortion sometimes is *approximated* by:

$$\text{Percentage Harmonic Distortion} = \sqrt{\frac{V_2^2 + V_3^2 + ... + V_n^2}{V_1^2}} \times 100.$$ **Equation 7.2**

To illustrate, the second column of Table 7–1 lists the voltages, in millivolts, for each of five harmonics listed in column one. The third column lists the squares of the voltages shown in column two. With the aid of Equation 7.1 we calculate that we have 0.1% harmonic distortion. The same answer is obtained if we use Equation 7.2 *for this example*, and the explanation for the equivalence should be obvious. With either equation, the numerator is the same, 0.002626. With Equation 7.1, the denominator for this example is 2,500.002626, whereas with Equation 7.2 the denominator is 2,500, which is not very different. Thus, we see for the example in Table 7–1, and for most instances that we are likely to encounter, Equation 7.2 provides a perfectly acceptable estimate of percentage harmonic distortion.

Table 7–1. Computation of percentage harmonic distortion

Harmonic	Voltage (V) in millivolts	V^2
1	50.0	2,500.0
2	.01	.0001
3	.05	.0025
4	.001	.000001
5	.005	.000025

$$\% = \sqrt{\frac{0.0001 + .0025 + .000001 + .000025}{2,500 + .0001 + .0025 + .000001 + .000025}} \times 100 = 0.1\%$$

Amplitude Response and Dynamic Range

In panel A of Figure 7–8 we show what happens if we define input-output functions for some system *for each of several input, or driving, frequencies*, not just one. Note that, for this example, the upper and lower limits of linearity are constant from about 500 Hz to 5000 Hz, and that the range of linearity diminishes for lower and higher frequencies. Next, we will decide on some *maximum permissible harmonic distortion*, say 0.1%, to accommodate whatever purpose we have in mind for the system that is being used.

We then locate the point of maximum permissible harmonic distortion on each of the functions in the figure, and those points are identified as filled dots in panel A of the figure. That means that if the input amplitude for that particular frequency exceeds the value

Figure 7-8. Input-output functions for each of several frequencies are shown in panel A. In panel B, the amplitude response (solid line), in relation to the maximum permissible harmonic distortion, is compared with the electrical noise floor (ENF) of a system. The distance between the ENF and the maximum amplitude response defines the **dynamic range** of a system.

corresponding to that point on the function, we will exceed the maximum permissible harmonic distortion that was agreed on. In other words, those points define the maximum driving amplitude as a function of frequency that we can utilize without producing an unacceptable amount of harmonic distortion.

The points of *maximum permissible harmonic distortion* (filled dots) are redrawn in the frequency domain as the upper curve in panel B of Figure 7–8. When the points are connected, the curve that results defines the **amplitude response** (or **frequency response**) of the system, just as we saw previously in panel C of Figure 7–1. As before, we see that the curve defines how the energy is attenuated selectively as a function of frequency *in relation to the maximum permissible harmonic distortion* that we have agreed can be tolerated.

Dynamic Range

When you examine the specifications for some electronic instrument, such as a tape recorder, you likely will see reference to the **dynamic range** of the system. The dashed curve in panel B of Figure 7–8 describes *the electrical noise floor* (ENF) of the hypothetical tape recorder. All electronic equipment generates a random time function, which as we learned in Chapter 5, is an aperiodic waveform, or *noise,* and the curve depicting the electrical noise floor shows how the level of the noise might vary as a function of frequency.

The amplitude response curve reflects the maximum signal level that the tape recorder can handle reliably without exceeding the maximum permissible harmonic distortion. If the input signal level is reduced, percentage harmonic distortion also will be lowered. We obviously, however, do not want a driving signal level that is so low that the signal is "buried" in the noise. Thus, to achieve an optimal signal-to-noise ratio, we want the driving signal to correspond to the highest possible amplitude without exceeding a tolerable amount of harmonic distortion.

Dynamic range is the distance in decibels between the electrical noise floor and the amplitude response curve. If, for example, the dynamic range is 60 dB, that means that you can record a signal with a signal-to-noise ratio of 60 dB or less without experiencing an intolerable amount of harmonic distortion. If signal level is reduced, percentage harmonic distortion is reduced, but at the expense of a less favorable signal-to-noise ratio. It should be obvious that because both the amplitude response curve and ENF vary with frequency, the dynamic range is also frequency dependent. If you examine the specifications for an instrument you are contemplating purchasing, however, the dynamic range probably will be expressed as a single value—perhaps even the most favorable one.

Intermodulation Distortion

Harmonic distortion is synonymous with **amplitude,** or **nonlinear, distortion** *when the driving signal is a simple sinusoid.* When the driving signal is a complex waveform, we still experience amplitude, or nonlinear, distortion, but the output spectrum is far more complicated than "simple" harmonic distortion. This kind of distortion is called **intermodulation distortion**, and it arises from the interactions among the various frequency components of the signal and from the interactions among their harmonics.

To illustrate the differences between intermodulation distortion and harmonic distortion, we will consider the simple case of a complex driving signal that has two components, $f_1 = 100$ Hz and $f_2 = 110$ Hz. The frequency components of the output signal contain two types of **distortion products**: harmonics and **combination tones**.

Harmonics

The output signal contains energy at **harmonics** of *each* of the frequency components of the driving signal. Thus, there will be energy at f_1 (100 Hz), $2f_1$ (200 Hz), $3f_1$ (300 Hz), and so forth, and there will be energy at f_2 (110 Hz), $2f_2$ (220 Hz), $3f_2$ (330 Hz), and so on. Each of those components of the output signal is harmonically related to one or the other of the two components of the driving signal, f_1 and f_2.

Combination Tones: Difference Tones and Summation Tones

A second type of distortion product, in addition to the harmonically related components listed above, comprises **combination tones**. Combination tones can be further subdivided into two types: **difference tones** and **summation tones**. For example, difference tones include $|f_1 - f_2|$ (10 Hz); $|2f_1 - f_2|$ (90 Hz); $|3f_1 - f_2|$ (190 Hz); and so on. Examples of summation tones include $|f_1 + f_2|$ (210 Hz); $|2f_1 + f_2|$ (310 Hz); $|3f_1 + f_2|$ (410 Hz); and so forth.

In theory, the combination tones comprise all possible sums (**summation tones**) and differences (**difference tones**) of the primary frequencies, f_1 and f_2, *and integer multiples of those primary components*. In practice, though, the amplitudes of many of the higher combination tones will be sufficiently small to render their contribution to the total energy in the output signal negligible. The general equation that defines the harmonics, summation tones, and difference tones produced by a nonlinear system is:

Equation 7.3

$$mf_1 \pm nf_2,$$

where **m** and **n** are assigned all integer values: 0, 1, 2, 3, 4, ... n.

If we apply Equation 7.3 to the example cited above where $f_1 = 100$ Hz and $f_2 = 110$ Hz, we generate the harmonics and combination tones listed in Table 7–2.

In this chapter we have learned how "ideal" sound waves are altered in various ways that, collectively, are called **distortion**. In the final chapter we will learn other ways in which sound waves are changed from the original state when transmitted through a medium.

Table 7–2. Examples of harmonics and combination tones produced for a complex wave with two frequency components, $f_1 = 100$ Hz and $f_2 = 110$ Hz

| Harmonics of | | Combination Tones | |
f_1	f_2	Difference Tones	Summation Tones
$\lvert 1f_1 + 0f_2 \rvert = 100$	$\lvert 0f_1 + 1f_2 \rvert = 110$	$\lvert 1f_1 - 1f_2 \rvert = 10$	$\lvert 1f_1 + 1f_2 \rvert = 210$
$\lvert 2f_1 + 0f_2 \rvert = 200$	$\lvert 0f_1 + 2f_2 \rvert = 220$	$\lvert 2f_1 - 1f_2 \rvert = 90$	$\lvert 2f_1 + 1f_2 \rvert = 310$
$\lvert 3f_1 + 0f_2 \rvert = 300$	$\lvert 0f_1 + 3f_2 \rvert = 330$	$\lvert 3f_1 - 1f_2 \rvert = 190$	$\lvert 3f_1 + 1f_2 \rvert = 410$
etc.	etc.	etc.	etc.

Sound Transmission

When sinusoidal waves were first discussed in Chapter 2, each cycle of sinusoidal motion *initially* was represented as being identical in every respect to every other cycle. That representation was appropriate when the sine wave was conceptualized from a strict mathematical perspective. We then learned that sound waves produced and transmitted in the real world encounter frictional forces that cause the amplitude of the sound wave to diminish over time. Thus, real sound waves are damped, and ultimately they fade away.

Furthermore, we know from experience that the amplitude of sound not only diminishes over time, but it also diminishes over distance traveled. All other factors being equal, if you are positioned too far from even an intense source of sound, the sound might be quite faint, if indeed it is audible, or even measurable.

It also was convenient to treat sound waves *initially* as if they were transmitted in a free, unbounded medium with no obstacles. When obstacles are present, or when certain conditions exist in the medium, important characteristics of sound waves and their transmission are altered.

In this final chapter we will learn how the characteristics of sound waves are altered in various ways during sound transmission. Although the factors that we will describe usually act in combination to affect the characteristics of sound waves in fairly complicated ways, for the sake of simplicity, we will consider them one at a time.

■ ATTENUATION OF SOUND INTENSITY OVER DISTANCE

Let us assume that a sound wave is propagated through a *free, unbounded medium* that contains no obstacles or conditions to affect the propagation or to affect the characteristics of the sound wave as it is transmitted through space. Suppose, for example, that a weapon is fired and that the resultant sound wave has a peak sound pressure level of 110 dB at a distance of 0.5 miles from the weapon. As the sound wave is propagated through the free, unbounded medium, the intensity of the sound wave diminishes in a lawful way.

The decrease in intensity in a free, unbounded medium behaves in accordance with the **inverse square law**. Could the shot be heard at a distance of 8,192 miles from the source if the listener's threshold of hearing (in the appropriate frequency range) is, for example, 20 dB SPL? We will subsequently demonstrate that the answer is "yes" for this example, even though the intensity of the sound wave does decrease with distance.

Think of a point source of sound, a spherically shaped source of vibration, or pulsation, with a very small diameter. We see in Figure 8–1 that when the point source is forced to pulsate by application of some external force, alternate regions of *increased density* (**compression**) and *decreased density* (**rarefaction**) are created. A "disturbance" is propagated through the medium, and sound, which is a form of energy, is transferred from the source through the medium. Thus, sound energy radiates away from the source in all directions, and four such "lines of propagation" are shown in the figure.

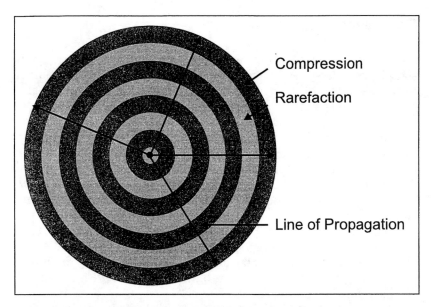

Figure 8–1. Alternate regions of compression and rarefaction in an air mass caused by pulsation of a point source of sound. Four lines of propagation from the source are shown. The compressions form a spherical shell around the spherical point source and the shell is called a **wave front** or, more precisely, a **spherical wave front.**

Spherical Waves

Let us also continue to assume that the medium has uniform properties and is unlimited in all directions, which is to say that the medium is free and unbounded. That defines a "free-field" condition. The **compressions**, or crests, form a **spherical shell** around the spherical point source. That spherical shell is called a **wave front**. The disturbance propagated through the medium is an ever increasingly larger **spherical wave front**.

Plane Waves

If the wave front is a considerable distance away from the point source, the radius of the sphere is sufficiently large that we can represent the wave front as a **plane wave front**, rather than as a spherical wave front, because the curvature of the sphere is negligible. Thus, sine waves also can be called **spherical waves**, or **plane progressive waves**, when they are propagated through a medium. A spherical wave can be visualized as being similar to a soap bubble that becomes larger and larger as it is blown at a constant rate, with the surface of the soap bubble representing a wave front.

The Inverse Square Law

As the wave front moves outward from the source, sound energy is spread over a larger and larger area. Thus, as we move from point **A** to point **B** to point **C** in Figure 8–1, the energy is dissipated over a progressively larger and larger area because the surface area of the sphere becomes progressively larger.

Recall from Chapter 4 that energy/unit time (energy/s) is **power**. The same amount of **power** is dissipated over the surfaces of the increasingly larger spheres at the distances represented by **A**, **B**, and **C** in Figure 8–1, but the energy/s/m^2 (**MKS** system) *must diminish* because the same amount of power is dissipated over a larger and larger area. Energy/s/m^2, sometimes called the **energy density**, is the **intensity** of a sound wave. Thus, if the energy/s (**power**) remains constant, but the **power** (energy/s) is dissipated over a larger and larger area as we move farther and farther away from the source, the **intensity**, or **energy density** (energy/s/m^2), must decrease with increasing distance from the point source.

Imagine that we place our eye at the point source and look away from the source at the increasingly larger area that is bounded by lines of propagation. Such a view is represented in Figure 8–2, and four lines of propagation are shown as we attempt to depict a three-

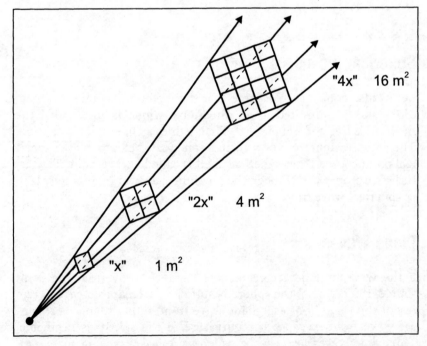

Figure 8–2. A three dimensional representation of the **inverse square law**. As the distance from the point source of sound increases from **X** to **2X** to **4X**, a finite amount of power is dissipated over a larger and larger area (from 1 m^2 at **X** to 4 m^2 at **2X** to 16 m^2 at **4X**). Hence, the intensity (energy/s/m^2) decreases inversely with the square of the distance from the source.

dimensional representation. We will assume that the distances of interest from the point source are so great that the wave front can be considered to be a **plane wave front**.

At distance **X** a finite amount of sound **power** (energy/s) is dissipated over an area of 1 m². That defines the **intensity** of the sound wave at distance **X** from the source, the energy/s/m². As we move twice as far away from the source to distance **2X**, the same finite amount of **power** is dissipated, but over a larger area. How much larger? The surface area of a sphere is given by Equation 8.1:

$$A = 4\pi r^2,$$

Equation 8.1

where **r** is the radius.

For example, if distance **X** is 1 m from the source, the area (**A**) of the sphere at distance **X** = 12.6 m² (4π1²). At distance **2X**, A = 50.3 m² (4π2²), and at distance **4X**, A = 201.1 m² (4π4²). From these calculations we should see that *each time the radius is increased by some factor, the surface area of the sphere is increased by the square of that factor.*

If the area of the sphere increases with increasing distance from the source, the energy/s/m² (the **intensity**) must decrease. The area (4 m²) bounded by lines of propagation at point **2X** is exactly four times the area at point **X** (1 m²). Because **intensity** is energy/s/m², we can see that the intensity is diminished as the sound wave travels between the two points. More precisely, the intensity at distance **2X** is only *one-fourth* the intensity at **X** because the power is dissipated over an area that is four times larger.

We have seen that when the distance from the source *increases* by a factor of 2:1, sound intensity *decreases*, and the ratio of the intensity at point **2X** to the intensity at point **X** is 1:4. Because 4 = 2², and because the relation is an inverse one, this phenomenon is called the **inverse square law**.

As we proceed farther and farther from the point source in the free, unbounded medium, we shall see that the **inverse square law** continues to hold. For example, at distance **4X**, which is twice as far from the source as distance **2X**, the **power** is spread over an area of 16 m² in comparison with an area of 4 m² at distance **2X**. Thus, the distance has increased by another factor of 2:1, the surface area of the wave front has increased by a factor of 2²:1, and the sound intensity, therefore, is changed once again by a ratio of 1:4.

The **inverse square law** can be expressed as:

$$I \propto \frac{1}{D^2},$$

Equation 8.2

where **D** refers to the ratio of two distances

from the sound source (**d$_i$/d$_r$**),

d$_i$ is the distance of interest,

and

d$_r$ is some reference distance.

For example, if we compare the intensities at two distances, 100 m ($\mathbf{d_r}$) and 200 m ($\mathbf{d_i}$), we should expect that the intensity at $\mathbf{d_i}$ will be inversely proportional to the square of the ratio of the two distances, $\mathbf{d_i/d_r}$.

Because $\mathbf{D} = (\mathbf{d_i/d_r})$ we can rewrite Equation 8.2 to obtain Equation 8.3:

Equation 8.3

$$I \propto \frac{1}{\left(\frac{d_i}{d_r}\right)^2},$$

which states that *the intensity is inversely proportional to the square of the ratio of two distances*, the ratio of distance of interest ($\mathbf{d_i}$) to some reference distance ($\mathbf{d_r}$).

The **inverse square law** applies to other physical phenomena in addition to transmission of sound. For example, the force of gravity also decreases over distance in accordance with the inverse square law.

Near the surface of the earth, a falling mass is accelerated at a rate of 9.8 m/s^2 because of *the attractive gravitational force exerted on the mass by the earth*. As we move farther and farther from the surface of the earth, the gravitational force varies inversely as the square of the distance from the earth's core. The radius of the earth, the distance from its center core to the surface, is approximately 6,400 km ($\mathbf{d_r}$). At a distance of 6,400 km from the earth's surface (12,800 km from the core, $\mathbf{d_i}$, a ratio of 1:2) the gravitational force is only one-fourth of what it was at the surface. The moon is a mass. How does the inverse square law inform us about the magnitude of acceleration on the moon? The distance from the surface of the earth to the surface of the moon is about 384,000 km ($\mathbf{d_i}$). Thus, the ratio, $\mathbf{d_i/d_r}$, is 384,000/6,400 = 60. In accordance with the inverse square law, $\mathbf{F_a}$ (the force of acceleration) is given by:

$$F_a = \frac{1}{60^2} = \frac{1}{3,600} = 0.00028 \text{ m/s}^2,$$

in contrast to 9.8 m/s^2 on earth. In other words, as Newton calculated, the gravitational attraction of the earth on any mass varies inversely with the square of the distance from the earth's center core.

One additional example should suffice to explain the generality of the inverse square law. Many will recall from a high school science class that *"like" electrostatic charges repel* with some force, whereas *"unlike" charges attract* with some force. Charles A. De Coulomb (1736–1806) demonstrated experimentally that the magnitudes of either repulsive or attractive forces vary directly with the product of the individual charges and *vary inversely with the square of the distance between the two charges*. With respect to generality of the law, the **inverse square law** applies to virtually all fields of force.

The Inverse Square Law and Decibels

As we learned in Chapter 4, we generally refer to the *level* of a sound in decibels rather than to its intensity in watts/m^2. To accomplish that transformation for applications involving the **inverse square law**, we simply calculate the log of the distance ratio and multiply by -20 to obtain Equation 8.4. Thus,

$$dB = 10 \log_{10} \frac{1}{\left(\frac{d_i}{d_r}\right)^2}$$

$$= -10 \log_{10} \left(\frac{d_i}{d_r}\right)^2 \qquad \textbf{(Log Law 4)}$$

$$= -20 \log_{10} \frac{d_i}{d_r}. \qquad \textbf{(Log Law 3)} \qquad \textbf{Equation 8.4}$$

If we return to Figure 8–2, we should gain an intuitive understanding of Equation 8.4. The area over which power is dissipated at distance **X** is 1 m^2. Thus, if we use Equation 8.4 to compare the intensity at distance **X** (d_i) with the intensity *at the same distance* **X** (d_r), we obtain 0 dB, because the ratio is 1:1 and the log of 1 is 0. If we instead compare the intensity at distance **2X** (d_i) with the intensity at a reference distance **X** (d_r), we calculate that:

$$dB = -20 \log \frac{2}{1}$$

$$= -6 \text{ dB.}$$

That answer agrees with what we discovered previously. The intensity at **2X** is one-fourth the intensity at **X**, and as we learned in Chapter 4, if intensity decreases by a factor of four, the *level* decreases by 6 dB (Equation 4.4). Obviously, therefore, between **2X** and **4X** the intensity decreases by another 6 dB because:

$$dB = -20 \log \frac{4}{2}$$

$$= -6 \text{ dB.}$$

Finally, between distance **X** and distance **4X** the intensity decreases by 12 dB because:

$$dB = -20 \log \frac{4}{1}$$

$$= -12 \text{ dB.}$$

The **inverse square law** is sometimes defined (incompletely) by saying that "the intensity decreases by 6 dB for each doubling of the distance." Although the statement is correct, it is an insufficient definition of the law because it does not describe the more general effect of distance ratios other than 2:1 on intensity. For that reason, the previous definition—the intensity varies inversely with the square of the distance—is preferable.

Sample Problems

Problem 1: If the sound pressure level is 80 dB at a distance of 100 m from the source, *by how much is the SPL decreased* at a distance of 200 m?

$$dB = -20 \log \frac{200}{100} = -6 \text{ dB.}$$

Note that the SPL at d_r (100 m) is irrelevant. The intensity at d_i will be attenuated by 6 dB re: the intensity at d_r regardless of the SPL at d_r.

Problem 2: If the sound pressure level is 80 dB SPL at a distance of 100 m from the source, *what is the SPL* at a distance of 200 m?

$$dB = 80 - 20 \log \frac{200}{100} = 74 \text{ dB SPL.}$$

It stands to reason that if the SPL decreases by 6 dB between the two distances, the SPL at the second distance is given by the SPL at the first, or reference, distance (80 dB) minus the amount by which the intensity is attenuated (6 dB).

Problem 3: If the SPL at a distance of 100 m is 80 dB, what is the SPL at a distance of 850 m?

$$dB = 80 - 20 \log \frac{850}{100} = 61.4 \text{ dB SPL.}$$

Problem 4: Finally, let us solve the problem that was posed at the outset. If the SPL of a gunshot is 110 dB at a distance of 0.5 miles from the weapon, could the shot be heard at a distance of 8,192 miles (*in a free, unbounded medium*) from the source if the observer's threshold of hearing in the appropriate frequency range is 20 dB SPL?

$$dB = 110 - 20 \log \frac{8,192}{0.5} = 110 - 84.2 = 25.8 \text{ dB SPL.}$$

Therefore, if the intensity of the sound is 25.8 dB SPL and the observer's threshold of hearing is 20 dB SPL, the shot should be heard. You should also note that if the distance from the source of the sound wave were doubled again to 16,384 miles, the SPL would only decrease by another 6 dB (to 0.2 dB below the postulated threshold) because, as we have seen, *the intensity varies inversely with the square of the distance.* Finally, you might wish to test your ability to still work problems such as those in Problem Set 8 of Chapter 4 by attempting to calculate just how far from the reference distance of 0.5 miles the observer would have to be positioned for the sound to just equal the observer's threshold of 20 dB SPL. The only difference is that now you are solving for d_i, a distance of interest, rather than p_x, a pressure of interest. You should calculate that the sound should just reach the observer's threshold of 20 dB SPL at a distance of approximately 15,811 miles, if the medium is free and unbounded.

The inverse square law only holds strictly when the sound waves are propagated through a free, unbounded medium. Such a medium, of course, is a theoretical construct and, in reality, the transmitting media of interest will have obstacles and other conditions that interfere with sound transmission in important ways.

If the sound wave encounters an obstacle, depending on the nature of the obstacle, the sound wave will be **reflected** (it will "bounce" back from the obstacle), **diffracted** (it will be scattered about the obstacle), **absorbed** (it will penetrate the obstacle), or **refracted** (it will be "bent").

■ REFLECTION

What happens when a rubber ball is thrown against a hard wooden wall? Obviously the ball does not penetrate the obstacle—it bounces off the wall. Moreover, many young children quickly learn the approximate path that the ball will take on its return so that they can get into position to catch it.

In Figure 8–3, a ball will be thrown toward a wall along a path marked by the dashed line that is perpendicular to the wall (90° angle). If, and only if, the ball is thrown toward the wall on a path that is precisely along the perpendicular, the ball will return to the thrower along the same perpendicular (dashed) line. If the ball is thrown more to the left along the path marked P_i, it will return along the path marked P_r. Why?

Let us call the path of the thrown ball the "incident path" (P_i) and the path of the bounced (reflected) ball the "reflected path" (P_r). From the point where the thrown ball strikes the wall, we have drawn another line (dashed) that also is perpendicular to the wall. *The angle of the reflected path (P_r) to the perpendicular equals the angle of the incident path (P_i) to the perpendicular.*

That rule applies to any angle of the incident path to the perpendicular, regardless of whether the ball is thrown to the left, the right, or straight ahead. The young child almost certainly cannot recite that rule of reflection, but most children "know" the rule or

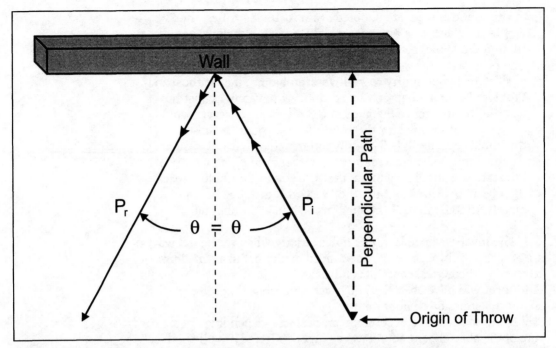

Figure 8–3. The paths of a ball thrown toward a wall and then reflected by the wall. When the ball is thrown straight at the wall along the dashed line, it bounces straight back to the thrower. When the ball is thrown at an angle along the path marked **P$_i$**, the ball bounces off the wall and away from the thrower along the path marked **P$_r$**. In both cases, and all others, the angle of the reflected path, **P$_r$**, to a line drawn perpendicular to the wall equals the angle of the incident path, **P$_i$**, to the same perpendicular line.

else learn it rather quickly. Unless that rule is mastered, attempts to participate in any sporting event in which reflection is part of the game (billiards, handball, etc.) will be futile.

Reflection of Sound Waves

Sound waves are affected by obstacles in the same way that the hard wall affects the path of the thrown ball. In Figure 8–4 we show spherical wave fronts moving from right to left. The wave fronts encounter a plane obstacle (a very thick wall of steel, for example). The sound wave moving from right to left *toward the wall* will be called the **incident wave**, and one *ray* of the incident wave (**i**) is shown pointing leftward toward the plane obstacle. A *ray* is simply a line perpendicular to the wave front. The point source of the sound wave is identified by **s**.

If there were no obstacle present, the wave would continue to move leftward toward point **s′**, which is shown to be as far to the left of the obstacle as point **s** is to the right of the obstacle. The obstacle, however, offers a large **acoustic impedance** to sound transmission. If the acoustic impedance is large, very little of the sound energy can

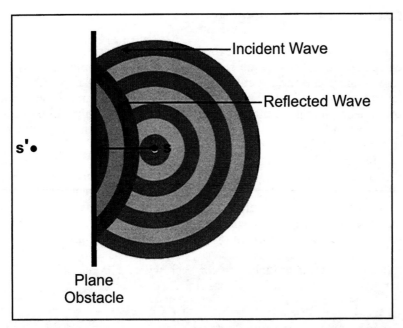

Figure 8–4. Sound wave **reflection**. A spherical wave front moving from right to left from a source **s** encounters a plane obstacle, such as a wall. The obstacle causes the sound wave to be **reflected** back toward the source with no change in speed of propagation. An observer will hear the reflected wave as having originated from point **s**', which is as far to the left of the obstacle as point **s** is to the right of the obstacle.

penetrate the wall. Instead, the sound wave is **reflected** back toward the source (**s**) *with no change in speed of propagation*, and the reflected wave that is moving from left to right toward the original point source also is shown in the figure. Because the speed of the **reflected wave** is identical to the speed of the incident wave, at any reference point in time the reflected wave will be just as far to the right of the plane surface as it would have been to the left of the plane surface had there been no obstacle.

The precise relation of reflected rays to incident rays conforms to the same rule that governed the path of the thrown ball in Figure 8–3; *the angle of reflected rays* (**r**) *to the perpendicular equals the angle of incident rays* (**i**) *to the perpendicular.* An observer located in the medium will perceive the reflected sound wave as having originated from point **s**', not point **s**. As a consequence of the sound wave being reflected, energy is retained in the medium. Because *energy is retained in the medium*, it should be apparent that the **inverse square law** does not hold for sound transmission in a medium with reflecting surfaces.

Reflection by Plane Surfaces

Figure 8–5 should serve to explain further the principle of sound wave reflection by a plane surface. In panel A, an incident ray (**i**) strikes the plane surface at an angle 45° to a line that is perpendicular to the plane surface. The incident ray is reflected, and the angle of the reflected ray (**r**) to the perpendicular also is 45°. In panel B of the figure, the angle of **i** to the perpendicular is 30°, and the angle of **r** to the perpendicular also is 30°.

In panel C, the angle of **i** is 0°. Therefore, the angle of **r** = 0° and the ray is reflected back on itself. Anyone who has successfully shot billiards or played pool in River City must be familiar with these concepts. The principle, therefore, is the same that we saw in Figure 8–3 for a ball thrown against a wall: *the angle of reflected rays to the perpendicular equals the angle of incident rays to the perpendicular.* That concept is important because, as you can see from Figure 8–4, there are a myriad of incident rays, each with a different angle to the perpendicular, that strike the obstacle.

Reflection by Convex Surfaces

The rule governing the relation of the angles of the reflected rays to the angles of the incident rays holds for other than plane surfaces. In panel A of Figure 8–6, a spherical wave moves from right to left toward an obstacle with a surface that is *convex* toward the source. As the wave fronts approach the obstacle at some considerable distance from the source, they are represented as plane waves rather than spherical waves. Two incident rays are shown, i_1 and i_2.

Because of the rule that specifies the angle of the reflected rays, we see that the reflected rays *diverge*. In a sense, the sound energy is scattered just as thrown balls would be scattered if they were thrown at various angles against a wall that is convex toward the thrower.

The divergence of the reflected rays in panel A of the figure describes what happens to a sound wave in air that strikes the *exterior* surface of a dome-shaped roof of a building. The rays of the reflected sound wave diverge. The intensity of the reflected sound wave at some distance from the surface will be less than the intensity of the incident sound wave at the same distance, because the sound energy in the reflected wave has been scattered.

Reflection by Concave Surfaces

In panel B of Figure 8–6, a plane progressive wave moves from right to left and encounters a surface that is *concave* toward the source. Four incident rays are shown and, as before, the angles of the reflected rays to the perpendicular equal the angles of the incident rays to the perpendicular. When the sound wave encounters the concave surface, the rays of the reflected wave *converge* toward a **focal point**, the point at which all reflected rays converge.

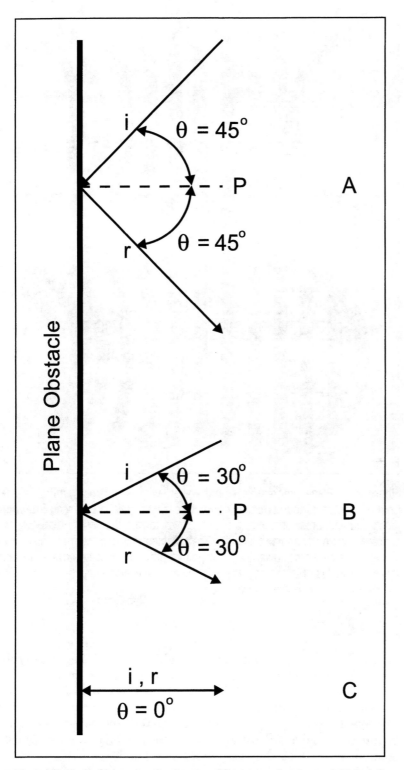

Figure 8–5. Incident rays, **i**, of a sound wave moving from right to left encounter a plane obstacle. The angles of the reflected rays, **r**, to the perpendicular are equal to the angles of the incident rays to the perpendicular.

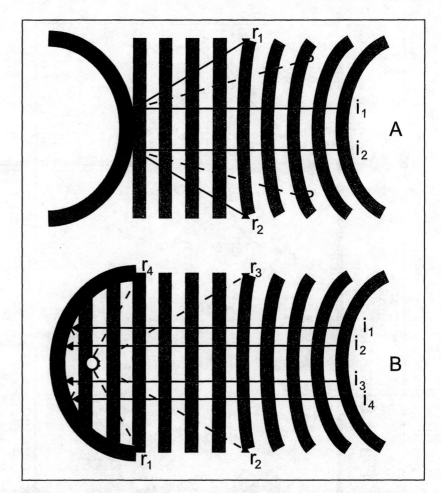

Figure 8–6. Plane progressive sound waves, with wave fronts sufficiently far from the source of sound that their curvature is negligible, are moving from right to left and encounter obstacles that are convex toward the source (panel A) and concave toward the source (panel B). The reflected rays diverge from the convex surface, but converge toward a focal point from the concave surface. In both cases, the angles of the reflected rays to the perpendicular equal the angles of the incident rays to the perpendicular.

Convergence of the reflected rays should help explain how "whispering galleries" work. Many readers will have had the experience of standing in a room that has a domed ceiling—a surface that is concave toward the floor. You try standing in several locations on one side of the room, and you discover that you cannot hear what someone is saying who is whispering from the other side of the room. If you then move to just the right point, which was previously marked on the floor, the same whispered speech is audible.

The point marked on the floor identifies the **focal point**, the point at which the rays of the whispered sound converge after having been reflected by the concave surface of the ceiling. The intensity of the reflected wave is greatest at the focal point, and, indeed, it is greater than the intensity of the incident wave because the sound energy, in a sense, has been "collected"; the **energy density**, or **intensity**, is maximal.

Perhaps you have observed a television crew at a sporting event such as a football game. The producer wants to enliven the audio portion of the broadcast by picking up the grunts, groans, and occasional profanities uttered by the players. The crew *does not point a microphone toward the playing field* to pick up the incident waves. Instead, the microphone is attached to a reflector (a "dish") that is held with its concave surface pointed toward the playing field. The microphone is pointed *away from the playing field and toward the reflector* so that it can pick up the reflected waves. If the microphone is mounted properly, the diaphragm of the microphone will be located at the focal point of the reflector where the intensity of the reflected sound waves will be greatest.

Echoes, Reverberation, and Reverberation Time

Reflected sound waves are sometimes called **echoes,** or **reverberating waves**, and rooms that have hard surfaces are called **reverberant rooms**. In contrast, rooms that are designed to minimize reverberation are called **anechoic rooms**, because they are designed to be nearly without echo, or reverberation.

If you have heard the echo of your voice bouncing from, for example, the walls of a canyon, you know that you can hear a few echoes, but finally they die away. The time required for the reflected wave to decay is called the **reverberation time**, which is defined as *the time required for a sound wave to be attenuated by 60 dB relative to its original level*. With the aid of Equation 4.4 from Chapter 4 you should be able to see why we also can say that **reverberation time** is defined as the time required for sound intensity to be attenuated to one-millionth of its original value.

One practical use of reflected waves was made in 1883 (Stewart, 1924). The explosion of a volcano in Krakatoa in the East Indies produced an intense compressional wave that progressed around the earth in all directions and converged at a point opposite Krakatoa. At that point, the wave was reflected back toward its source. From inspection of barometric records, the speed of propagation was measured to be 320 m/s, which stands in close agreement to modern, more technically accurate measures of the speed of sound.

Standing Waves

We have learned that when a sound wave is reflected by a surface, sound energy is retained in the medium. This gives rise to what are called **standing waves**. Standing waves occur when *two progressive* *waves, the incident wave and the reflected wave, of the same frequency and amplitude travel through the same medium in opposite directions.*

Transverse Wave Motion and Standing Waves

Transverse standing waves are illustrated in Figure 8–7. A string or wire is stretched tautly and is anchored at both ends. Dots have been painted on the string at equal intervals to help us observe their motion over time.

In panel A of Figure 8–7, the string is stretched with some fixed tension and the identifying points are labeled **a** through **k**. In panel B, a source of sound causes a transverse sound wave of some fixed frequency and amplitude to travel from *left to right* (the dashed line). At the same time, another sound source produces a second transverse wave *of identical amplitude and frequency* that travels in the opposite direction, from *right to left* (the solid line).

We learned in Chapter 1, with an unanchored stretched rope and only one transverse wave present, that each identifying point on the rope moves up and down with identical frequency. Now, because the string in Figure 8–7 is anchored, and because we have two identical transverse waves traveling in opposite directions, the pattern of movement of the points along the string is different from what we observed previously.

Points **b**, **d**, **f**, **h**, and **j** on the string move alternately upward and downward. Those points identify **displacement antinodes**, which are *points of maximum displacement* upward and downward. For example, at point **h**, the wave traveling from right to left shows a maximum downward displacement, whereas the wave traveling from left to right shows a maximum upward displacement. The other marked points on the string, **a**, **c**, **e**, **g**, **i**, and **k**, *remain stationary* at the equilibrium position. The string does not vibrate at those points, and points of "no vibration" are called **displacement nodes**. In summary, points of no vibration are called **displacement nodes** and points of maximum displacement, upward and downward, are called **displacement antinodes**.

Successive antinodes and nodes are spaced at equal intervals along the string, and between each pair of nodes, **loops** in the string are formed. The center of each loop corresponds to a **displacement antinode.** In panel C of Figure 8–7 we show just one cycle of each of the two transverse waves from panel B. Two loops have been formed and the locations of the displacement antinodes (**A**) and displacement nodes (**N**) are identified.

As we learned in Chapter 2, the distance traveled during one cycle defines the wavelength. Therefore, we can see that *the distance between successive antinodes (**A** to **A**) or between successive nodes (**N** to **N**) corresponds to one-half the wavelength of the moving waves.* For example, if the wavelength of each of the two waves is 1 m, the nodes will be spaced at intervals of 0.5 m and the antinodes

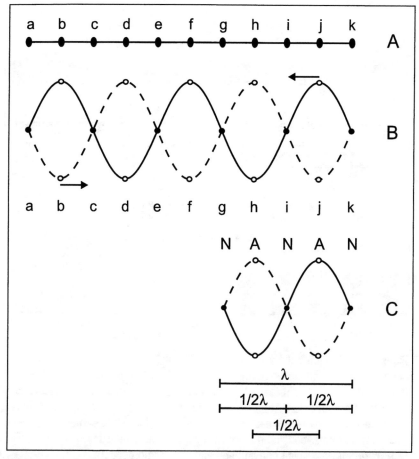

Figure 8–7. Creation of **standing**, or **stationary**, **waves** on a vibrating string that is stretched tautly and is anchored at both ends. Two trains of waves of identical amplitude and frequency are moving in opposite directions along the string. The wave shown by the solid line is moving from right to left and the wave shown by the dashed line is moving from left to right. Points b, d, f, h, and j on the string move alternately upward and downward over time and are called **displacement antinodes**, which are points of maximum vibratory movement. Points a, c, e, g, i, and k remain stationary and are called **displacement nodes**, which are points of no vibration. The distance between successive antinodes or between successive nodes is equal to one-half of the wavelength of the two waves moving in opposite directions.

also will be spaced at intervals of 0.5 m. Although each of the two waves in Figure 8–7 is moving, *the resultant wave is stationary,* which is why it is called a **standing wave**.

Longitudinal Wave Motion and Standing Waves

Standing waves also can be created with **longitudinal wave motion**. Panel A of Figure 8–8 shows an air-filled tube of uniform cross-sec-

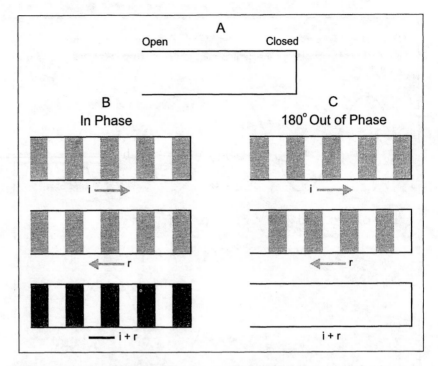

Figure 8–8. Creation of standing waves with longitudinal wave motion in a tube open at one end and closed at the other (panel A). Panel B shows incident waves moving from left to right toward the closed end of the tube and reflected waves moving from right to left. At that moment in time, the incident and reflected waves are precisely *in phase* with each other, which results in reinforcement. In panel C (one-fourth of a period later in time) the incident and reflected waves are precisely 180° *out of phase* with one another, and cancellation occurs.

tional area that is open at one end and closed at the other. Incident waves that travel from left to right in the tube will be reflected by the hard-surfaced closed end and travel in the air-filled tube in a direction opposite (right to left) to the direction of the incident wave. Therefore, we should expect that the incident waves and the reflected waves will interact all along the length of the tube. Both waves are characterized by alternate regions of **compression** (high density) and **rarefaction** (low density) and both move along the length of the tube, but in opposite directions.

Panel B of Figure 8–8 illustrates that, at a particular moment in time, the **compressions** (darker regions) of the *incident wave* moving from left to right are precisely aligned with—in phase with—the **compressions** of the *reflected wave* moving from right to left. One wave serves to maximally *reinforce* the other wave because the air particles are displaced maximally, and the result is a maximal increase in intensity. This also is called **constructive interference**.

In panel C of Figure 8–8, we see what happens one-fourth of a period later. At that moment in time, the compressions of the incident wave are 180° *out of phase* with the compressions of the reflected wave all along the length of the tube. The air medium in the tube cannot simultaneously, at that moment, be in a state of high density and a state of low density. Thus, the waves are said to "cancel" one another, and **cancellation** means that at that moment, the medium is not vibrating. This also is called **destructive interference**. At given points along the length of the tube, the medium will alternate over time from reinforcement (**constructive interference**) to cancellation (**destructive interference**) and the intensity of the sound wave at those points will alternately increase and decrease.

There are certain points (whose locations depend on the length of the tube and the wavelength of the sound waves) where the incident and reflected waves *are always in phase* with one another, and other points where the incident and reflected waves *are always 180° out of phase*. The interactions of the two waves produce **standing waves**. They are called standing waves because they appear to be "standing still" rather than to be moving along the tube. Both the incident wave and the reflected wave *are moving* along the tube in opposite directions. It is the resultant wave—the sum of the incident and reflected waves—that *is stationary*.

Figure 8–9 provides a further illustration of the interactions of incident and reflected waves. In each panel of the figure, the dotted line represents the incident wave moving from right to left and the dashed line represents the reflected wave moving from left to right. The solid line shows the resultant wave, which is the point-by-point summation over time of the incident and reflected waves. Each panel of the figure shows the status of events at a particular point in time, and each successive panel from top to bottom is separated by an interval equal to one-eighth of a period. Thus, if the frequency of the waves is 125 Hz, the period is 8 ms, and each successive group from panel A to panel F would be separated by an interval of 1 ms.

Consider what happens at a given location from moment to moment at, for example, the locations marked by the three *solid* vertical lines. The solid lines are positioned on **displacement antinodes**, which is similar to what was observed for point **b** in Figure 8–7. At those locations in panel A of Figure 8–9, the two waves are partially in phase with each other, and the displacement of the resultant wave (solid line) is greater than the displacement of either the incident or the reflected wave alone. That represents a **partial reinforcement**. In panel B (one-eighth of a period, or 1 ms, later), the two waves are in phase. The result is **maximal reinforcement**, and therefore maximal intensity, because the amplitudes of both the incident and the reflected waves are maximal and the amplitude of the resultant wave is the sum of those two waves.

In panel C of Figure 8–9, the resultant wave is identical to that observed in panel A. In panel D, the two waves are 180° out of phase, and the result is **cancellation**. In panel E, the displacements are identical to those in panel C, but in the opposite direction, and in panel F, maximum displacement in the opposite direction occurs.

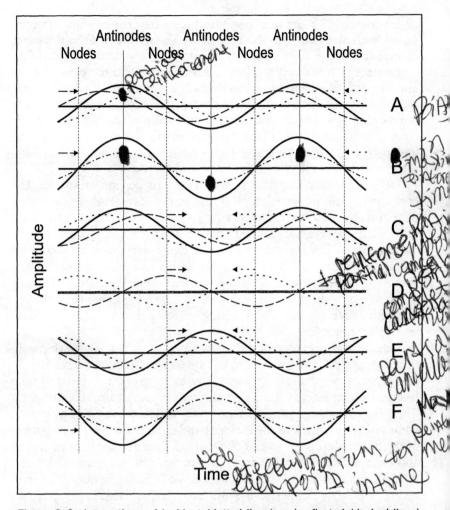

Figure 8–9. Interactions of incident (dotted lines) and reflected (dashed lines) waves of identical frequency and amplitude moving in opposite directions to produce resultant waves (solid lines) that vary in amplitude over time (from panel to panel). At the points indicated by the three solid vertical lines, we see that the resultant wave, over time, ranges from **partial reinforcement**, to **maximal reinforcement**, to **cancellation**, to **partial cancellation**. The points along the four dashed vertical lines represent nodes—points of no vibration. The resultant sound wave is a standing, or stationary, wave.

Next, note what happens at all of the locations that fall on the four *dashed* vertical lines in Figure 8–9. In a sense, nothing happens. The resultant wave (solid line) is always located on the time axis, regardless of whether it is part of a positively going displacement or of a negatively going displacement. Those points are **displacement nodes**, and as we can see, there is no vibratory motion at those locations. Thus, the dashed vertical lines identify **displacement nodes**, whereas the solid vertical lines identify **displacement antinodes**. **Displacement antinodes** are locations at which the amplitude of displacement alternates from maximally positive to maximally negative, and displacement nodes are points at which there is no upward and downward displacement.

Standing Waves and Resonant Frequency

Finally, let us examine the relation between sound wave reflection in an air-filled circular tube and the **resonant frequency** (actually resonant frequencies) of the tube. We will consider first a tube that is *open at one end and closed at the other end*, and begin with the most simple case where there is only one **displacement node** and one **displacement antinode**.

Panel A of Figure 8–10 shows the *displacement pattern* of an air mass in a tube that is *open at one end and closed at the other*. The solid horizontal line in the middle of the tube represents equilibrium (0°). All along the length of the tube, displacement of the air mass progresses upward in the tube through 45° (70.7% of maximum upward displacement) to maximum displacement at 90° (dashed line),

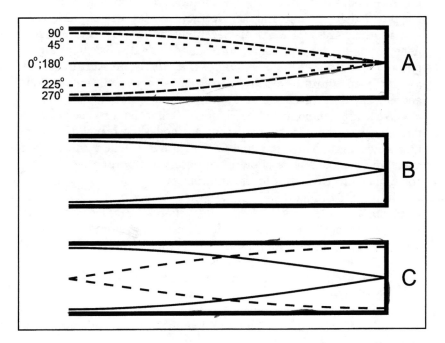

Figure 8–10. A tube open at one end and closed at the other. Panel A shows the changing displacement pattern over time from 0° through 360°. Panel B displays only the maximum displacements at 90° and 270° from panel A. In both panels A and B, a **displacement node** is located at the closed end of the tube, and a **displacement antinode** is located at the open end of the tube. In panel C, the displacement pattern is redrawn from panel B (solid lines) and contrasted with the pressure pattern for the tube (dashed lines). A **pressure node** is located at the open end of the tube, and a **pressure antinode** is located at the closed end.

then downward through equilibrium (solid line), on through 225° (70.7% of maximum downward displacement), to maximum displacement in the opposite direction at 270° (dashed line), and then returns upward to equilibrium. The two dashed lines (90° and 270°) thus display the *maximum displacement pattern* at 90° (upward) and 270° (downward), and they are redrawn in panel B of Figure 8–10 with solid lines, without showing the intermediate displacements between 90° and 270°. Thus, throughout the length of the tube, the air particles are displaced upward and downward over time, and panel B of Figure 8–10 shows only the envelopes (maximum displacements in either direction) of that displacement pattern.

A **displacement node**, a point of no vibration, *is always located at the closed end of the tube* because the air is not free to move at that location. A **displacement antinode**, a point of maximum displacement of air particles, *is always located at the open end* where the air can move freely.

We can also talk about **pressure nodes** and **pressure antinodes**. Both the *displacement pattern* (solid lines) and the *pressure pattern* (dashed lines) along the length of the tube are shown in panel C of Figure 8–10. To understand the relation between displacement and pressure nodes and antinodes, we should recall from Figure 2–11 in Chapter 2 that pressure and displacement are 90° out of phase with one another; pressure leads displacement by 90°. Thus, a **pressure node**, a point of zero pressure, corresponds to a **displacement antinode** and is located *at the open end of the tube*. A **pressure antinode**, a point of maximum pressure, corresponds to a **displacement node** and is located *at the closed end of the tube*.

We learned previously (see Figure 8–7) that the distance between two adjacent nodes (or two adjacent antinodes) corresponds to one-half wavelength. Thus, in panel C of Figure 8–7, where three nodes and two antinodes were shown, we observed that *one wavelength corresponds to two loops in the standing wave*.

In panel B of Figure 8–10 we see that *there is only one **displacement node** (located at the closed end) and one **displacement antinode** (located at the open end)*. Therefore, we have only one-half of one loop. Thus, in this simple case where there is only one node and one antinode, a standing wave pattern is created that has a wavelength that is *one-fourth the length of the wavelength of the incident wave*. If the frequency of the incident wave is four times the length of the tube (4L), a standing wave pattern is created.

Recall from Equation 2.12 in Chapter 2 that wavelength (λ) is given by:

$$\lambda = \frac{s}{f}.$$

By rearranging Equation 2.12 to solve for frequency (**f**), we see that:

Equation 8.5

$$f = \frac{s}{\lambda}.$$

In the case of the tube that is open at only one end, a standing wave pattern with only one node and one antinode is created when the frequency of the sound wave has a wavelength that is four times the length of the tube. Therefore, Equation 8.5 can be modified to read:

$$F_1 = \frac{s}{4L},$$

Equation 8.6

where **L** is the length of the tube

and

F₁ refers to the *center frequency of the first of a series of resonances.*

We say a "series of resonances" because a tube that is open at one end does not have just one node and one antinode. Instead, there are, in theory, an infinite number of nodes and antinodes and an infinite number of resonances. But to complete the discussion, we will refer to only three such resonances. What will be their resonant frequencies? We shall see that they are *odd integer multiples of the lowest resonant frequency,* **F₁.**

Panel A of Figure 8–11 shows the *lowest resonant frequency* for a tube that is open at one end and closed at the other. The pattern is

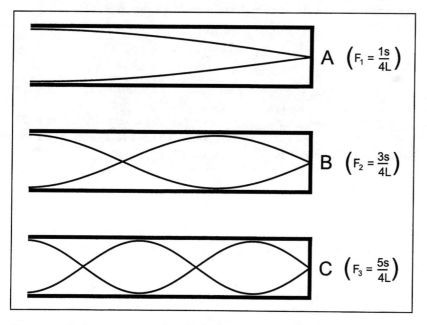

Figure 8–11. Panel A shows the displacement pattern again from Figure 8–10. One **displacement node** and one **displacement antinode** form one-half of a **loop**, which corresponds to the lowest resonant frequency of the tube, **F₁**. In panel B, two **nodes** and two **antinodes** form one and one-half **loops**, which corresponds to the next higher resonant frequency, **F₂**. A third standing wave pattern is shown in panel C; three **nodes** and three **antinodes** form two and one-half loops, which corresponds to **F₃**. All resonant frequencies are odd integer multiples of **F₁**.

identical to what was seen in panel B of Figure 8–10. Panel B of Figure 8–11 shows the next higher resonant frequency. In fitting this displacement pattern in the tube, we still must follow the rules that (1) a **displacement node** must be located at the closed end where the air is not free to move, and (2) a **displacement antinode** must be located at the open end of the tube where the air can move freely. As with the lowest resonant frequency in panel A, *the distance between a node and an adjacent antinode corresponds to 1/4 λ.*

Thus, in panel B of Figure 8–11, the next higher resonant frequency that will fit in the tube and obey those two rules has two nodes and two antinodes. Importantly, instead of one-half of one loop like we see in panel A, the displacement pattern in panel B has one and one-half loops. If one-half loop corresponds to 1/4 λ, then one and one-half loops must correspond to 3/4 λ. Thus, the equation for this next higher mode of vibration is:

Equation 8.7

$$F_2 = \frac{3s}{4L}.$$

In panel C, the third standing wave pattern still is constrained by restriction that there must be a displacement node at the closed end and a displacement antinode at the open end, and the resulting displacement pattern is shown to have two and one-half loops. Thus, the equation for this next higher mode of vibration is:

Equation 8.8

$$F_3 = \frac{5s}{4L}.$$

Thus, we see that the two higher modes of vibration, F_2 and F_3, *are odd integer multiples of the lowest resonant frequency, F_1.*

Suppose, for example, that the length of the tube in Figure 8–11 is 0.2 m. If we accept the speed of sound to be 340 m/s, with Equation 8.6 we calculate that the lowest resonant frequency, F_1, is 425 Hz:

$$F_1 = \frac{340}{4 \times .2} = 425 \text{ Hz}.$$

Next, with Equations 8.7 and 8.8, we see that the next two resonant frequencies, F_2 and F_3, are indeed odd-integer multiples of F_1:

$$F_2 = \frac{3 \times 340}{4 \times .2} = 1275 \text{ Hz, which} = 3 \times 425 \text{ Hz,}$$

and

$$F_3 = \frac{5 \times 340}{4 \times .2} = 2125 \text{ Hz, which} = 5 \times 425 \text{ Hz.}$$

Finally, equations 8.6, 8.7, and 8.8 can be consolidated to form Equation 8.9 so that it will apply more generally to *all resonances,* F_n, of an open-closed tube:

$$F_n = \frac{[(2n) - 1]s}{4L},$$

Equation 8.9

where **n** refers to the nth resonance.

Why are the resonant frequencies of a tube open at one end and closed at the other end restricted to odd-integer multiples of F_1 rather than odd *and* even integer multiples? Recall that a **displacement node** must be located at the closed end of the tube, and that a **displacement antinode** must be located at the open end of the tube. It would be impossible for waves that *are even integer multiples* of F_1 to have a node at the closed end and an antinode at the open end. For example, if F_1 corresponds to 1/4 λ, then $2 \times F_1$ must correspond to 1/2 λ. To fit a wave that is 1/2 λ into the tube, we would have to have either antinodes at both ends with a node in the middle, or nodes at both ends with an antinode in the middle. Neither circumstance is possible. For that reason, standing waves that are even integer multiples of the lowest resonant frequency *cannot exist* in a tube that is open at one end and closed at the other.

A tube that is either *open at both ends* (panel A of Figure 8–12) or *closed at both ends* (panel B of Figure 8–12) behaves differently from the tube that is open at only one end. If the tube is open at both ends (panel A), a **displacement antinode** is located at each end where the air can move freely. There must be at least one **displacement node** within the tube if there is to be a standing wave, and in Panel A we see a node located midway in the tube.

If the tube is closed at both ends (panel B), a **displacement node** is located at each end and a **displacement antinode** is located midway in the tube. In either case, an open-open or closed-closed tube, a standing wave pattern is created that has a wavelength that is 1/2 λ instead of 1/4 λ. Therefore, if the frequency of the incident wave is

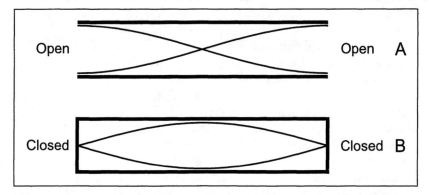

Figure 8–12. Standing wave patterns for the lowest resonant frequency in tubes open at both ends (panel A) or closed at both ends (panel B). In each case, the lowest resonant frequency corresponds to one full **loop**, 1/2 λ, that is formed either by two **antinodes** and one **node** (panel A) or two **nodes** and one **antinode** (panel B).

two times the length of the tube (2L), a standing wave pattern is created. Thus, for either of these tubes,

Equation 8.10
$$F_1 = \frac{s}{2L}.$$

If **L** is set at a fixed length such as 0.2 m, F_1 will be twice as high in frequency (850 Hz) for tubes closed at both ends or open at both ends as it would be for a tube that is open at only one end (425 Hz). Moreover, if the tube is either closed at both ends or open at both ends, successively higher resonant frequencies will be *odd and even* integer multiples of F_1. Thus, in Figure 8–12, the first three resonant frequencies for panel A and for panel B are 850 Hz, 1700 Hz, and 2550 Hz (odd and even integer multiples).

Equation 8.10 for F_1 is rewritten as Equation 8.11 to apply more generally to all resonant frequencies for open-open or closed-closed tubes:

Equation 8.11
$$F_n = \frac{ns}{2L},$$

where **n** is the nth resonance.

For those who are interested in the acoustics of speech production, the relation between standing wave patterns and resonant frequencies is quite important. During vowel production, for example, the vibratory movement of the vocal folds produces a complex quasiperiodic waveform that resembles a sawtooth wave in shape. The vocal tract, the cavity that extends from the vibrating vocal folds at one end to the mouth opening at the other end, is an air-filled resonator.

If the opening to the nasal cavity is closed by elevation of the soft palate, the vocal tract can be modeled, as a first approximation, to be a circular tube with uniform cross-sectional area that is open at one end (the mouth opening) and closed at the other end (the vibrating vocal folds). This configuration of the vocal tract is approximated when the talker utters what is called the *schwa* vowel, the first sound in the word "*a*bout." Suppose the talker is an adult male. The average length of the vocal tract for an adult male is .17 m.

With the aid of Equations 8.6, 8.7, and 8.8, or with the more general Equation 8.9, we calculate that the frequencies of the first three resonances for the tube with a length of .17 m are: F_1 = 500 Hz, F_2 = 1500 Hz, and F_3 = 2500 Hz. Note that each of the resonant frequencies is an odd integer multiple of F_1. If the vocal tract is shorter than .17 m, the frequencies of the resonances increase and, of course, if the vocal tract is longer, the frequencies of the resonances decrease because *resonant frequency is inversely proportional to the length of the tube*. In speech acoustics, and sometimes in musical acoustics, the resonances are called **formants**, and the center frequency of a formant is called the **formant frequency, F_n**.

Vibration of Strings

Equation 2.10 (Chapter 2) informed us that "the frequency" of a vibrating string is given by:

$$f = \frac{1}{2L}\sqrt{\frac{t}{m}},$$

where **L** = length, **t** = tension, and **m** = cross-sectional mass.

Thus, we learned that frequency of vibration of a string is inversely proportional to twice the length of the string, directly proportional to the square root of the tension, and inversely proportional to the square root of the mass. We placed "the frequency" in quotation marks because the string actually vibrates in many modes simultaneously (with many different frequencies of vibration), and Equation 2.10 provides the solution for only *the lowest of those frequencies*, which is the **fundamental frequency** of the vibrating string.

The string also vibrates at frequencies that are **harmonics** of the fundamental frequency, and we shall see that *the harmonic frequencies are odd and even integer multiples of the fundamental, or lowest, frequency in the series*. By examining the displacement pattern of the string during vibration, we can learn why there is energy at harmonic frequencies as well as at the fundamental frequency.

The string is a low-damped, narrowly tuned elastic system, and, after having been displaced from equilibrium, it continues to vibrate at its **natural frequency** for some considerable amount of time. When the string is displaced, waves travel along the string in both directions, and after reaching the ends where the string is fixed on pegs, the waves are reflected back in the opposite direction. Many of those reflected waves interfere (**destructive interference**) with one another, and their energy is dissipated. On the other hand, waves with a frequency corresponding to the **natural**, or **resonant**, **frequencies** of the string continue to travel.

The solid line of Panel A of Figure 8–13 shows a string that is attached at either end to pegs, and then stretched to be rather taut. The dashed line in panel A shows the string after it has been displaced from equilibrium.

The array of dashed lines in panel B of Figure 8–13 shows a series of displacement patterns over time after the string has been displaced and then released. The string is displaced over its full length from equilibrium (0°) upward to some maximum displacement (90°), downward through equilibrium (180°) and beyond to some maximum displacement in the opposite direction (270°), and then back to equilibrium (360°). That describes *one cycle of vibration*, and as we learned previously, the time required to complete one such cycle of vibration defines the **fundamental period**, **T**. The reciprocal of **T**, **1/T**, yields the **fundamental frequency**, **f₀**.

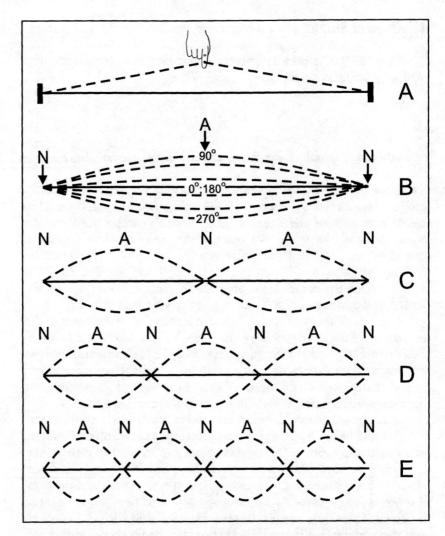

Figure 8–13. Displacement pattern of a vibrating string. In panel A, a stretched string is displaced. Panel B shows the displacement pattern over time from 0° through 360° for the lowest resonant frequency; one **loop** is formed by two **displacement nodes** and one **displacement antinode**. Panels C, D, and E show higher modes of vibration of the string (higher resonant frequencies) as more and more **loops** are formed by an increasing number of **nodes** and **antinodes**. All resonant frequencies of the string are odd and even integer multiples of F_1, which for a string is usually called f_0, the **fundamental frequency**.

In panel B of Figure 8–12 we see that there are **displacement nodes (N)** at the two fixed ends of the string where the string is not free to vibrate, and a single **displacement antinode (A)** midway between the fixed ends where the string can vibrate freely. As we learned previously, **standing waves** occur when two progressive waves, an **incident wave** and a **reflected wave**, of the same frequency and amplitude travel through the same medium in opposite directions. Importantly, *those standing waves occur at more than a single frequency*, and panel B of Figure 8–12 shows only the *lowest* frequency at which a standing wave is created: the **fundamental frequency, f_0, or first frequency, f_1**.

With two displacement nodes and one displacement antinode in panel B of Figure 8–12, a single **loop** is formed. Recall that one loop corresponds to one-half wavelength. Because the single loop in panel B corresponds to one-half wavelength, the equation for the **fundamental**, or **lowest, frequency** is:

$$f_0 = \frac{s}{2L},$$

Equation 8.12

where f_0 is the fundamental frequency,

s is the speed of sound along the string $\left(s = \sqrt{\frac{t}{m}}\right)$,

and

L is the length of the string.

Thus, the standing wave pattern for a vibrating string that is fixed at both ends behaves likes the standing wave pattern for a tube that is either open at both ends or closed at both ends. Therefore, we should expect that the higher modes of vibration for the vibrating string would be *both odd and even integer multiples of the lowest frequency*.

Finally, we can modify Equation 8.12 so that it will apply more generally to situations in which more than a single loop appears on the string:

$$f_n = \frac{ns}{2L},$$

Equation 8.13

where **n** is the nth frequency, which corresponds to

the number of **loops** that are formed on the string.

By way of example, if the length (**L**) of the string is 1.68 m, and the speed (**s**) of wave transmission along the string is 420 m/s, the frequency of the first harmonic (h_1 or f_0) is:

$$f_0 = \frac{ns}{2L}$$

$$= \frac{(1 \times 420)}{(2 \times 1.68)}$$

$$= 125 \text{ Hz}$$

Why does the sound wave generated by a string have energy at odd and even harmonics of the fundamental frequency? Because the string vibrates in many modes and, as a consequence, additional displacement nodes and antinodes are located along the length of the string. Hence, *more than one single loop is formed.* In panel C of Figure 8–13, there are three **displacement nodes** and two **displacement antinodes**, which combine to form *two loops*. In panel D, *three loops* are formed by the presence of four **displacement nodes** and three **displacement antinodes**. Finally, in panel E, five **displacement nodes** and four **displacement antinodes** result in the formation of *four loops*. As before, each loop corresponds to one-half wavelength, and with Equation 8.13 we calculate that the frequencies of vibrations for the same string in panels C, D, and E are, respectively:

$$f_2 = \frac{(2 \times 420)}{(2 \times 1.68)} = 250 \text{ Hz,}$$

$$f_3 = \frac{(3 \times 420)}{(2 \times 1.68)} = 375 \text{ Hz,}$$

and

$$f_4 = \frac{(4 \times 420)}{(2 \times 1.68)} = 500 \text{ Hz,}$$

The coefficients (**n**) are integers. Because all other terms in Equation 8.13 for a given string are constant, we see that each of the frequencies of vibration is an integer multiple of the lowest frequency. Thus, the second harmonic $(2f_0)$, the third harmonic $(3f_0)$, the fourth harmonic $(4f_0)$, and so forth are created.

The important concepts are that (a) the string vibrates in a complex manner, (b) standing waves are created that correspond to the natural frequencies of the string, (c) the natural frequencies (and the corresponding standing waves) are dependent on the length of the string and the speed of wave transmission along the string, and (d) when the string is displaced, it vibrates in all of its modes. The actual displacement pattern of the string on a musical instrument depends on whether the string is plucked or bowed, and the student who is interested in more details concerning musical acoustics might wish to consult Backus (1977), among others.

■ REFRACTION

We observed previously in our discussion of sound wave **reflection** that when an incident wave strikes an obstacle with a large acoustic impedance, the wave is reflected by the obstacle *with no change in speed of propagation.* Because there is no change in speed, at any given moment, the **reflected wave** is just as far from the obstacle in one direction as the **incident wave** would have been in the other direction if the obstacle had not been present.

Suppose, instead, that the sound wave passes from one medium of transmission, **M₁**, to another medium, **M₂**, *and* suppose that the speed of sound for M_1 (s_{M_1}) *does not equal* the speed of sound for M_2 (s_{M_2}). When this happens, the ray is bent and the direction of wave propagation changes.

Consider the light waves depicted in Figure 8–14. A stick is held in air, M_1, and is pointed at the surface of water, M_2, at various angles to the surface. Some of the light energy will penetrate the surface of the water. The speed of light is different in the two media and, for light, $s_{M_1} > s_{M_2}$. The stick is not really "bent," but because of the differences in speed of propagation of light waves in air and water, the *image* of the stick appears to be bent at the surface of the water because the ray bends toward the perpendicular (dashed line) when the ray enters the water. That perception is due to a change in speed of wave propagation in accordance with Snell's law.

As we move from left to right in Figure 8–14, the angle of the **incident ray** (the stick) to the surface decreases, and the appearance of bending is lessened. At the far right, the incident ray is perpendicular to the surface, and under this circumstance, the angle of the **refracted ray** to the surface, the image of the stick in water, equals the angle of the **incident ray** to the surface.

The phenomenon shown in Figure 8–14 for light waves also happens when a sound wave penetrates a new medium (for example, air to water) or encounters a change in the "conditions" of a medium that causes *the speed of wave propagation* to be changed. The rays of the incident wave are bent; they are **refracted**. Thus, **refraction** can be defined as *a bending of the sound waves, or a change in the direction of sound-wave propagation, due to a change in speed of propagation.*

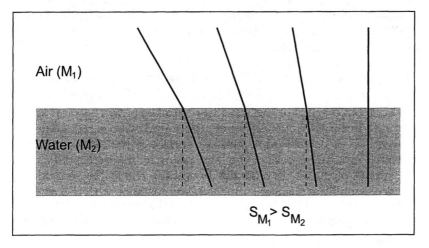

Figure 8–14. Refraction. A stick is pointed at the surface of a body of water at various angles. The ray of light corresponding to the image of the stick in the water appears to be bent as it passes from one medium (air) to a different medium (water) because the speeds of propagation are different in the two transmitting media. The bending of the light rays is called **refraction**.

Examples of Refraction and Reflection

We can use our understanding of wave **reflection** and wave **refraction** to explain some natural occurrences in sound transmission. For example, why does sound "carry better," that is, travel over a greater distance, when it travels *with the wind* as opposed to when it travels *against the wind*. It is tempting to assume that when traveling with the wind, the wind somehow "carries the sound wave along," and that when traveling against the wind, the wind "pushes the sound wave back" toward the source. Actually, the effect of the wind in that sense is negligible.

The answer comes from a combination of wave reflection and wave refraction as is shown in Figure 8–15. In panel A of the figure, we show a series of **spherical wave fronts** being propagated from left to right toward some receiver, **R**. If there were no wind, and if wave reflection and refraction did not occur, the wave would look much like you see in panel A. We see one ray of the wave that is parallel to the surface of the ground and progressing toward the receiver.

Now suppose we introduce a windy condition. First we must note that *wind speed normally increases with increasing height above ground*. Therefore, in panel B wind speed is shown as a vector quantity in which the lengthening of the vectors with increasing height reflects the increasing wind speed blowing from left to right in the direction of the arrows.

In panel C of Figure 8–15, the sound wave is propagated from left to right *against the wind* that is blowing from right to left. The greater wind speeds at the higher elevations serve to impede sound wave propagation more than the lesser wind speeds at the lower elevations near the ground. Thus, the higher the elevation, the less the speed of wave propagation. Because of the change in speed with elevation above the surface, the sound wave is **refracted** (bent) upward and the sound energy is directed upward into the atmosphere and well above the receiver.

The opposite occurs when sound is propagated *with the wind*. Thus, we see in panel D of Figure 8–15 that when traveling with the wind, the greater wind speed at increasingly higher elevations causes the upper reaches of the wave fronts to travel with greater speed than the lower portions. As before, the sound wave is **refracted**, but now it is bent downward toward the surface of the earth. It then is **reflected** upward because of the large **acoustic impedance** offered by the surface of the earth, **refracted** downward, and so on. As a consequence, sound travels over a much greater distance with the wind. If you are lost and shout for help, you should hope that there will be someone who is downwind from you who has a chance of hearing your plea.

Consider one final example of what might be called "environmental influences" on sound transmission. Why does sound (typically) travel farther early in the morning than at midday? Normally, the air near the ground has cooled overnight so that in the early morning, the air is warmer at higher elevations above the surface of

Figure 8–15. Sound wave **refraction**. Differential effects of a sound wave being propagated against the wind and with the wind. In panel A there is no wind, and the wave fronts progress from left to right unaltered. Because wind speed varies as a function of height above the ground (panel B), the wind offers different amounts of resistance to different portions of the wave front. Against the wind (panel C), the wind offers greater opposition to the upper reaches of the wave fronts, and the sound wave is refracted over the receiver and into the atmosphere. With the wind (panel D), the wind causes the upper reaches of the wave fronts to be propagated with greater speed, and the sound wave is refracted toward the surface of the earth, reflected by the earth's surface, refracted downward, reflected upward, and so on. As a consequence, sound travels over a greater distance with the wind.

the earth. We know from Chapter 1 (Equation 1.16) that the speed of sound is directly proportional to the square root of elasticity of the medium and inversely proportional to the square root of the density of the medium. As temperature increases, density decreases, and therefore the speed of sound is directly proportional to the temperature.

Suppose you and your partner are sitting in a canoe on a lake early in the morning. To keep matters simple, also suppose there is virtually no wind and that the surface of the water is glassy. You notice that a couple is sitting in another canoe at some considerable distance across the lake. To your surprise, you can hear them fairly easily, which means that the sound has traveled a long way.

The explanation is given by refraction and reflection, as is illustrated in panel A of Figure 8–16. The speed of sound increases with increasing distance above the surface because of the presence of warmer air. As a consequence, the sound wave is **refracted** downward, **reflected** by the surface of the water, **refracted** downward, and so on. The result is that the sound wave travels over a long distance.

You return to the same spot on the lake later in the day and see the same couple across the lake. You have a hunch that they are talking again, but this time you cannot hear them. As we see in panel B of Figure 8–16, by now the sun has warmed the air near the surface of the water so that the air *is cooler with increasing height* above ground. Thus, the speed of sound is greater at the lower elevations, and the sound waves created by the couple are **refracted** upward into the atmosphere.

Note, that when we described the early morning condition in panel A of Figure 8–16, we said that sound travels farther early in the morning because the sound wave is refracted downward toward the surface of the water, *reflected upward by the surface,* and so forth. Why doesn't the sound that is refracted downward simply penetrate the water and travel as a sound wave in water?

Figure 8–16. Sound wave **refraction**. Differential effects of a sound wave in air propagated in the early morning (panel A) when the surface of the earth has cooled over night and later in the day (panel B) when the surface of the earth has been warmed. Because temperature of the air varies with height above ground (warmer in the morning; cooler later in the day) and speed of propagation is directly proportional to temperature of the transmitting medium, the sound wave is refracted. Early in the morning, the sound wave is refracted toward the surface, reflected by the surface, and so on. Hence, sound travels over a great distance. Later in the day, the sound wave is refracted upward into the atmosphere.

The **acoustic impedance** of water is much greater than the acoustic impedance of air. Thus, there is an *impedance mismatch* between the two media. About 0.1% of the incident sound energy penetrates the surface and travels as a sound wave in the water, and approximately 99.9% of the sound energy *is reflected by the surface of the water* and retained in the air medium. With the aid of Equation 4.4 in Chapter 4, we can calculate that the intensity of sound in air is attenuated by approximately 30 dB when it penetrates the surface of the water because,

$$dB = 10 \log \frac{I_x}{I_r}$$

$$= 10 \log \frac{1 \times 10^{-3}}{1 \times 10^0}$$

$$= 10 \log (1 \times 10^{-3})$$

$$= -30 \text{ dB}.$$

■ DIFFRACTION

Most of us have observed that when water waves encounter a pier, a dock, or some other obstacle, the water is not "parted" (unless it is the Red Sea). Instead, it "bends" around the obstacle and the wave motion continues as if the obstacle had not been present. Sound waves behave in the same way, and the bending or scattering of a sound wave around an obstacle is called **diffraction**.

The amount of **diffraction** that occurs depends on *the size of the obstacle relative to the wavelength of the wave*. **Diffraction** is more efficient when the wavelength of the sound wave is much larger than the size of the obstacle. Thus, it should be apparent that diffraction varies with frequency, because as wavelength increases, frequency decreases.

Consider, for example, a water wave. If the wave encounters a small obstacle such as a reed, the wave will be diffracted around the reed almost as if the reed were not there. If the wave encounters a larger object such as a floating log or an anchored boat, the wave will be diffracted, but there will be a "shadow region" immediately behind the object that shows no evidence of wave motion. More distant from the obstacle, the wave will reform and continue on.

In panel A of Figure 8–17 a plane progressive sound wave is traveling from left to right in a large room and encounters a barrier. If the size of the barrier is large relative to the wavelength of the sound wave, most of the energy will be reflected back toward the source. In this case, however, the size of the barrier is small relative to the wavelength of the incident wave. Of course, some of the sound energy will be reflected from right to left by the barrier as the leftward pointing *dashed* arrows represent.

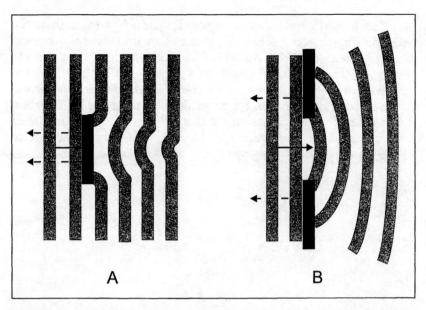

Figure 8–17. Diffraction of waves around an obstacle (panel A) and diffraction of sound waves through an opening (panel B).

We also can see that the wave fronts are **diffracted** and they then converge at the right side of the barrier. At some distance away from the obstacle the shape of the wave fronts is nearly identical to the shape that we would have seen had the obstacle not been present. A person sitting some distance to the right of the obstacle will hear the sound in a nearly unaltered state.

The sound wave, after bending around the obstacle, continues as a plane progressive wave from left to right until finally, in panel B of the figure, it encounters an opening in the wall (a window). Again, some of the sound energy will be reflected by the wall. In addition, the portion of the wave front "striking" the opening will pass through and re-form on the outside of the room. The implication should be obvious. A person standing near the window on the outside of the room can hear the sound that was transmitted in the room.

Think about another experience that you might have had. You are relaxing in a living room while listening to music emanating from a good sound system. You can appreciate the full range of the music from the bass to the treble. Then, you leave the room, walk down a hallway, and turn off into another room. You can still hear the music, but now it "sounds different." The bass notes are more prominent than the treble. That occurs because the long wavelengths of the bass notes are more likely to be diffracted (scattered around) the obstacles (walls of the hallway and rooms) than the shorter wavelengths of the treble notes.

■ ABSORPTION

When the concept of sound wave **reflection** was introduced, we said that when obstacles in the medium offer a large acoustic impedance to the propagation of the wave, much of the sound energy is **reflected** back toward the source. The sound wave need not encounter a dense, rigid obstacle such as a steel wall to encounter impedance that causes the sound wave to be reflected.

Opposition to sound transmission will exist at *any* boundary between different transmitting media that have different impedances. We have already seen, for example, that sound waves traveling in air are impeded by the surface of water, and when that occurs, transmission of sound is affected. Very little of the sound energy is absorbed by the medium, and most (99.9%) of the energy is reflected by the surface of the water and retained in the air medium.

If the impedance offered by the obstacle is *infinite*, the intensity of the reflected wave will equal the intensity of the incident wave. It should be apparent, however, that different materials will offer different amounts of acoustic impedance. For example, a wall made of steel impedes sound transmission more than a wall made of wood, which, in turn, impedes the transmission of sound more than a wall made of cotton batting.

If the impedance offered by the obstacle *is not infinite*, some of the sound energy will penetrate the material of the obstacle, and that defines **sound wave absorption**. Some of the energy is **absorbed** by the obstacle that the sound wave encounters. In that case, it stands to reason that the intensity of the reflected wave will be less than the intensity of the incident wave because some of the sound energy has been absorbed.

The Absorption Coefficient (α)

Sound wave absorption is quantified in a very simple way. The magnitude of absorption is given by the **absorption coefficient** (α), and the absorption coefficient is the ratio of the sound energy absorbed (I_a) to the sound energy contained in the incident wave (I_i),

$$\alpha = \frac{I_a}{I_i}.$$

Equation 8.14

Let us return to the situation in which a sound wave traveling in air encounters the surface of a water medium. Approximately 99.9% of the sound energy is reflected by the surface of the water and 0.1% is absorbed by the water medium. Suppose the sound pressure level of the incident wave is 70 dB. That means that its intensity is 10^{-5} watt/m^2 (Equation 4.4 from Chapter 4). If only 0.1% of the sound energy is absorbed by the water medium, that means that the intensity of the sound wave in water will be 40 dB SPL and that the absorption coefficient is 0.001 (10^{-3}).

Thus, the **absorption coefficient** is simply the *proportion* of energy in the incident wave that is absorbed by the material of the obstacle. From the calculation above, we have seen that because 0.1% of the sound energy is absorbed by the water medium, the intensity of the sound wave traveling in water will be attenuated by 30 dB. If 99.9% of the sound energy is reflected back into the air by the surface of the water, by how much would the reflected wave be attenuated?

$$dB = 10 \log 0.999 = 0.0043 \text{ dB}.$$

As with any proportion, the absorption coefficient can, in theory, vary between 1 (all of the energy is absorbed; none is reflected) and 0 (all of the energy is reflected; none is absorbed). In the example above, an absorption coefficient of 0.001 means that very little (0.1%) of the energy of the sound wave is absorbed by the water.

It is important to note that the absorption coefficient *is independent of the intensity of the incident wave*. Thus, if the SPL of the incident wave had increased from 70 dB SPL to 90 dB SPL, the absorption coefficient would still be 0.001, 99.9% of the sound energy would be reflected by the surface of the water and retained in the air medium, and the SPL of the sound wave in water would then be approximately 60 dB SPL.

Sound-Treated Rooms

Rooms that are designed to minimize reverberations, or sound wave reflections, are called **anechoic** rooms. If a room is to approach being **anechoic**, nearly all of the sound energy transmitted within the room must be absorbed; that is, the room must have a very high **absorption coefficient**.

To create an **anechoic** room, fiberglass wedges are fixed to all six surfaces of the room. Because fiberglass has a high absorption coefficient, it acts as an "acoustic sponge." If the exterior surfaces of the room are made of steel or some other material with a very low absorption coefficient, then, in addition to being **anechoic**, the room is also **sound isolated** because virtually no sound exterior to the room will penetrate the steel walls and be transmitted as sound waves within the room.

Rooms that are **sound isolated** and reasonably **anechoic** are commonly used to test the status of a person's hearing and to conduct experiments in hearing. Thus, the person being tested is isolated from sound outside the room to minimize interference with the sound waves generated inside the room for the test or experiment. Moreover, if the sound waves in the room are transduced by a loudspeaker instead of earphones, very little of the sound energy will be reflected by the highly absorbent walls and be retained in the medium to interfere with the incident waves.

Absorption and Reflection

It should be apparent that sound wave **absorption** *is inversely proportional to sound wave **reflection***. Thus, as the absorption coefficient increases, sound wave reflection decreases and reverberation time decreases. Although the absorption coefficient of different materials varies with the frequency of the incident wave, we will choose a single mid-range frequency of 1000 Hz and see how the proportion of sound energy absorbed varies among common materials in a room (Backus, 1977).

Walls made of unpainted concrete, marble, or glazed tile have an absorption coefficient of about 0.01. Thus, those materials absorb about 10 times as much sound energy as we saw with the surface of the water where the absorption coefficient was about 0.001. If we fix a heavy carpet to the walls, the absorption coefficient increases from 0.01 to about 0.37, and approximately one-third of the energy is absorbed by the material. But, of course, there might be other materials in the room that would contribute to the absorption of sound: upholstered seats, clothing apparel, and people's skin. Some sound energy is even absorbed by the air medium itself, and the amount of energy absorbed depends on the temperature and humidity of the air and the frequency of the sound wave.

We noted above that *the absorption coefficient covaries with the nature of the material and the frequency of the incident sound wave*. The relation, however, is not a simple one. With some materials, the absorption coefficient *increases* with increasing frequency. For example, in the frequency range from 125 Hz to 4000 Hz, the coefficient for thick carpeting installed over concrete increases from .02 (2% of the energy is absorbed) at 125 Hz, to .37 (37% of the energy is absorbed) at 1000 Hz, to .65 (65% of the energy is absorbed) at 4000 Hz. If the same carpeting is installed over a felt pad laid on the concrete, the coefficient increases at some frequencies (e.g., from .06 to .27 at 125 Hz, and from .14 to .39 at 500 Hz), decreases at some frequencies (e.g., from .60 to .48 at 2000 Hz), and remains essentially the same for other frequencies (e.g., from .37 to .34 at 1000 Hz, and from .65 to .63 at 4000 Hz).

With other materials, the absorption coefficient *decreases* with increasing frequency. Plywood (1/4 in.) is an example of this inverse relation. The absorption coefficient is .60 at 125 Hz, .30 at 250 Hz, and ranges from .09 to .10 for frequencies from 500 Hz to 4000 Hz. Finally, there are some materials for which the absorption coefficient is largely *independent* of frequency. The coefficients range from .01 to .02 for glazed tile, from .01 to .03 for unpainted concrete, and from .02 to .03 for asphalt tile laid on concrete. One of the very best sound-absorbing materials is suspended acoustical tiling for which the absorption coefficients range from a low of .76 at 125 Hz to a high of .99 at 1000 and 2000 Hz.

In the foregoing discussion of absorption, we called attention only to the absorption of sound energy by materials in, for example, a room. The *total* sound energy absorbed in a room, however, depends not only on the absorption coefficients of the materials in the room, but also on *the volume of the room*. Total absorption is usually quantified in **absorption units**, and the unit of measure is the **sabine** (fps) or **metric sabine** (MKS) in honor of Wallace C. Sabine who performed pioneering empirical studies on architectural acoustics at Harvard University near the turn of the 19th century.

Imagine a large, bare room with hard interior surfaces and an opening (window) in one wall with an area of 1 m^2. There is no carpeting, upholstery, or other sound-absorbing materials in the room. The opening can effectively "absorb" all of the sound energy that strikes it, and it therefore has an **absorption coefficient**, α, of 1.0 (100% of the sound energy is absorbed). That defines one **absorption unit**, which is expressed as one **sabine** (fps) or one **metric sabine** (MKS). Thus, a **sabine** is the total absorption for one square foot of window opening, and a **metric sabine** is the total absorption for a window with an area of one square meter.

How do **absorption** and **reflection** interact? In the room described above, each of the six surfaces can be assumed to absorb the same amount of sound energy. The theoretical **reverberation time**, T_{60}, for such a room is *directly proportional* to the volume of the room, **V**, and *inversely proportional* to the area of the opening, **A**:

Equation 8.15

$$T_{60} = k\frac{V}{A},$$

where **k** is a constant.

The value of **k** is .049 in the fps system, where volume is expressed in cubic feet and area in square feet, but .161 in the MKS system, where volume is expressed in cubic meters and area in square meters.

We can see from Equation 8.15 that if room volume increases by same factor, with area of the window held constant, T_{60} increases by the same factor, and sound energy is retained in the room for a longer time. If room volume is held constant, but the area of the opening is increased by some factor, T_{60} decreases by the same factor, and sound energy escapes from the room more quickly.

Suppose we cover the opening (1 m^2) with an "ideal" material that also has an **absorption coefficient** of 1.0. Sound energy, of course, would now dissipate at the same rate that it did with the uncovered opening. If another material is substituted that has an **absorption coefficient** of 0.5, what will be the **total absorption**? **Total absorption** is given by *the product of the surface area of the covered opening and the absorption coefficient of the material*. Thus,

Equation 8.16

$$A \text{ (sabine or metric sabine)} = S\alpha,$$

where **A** is total absorption, **S** is surface area, and

α is the absorption coefficient.

For example, if **S** = 1 m^2 and α = 0.5, we have 0.5 **metric sabines**. Then, if α remains 0.5, but **S** is increased to 2 m^2, we have 1 **metric sabine**.

Equation 8.16 enables us to calculate the **total absorption** where there is only one absorbing surface, in this case, one covered opening. Equation 8.17 applies to the more general case where the room has multiple absorbing surface:

$$A' = S_1\alpha_1 + S_2\alpha_2 + ... + S_n\alpha_n.$$

Equation 8.17

Thus, the **total absorption** for multiple absorbing surfaces *equals the sum of the total absorption of the individual surfaces*. For example, for four absorbing surfaces with different values of **S** and α, with each expressed in metric units (MKS), A′ would be

$$A' = (1.0 \times 0.5) + (2.0 \times 0.5) + (1.0 \times .68) + (2.0 \times .39)$$

$$= 2.96 \text{ metric sabines}.$$

Recall that *sound absorption is inversely proportional to sound reflection*. Too much absorption, with correspondingly decreased reverberation, results in a "dead" room, and at the extreme, an **anechoic room**. Too little absorption, with correspondingly increased reflection, results in a "live" room, and at the extreme, a **reverberant room**.

What is the optimum **reverberation time**, T_{60}? The optimum **reverberation time** for a large room, such as an auditorium, becomes a compromise between satisfactory clarity on one hand (clarity decreases as T_{60} increases) and satisfactory sound intensity (maximum intensity increases as T_{60} increases) on the other hand. Moreover, the optimal reverberation time is different for speech and music, and, in some instances, the optimal value varies with room volume. For speech in a conference room, optimal T_{60} ranges between 400 ms and 800 ms, whereas optimal T_{60} ranges between 900 ms and 1400 ms for chamber music, and ranges between 1500 ms and 2400 ms for organ music (Backus, 1977).

Sample Computations

Suppose we have a classroom with the dimensions 8 m wide, 15 m long, and 3 m high. Reverberation time varies with frequency, but we will compute T_{60} only for 500 Hz. If the floor is covered with a heavy carpet ($\alpha = 0.4$) and the walls and ceiling are constructed with plaster ($\alpha = 0.1$), the total absorption, **A′**, is computed as follows with Equation 8.17:

	Surface Dimensions	*Surface Area* (**S**)	α	**A**
Side wall 1	15 × 3	45	0.10	4.5
Side wall 2	15 × 3	45	0.10	4.5
End wall 1	8 × 3	24	0.10	2.4
End wall 2	8 × 3	24	0.10	2.4
Floor	8 × 15	120	0.40	48.0
Ceiling	8 × 15	120	0.10	12.0
			A′ =	**73.8.**

The volume of the room is 360 m^3 (15 × 3 × 8). Finally, with Equation 8.15, but with A' instead of A in the denominator, we calculate T_{60} to be:

$$T_{60} = k \frac{V}{A'}$$

$$= .161 \frac{360}{73.8}$$

$$= 785 \text{ ms.}$$

Thus, with a room volume of 360 m^3 and a **total absorption** of 73.8 **metric sabines**, the **reverberation time**, T_{60}, is about 785 ms. That might be longer than is desirable. Suppose, then, that we place acoustical tile with $\alpha = 0.76$ on the ceiling and on one wall at the end of the room toward which the instructor is facing. The **total absorption, A'**, is increased from 73.8 to 168.8 **metric sabines**. Then we compute the new value of T_{60} to be

$$T_{60} = k \frac{V}{A'}$$

$$= .161 \frac{360}{168.8}$$

$$= 343 \text{ ms.}$$

Thus, the addition of the acoustical tile on the ceiling and one end wall decreased T_{60} from 785 ms to 343 ms.

We all know, of course, that installing carpeting in a classroom is problematic because of the potential for stain from spillage. Now that acoustical tile has been placed on the ceiling and one end wall, if we decide to install asphalt tile on the floor with an absorption coefficient, α, of .03 instead of a heavy carpeting with an absorption coefficient of .40, what will happen to T_{60}? We know that the reverberation time will increase, but will it lie in an acceptable range?

The **total absorption, A'**, is decreased from 168.8 to 124.4 **metric sabines**. Finally, we compute the new value of T_{60} to be:

$$T_{60} = k \frac{V}{A'}$$

$$= .161 \frac{360}{124.4}$$

$$= 466 \text{ ms.}$$

Thus, when the carpeting is replaced with asphalt tile, we should expect T_{60} to be approximately 466 ms, and that lies in the acceptable range of 400–800 ms.

There are several caveats that should be noted. One, the sample computations were made for only a single frequency, 500 Hz, and different results would be obtained for other frequencies. Two, the room did not contain seats or people. Even wooden chairs absorb sound energy, and each person in the room might add as many as 3 to 5 absorption units. Beranek (1960), however, has claimed that total absorption for a half-filled auditorium is the same as for a full auditorium, if the people are distributed uniformly throughout the room. Finally, the equations for calculation of **reverberation time** and **total absorption** are susceptible to some error because of certain assumptions that are made. The computations do provide, however, a useful starting point.

Absorption and Diffraction

The air medium in which sound is transmitted also absorbs sound energy, and that helps explain why the foghorn on a ship at sea emits a very low-frequency sound rather than a high-frequency whistle. When the conditions are foggy, the air contains water droplets with a size that is very small relative to the long wavelength of the sound emitted by the foghorn. The sound energy is **diffracted**; it bends around the small objects, reforms, and then continues to be transmitted as an effective warning signal. If a high-frequency whistle with a very short wavelength approaching the diameter of the water droplets were used, too much of the sound energy would be **absorbed** by the water droplets, and the effectiveness of the alerting signal would be diminished.

■ OTHER PHENOMENA IN SOUND TRANSMISSION

Beats

Suppose two people are walking along a path, but they are walking at different rates. If one is walking at a rate of 60 steps per minute, and the other at a rate of 56 steps per minute, there will be moments when they are "in-step" (in phase) with each other and moments when they are "out-of-step" (out of phase) with each other.

The one who is walking with the faster pace gains 4 steps each minute on the other person, and they will be "in-step" 4 times each minute. Thus, the number of times that the two people are "in-step" equals the difference between their two walking rates: 60 steps/min minus 56 steps/min = 4 steps/min.

The same principle can be applied to understand what happens when two sine waves with slightly different frequencies coexist in the same medium. As we learned in Chapter 2, because their frequencies are different, they will move in and out of phase just as our two walkers did. If we have two sine waves, one with a frequency of 55 Hz and a second with a frequency of 50 Hz, at a given place in the medium the compressions of the two waves will be in phase 5 times each second. When that happens, the two waves maximally *reinforce* (**constructive interference**) each other and the result is an *increase* in intensity.

Similarly, five times each second the compressions of one sine wave will be 180° out of phase with the compressions of the second wave. When that happens, the two waves maximally *interfere* (**destructive interference**) with each other and the result is a *decrease* in intensity. The consequence of alternating between reinforcement and interference is *a periodic increase and decrease in amplitude of the resultant wave*, and those changes in amplitude are called **beats**.

The **beat frequency**, the rate at which the periodic increases and decreases in *amplitude* occur, is given by $f_2 - f_1$. In the case of the two waves mentioned above, a listener will hear a single sound wave with a frequency equal to $(f_2 + f_1)/2$ (57.5 Hz) and with an intensity that changes at a rate given by $f_2 - f_1$ (5 Hz). Thus, even though there are two sine waves with frequencies of 55 Hz and 50 Hz traveling in the medium, the listener hears a single sound wave with a frequency of 57.5 Hz whose intensity waxes and wanes at a rate of 5 times per second.

Panels A and B of Figure 8–18 shows two sine waves with equal amplitude, but different frequencies: $f_1 = 50$ Hz ($T = 20$ ms) and $f_2 = 55$ Hz ($T = 18.2$ ms). Panel C of the figure shows the resultant wave, which is the sum over time of f_1 and f_2.

At $t = 0$, f_1 and f_2 are in phase and reinforce each other (**constructive interference**). By time $t = 100$ ms, f_1 has completed 5 cycles (100 ÷ 20), f_2 has completed about 5.49 cycles (100 ÷ 18.2), and f_1 and f_2 are 180° out of phase (**destructive interference**); **cancellation** occurs. The two sine waves are next in phase at $t = 200$ ms, by which time f_1 has completed 10 cycles and f_2 has completed about 10.99 cycles. Maximum reinforcement occurs. Thus, between $t = 0$ and $t = 200$ ms, the resultant wave changes from maximum reinforcement ($t = 0$), to cancellation ($t = 100$ ms), and to maximum reinforcement ($t = 200$ ms). Why are the two maxima separated by an interval of 200 ms? The **beat frequency** $(f_2 - f_1) = 5$ Hz, and the **beat period** $(T = 1/f) = 200$ ms.

A guitarist, for example, can use the perception of beats to help tune an instrument. Suppose the lowest (6th) string (E_3) has previously been tuned to approximately 165 Hz and one now wishes to tune the 5th string (A_3) to approximately 220 Hz. First, one presses the 6th string against the 5th fret, which means that it will produce A_3 (220 Hz) rather than E_3 (165 Hz). Then, one alternately plucks the 6th *fretted string* and the 5th *unfretted string*, and systematically adjusts the tension on the 5th string until the two produce the same perception of pitch.

When the tension of the 5th string is not adjusted properly, you hear a single pitch that alternately increases and decreases in loudness because of a change in intensity. You are hearing beats, and the rate at which the *intensity* increases and decreases defines the **beat frequency**. If you count the rate at which the beats are occurring, the beat frequency, you can estimate just how mismatched the two strings are in frequency.

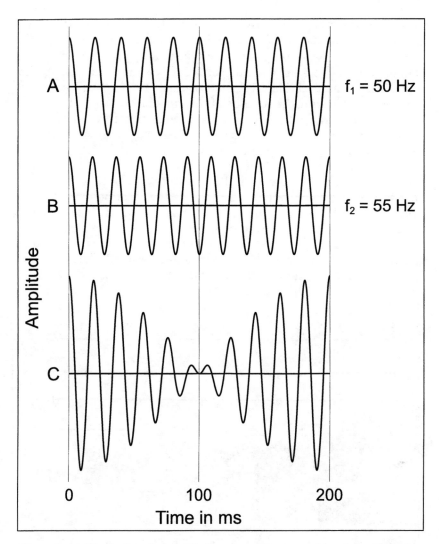

Figure 8–18. Beats. Panels A and B show two sine waves of equal amplitude, but different frequency. Panel C shows the resultant wave, a point-by-point summation of f_1 and f_2. The *amplitude* of the resultant wave increases and decreases periodically, and the rate at which those periodic changes in *amplitude* occur is called the **beat frequency**.

The Doppler Effect

We learned in Chapter 1 that the frequency of a sound wave is governed by properties of the source and that the speed of sound wave propagation is governed by properties of the medium. Thus, if the sound source vibrates with a frequency of 250 Hz, the air particles are displaced at a rate of 250 Hz (the same frequency as the source), and a disturbance is propagated through an air medium at a rate of about 340 m/s. If the resulting sound wave penetrates the surface of, for example, water and then travels as a sound wave through the water medium, the frequency of particle displacement will still be 250 Hz, but the speed of wave propagation will be different because of the different values of elasticity and density of the two transmitting media.

There is an exception. Position yourself at a certain location at the race track during the running of the Indianapolis 500. As the Indy cars approach, the pitch of their whining engines increases and reaches a highest pitch as the cars pass you. As they then speed farther away, the pitch of the sound decreases.

The explanation for this phenomenon, known as the **Doppler effect**, is shown in Figure 8–19. Point **A** marks *a location of a moving source* of a sound wave and **C** marks the location of a receiver, which is positioned 340 meters from the source, **A**. The speed of sound is represented by a vector **s**, and the vector s_s represents the speed of the moving source. The length **AC** corresponds to a *distance* equal to the speed of sound (340 m/s), and length **AB** corresponds to a *distance* equal to the speed of the moving source (85 m/s).

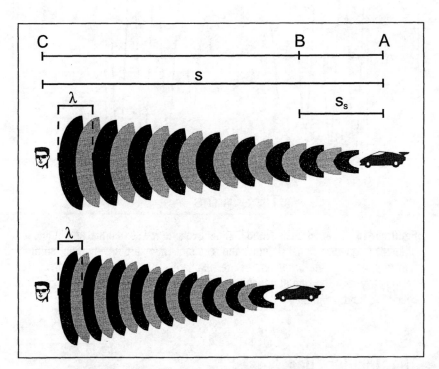

Figure 8–19. The Doppler effect. Point **A** is the location of a moving source of sound, point **C** is the location of a receiver, distance **s** is the speed of sound, and distance s_s is the speed of the moving source. If the source were stationary, after 1 s the compressions and rarefactions would be spread over distance **AC**. But, the source is moving, and after 1 s it has moved to location **B**. Thus, the same number of compressions and rarefactions now will be crowded into distance **BC**. The wavelength, the distance from one compression to another, must be decreased, and the frequency with which wavefronts move by the receiver **C** must be increased.

If the source **A** remains stationary, after 1 second the waves of compressions and rarefactions will be spread over distance **AC**. The wavelength, λ, is shown as the distance between two compressions.

Suppose that during that 1 second of time, the source **A** moves to location **B** at speed s_s. Now, the same number of compressions and rarefactions will be crowded into distance **BC** rather than distance **AC**, as is shown in the bottom row of the figure. If the same number of compressions are crowded into a smaller distance, *the wavelength must be decreased.* Thus, the number of compressions that pass by the receiver **C** each second must be increased because frequency is inversely proportional to wavelength, $f \propto 1/\lambda$.

By how much will the frequency change? The magnitude of change in frequency *is directly proportional* to both frequency and the speed of the moving source. If the source of sound is moving *toward* the observer, the altered frequency (**f'**) is given by Equation 8.18

$$f' = f\left(\frac{s}{s - s_s}\right) ,$$

Equation 8.18

where **f'** is the altered frequency,

f is the frequency produced by the source,

s is the speed of sound wave propagation,

and

s_s is the speed of the moving source.

For example, if frequency = 400 Hz, speed of sound = 340 m/s, and the speed of the moving source = 85 m/s, the altered frequency would be:

$$f' = 400\left(\frac{340}{340 - 85}\right) = 533 \text{ Hz}.$$

Thus, if the source is moving toward the observer, the observer will hear the pitch rise to a maximum that corresponds to a frequency of 533 Hz instead of 400 Hz.

If the source moves *away* from the observer, the pitch of the sound will decrease, and the altered frequency is given by:

$$f' = f\left(\frac{s}{s + s_s}\right).$$

Equation 8.19

Therefore, in this case, the frequency would decrease from 400 Hz to 320 Hz because:

$$f' = 400\left(\frac{340}{340 + 85}\right) = 320 \text{ Hz}.$$

Sonic Booms

Why is a "sonic boom" created when an airplane exceeds the speed of sound? An airplane traveling with a speed greater than the speed of sound is moving at supersonic speed. Supersonic speeds can be rated in "Mach numbers," and a Mach number is simply the ratio of the speed of the plane to the speed of sound. Thus, if the airplane's speed is 680 m/s and the speed of sound is 340 m/s, the airplane has achieved Mach 2.

Before the airplane achieves Mach 1, the point at which the speed of the airplane would equal the speed of sound, it behaves as a moving source. An observer will hear a change in pitch in accordance with the Doppler principle. The pitch will be heard to rise if the plane is moving toward the observer or to fall if the plane is moving away from the observer. We can imagine that circumstance to mean that the plane with a speed < 340 m/s, in effect, "is chasing its own sound waves" because the speed of sound exceeds the speed of the moving source, the airplane.

When the airplane is accelerated until its speed approaches Mach 1, the sound waves in front of it serve to impede the flight of the airplane, and additional thrust is required to achieve Mach 1. That is called "breaking the sound barrier." When the barrier is broken and Mach 1 is achieved and exceeded, the airplane will have moved out in front of its own sound wave. The successive compressions of the sound wave actually pile upon one another, rather than be separated by rarefactions, to form a very *large compression* that contains considerable sound energy. The energy may even be sufficiently great to break a window. The sound that we hear is called the "sonic boom."

■ A CLOSING COMMENT

We have now gone full circle. Initially, sound waves were treated as if their durations were infinite, as if the distance traveled had no effect on the properties of the sound waves, as if there were no obstacles in the transmitting medium to interfere with sound wave propagation, and as if the characteristics of the waveform were preserved in all respects for an infinity of time. Those assumptions were convenient to help us build a foundation for understanding sound. Subsequently, we have seen that none of those four assumptions holds completely, and we now should have a more complete understanding of how sound is generated and propagated by taking those factors into account.

■ FREQUENTLY MISUNDERSTOOD CONCEPTS

1. A tube with length = 0.5 m, open at one end and closed at the other end, is filled with air at a temperature of 15°C. Calculate the first three resonant frequencies of the tube.

Before using Equations 8.6, 8.7, and 8.8 (or Equation 8.9) to calculate F_1, F_2, and F_3, each of which have speed of sound (s) in the numerator, we must first consider the effects of temperature on s. We learned in Chapter 1 that the speed of sound at 0°C is 331 m/s, and that the speed of sound increases by 0.61 m/s for each 1°C increase in temperature. Therefore, the speed of sound at 15°C will be given by:

$$s = 331° + (0.61 \times 15°) = 340 \text{ m/s.}$$

Next, the frequencies of the three lowest resonant frequencies will be given by:

$$F_1 = \frac{s}{4L} = \frac{340}{2} = 170 \text{ Hz} \qquad \textbf{Equation 8.6}$$

$$F_2 = \frac{3s}{4L} = \frac{1,020}{2} = 510 \text{ Hz} \qquad \textbf{Equation 8.7}$$

$$F_3 = \frac{5s}{4L} = \frac{1,700}{2} = 850 \text{ Hz} \qquad \textbf{Equation 8.8}$$

Thus, the higher resonant frequencies are *odd integer multiples* of F_1 (F_2 = 170 × 3 = 510 Hz; F_3 = 170 × 5 = 850 Hz; and so forth).

2. The air in the tube described in #1 is replaced with helium at a temperature of 20°C. The speed of sound is 927 m/s under these conditions. Calculate the first three resonant frequencies of the tube.

In this case, we should *not* correct for the fact that the temperature of the helium is 20°C because the speed of sound in helium at 20°C is already given as 927 m/s. Because the resonant frequencies are *directly proportional* to the speed of sound propagation, and because speed in helium at 20°C is 2.73 times faster (927/340 = 2.73) than speed in air at 15°C, we can simply multiply the three frequencies calculated for #1 by 2.73 to find the correct answers: F_1 = 170 × 2.73 = 464 Hz; F_2 = 510 × 2.73 = 1391 Hz; and F_3 = 850 × 2.73 = 2318 Hz. Alternatively, we can compute the resonant frequencies and obtain the same results by using Equations 8.6, 8.7, and 8.8 (or Equation 8.9).

3. The tube described in #2 is replaced with one that is open at both ends. By how much will the *lowest* resonant frequency increase?

It will increase by a factor of 2:1 (464 × 2 = 928 Hz), subject to rounding error, because F_1 in a tube open at both ends is given by:

$$F_1 = \frac{s}{2L} = \frac{927}{1} = 927 \text{ Hz}.$$

4. When two sound waves with slightly different frequencies co-exist in the same medium, what does the beat frequency reveal?

The **beat frequency** corresponds to the rate at which the *amplitude* increases and decreases. Suppose the frequencies are 256 Hz and 260 Hz. The **beat frequency**, the rate at which the periodic increases and decreases in *amplitude* occur, is given by $f_2 - f_1$, which in this case would be 4 Hz (260 − 256 = 4 Hz). The listener should hear a single sound wave with a pitch corresponding to a frequency of 258 Hz ($f_1 + f_2 / 2 = 258$ Hz) whose intensity waxes and wanes at a rate of 4 Hz, the **beat frequency**.

5. If intensity level decreases by 6 dB with each doubling of distance from the source, sound pressure level decreases by how many dB?

6 dB. A common, but *incorrect*, answer is 12 dB. If it is not clear why 12 dB is incorrect, review **The Relation Between dB IL and dB SPL** in Chapter 4. We learned that 2×10^1 µPa, the reference pressure for dB SPL, is the pressure equivalent of the reference intensity for dB IL, 10^{-12} watt/m². As long as equivalent references for pressure and intensity are used, dB IL = dB SPL. Strictly speaking, of course, this was not really an inverse square law problem.

6. If sound intensity level is 85 dB at a distance of 200 m from the source, by how many dB will the level be *decreased* at a distance of 2,000 m from the source?

20 dB, not 65 dB SPL. Solution of this problem is fairly straightforward with Equation 8.4:

$$dB = -20 \log \frac{d_i}{d_r}$$

$$= -20 \log \frac{2,000}{200}$$

$$= -20 \text{ dB}$$

It is true that the SPL at 2,000 m will be 65 dB SPL (85 − 20), but the question asked, "by how many dB will the level be *decreased*?"

References

Albers, V. M. (1970). *The world of sound*. New York: A. S. Barnes and Company.

American National Standards Institute. (1984). *Preferred frequencies, frequency levels, and band numbers for acoustical measurements* (ANSI S1.6-1984, Revised 1997). New York: ANSI.

American National Standards Institute. (1989). *Specifications for audiometers* (ANSI S3.6-1989). New York: ANSI.

Backus, J. (1977). *The acoustical foundations of music*. New York: W. W. Norton.

Beranek, L. (1960). Audience and seat absorption in large halls. *Journal of the Acoustical Society of America, 32*, 661–670.

Daniloff, R., Schuckers, G., & Feth, L. (1980). *The physiology of speech and hearing*. Englewood Cliffs, NJ: Prentice-Hall.

Feth, L. L. (1977). Letter-to-the-Editor. *Asha, 19*, 225–226.

Hirsh, I. J. (1952). *The measurement of hearing*. New York: McGraw-Hill.

Kramer, M. B. (1977). Letter-to-the-Editor. *Asha, 19*, 225.

Rosen, S., & Howell, P. (1991). *Signals and systems for speech and hearing*. San Diego: Academic Press.

Senders, V. L. (1958). *Measurement and statistics*. New York: Oxford University Press.

Stevens, S. S. (1951). Mathematics, measurement, and psychophysics. In S. S. Stevens (Ed.), *Handbook of experimental psychology* (pp. 1–49). New York: John Wiley and Sons.

Stewart, O. M. (1924). *Physics*. New York: Ginn and Company.

Ward, W. D. (1977). Letter-to-the-Editor. *Asha, 19*, 226.

Yost, W. A., & Nielson, D. W. (1977). *Fundamentals of hearing*. New York: Holt, Rinehart, and Winston.

Alphabetical Listing of Selected Equations

TERM	EQUATION	NO.	PAGE
absorption coefficient	$\alpha = I_a / I_i$	8.14	287
absorption (total)	$A' = S_1\alpha_1 + S_2\alpha_2 + \ldots = S_n\alpha_n$	8.17	291
acceleration	$a = \Delta c / t$	1.3	21
angular velocity	$\omega = 2\pi f$	2.11	75
bandwidth	$\Delta f = f_U - f_L$	6.1	199
combining sound intensities from equal sources	$dB_N = dB_i + 10 \log_{10} N$	4.9	146
compliant reactance	$X_c = 1/2\pi fc$	2.15	87
constant percentage bandwidth filter	$f_L = \text{antilog}_{10} \left(\log_{10} f_c - 0.3/2n\right)$	6.6	210
	$f_U = \text{antilog}_{10} \left(\log_{10} f_c + 0.3/2n\right)$	6.7	210
	$\Delta f = f_U - f_L$	6.8	210
1/1-octave filter	$\Delta f = 0.707 \,(f_c)$	6.2	208
1/2-octave filter	$\Delta f = 0.346 \,(f_c)$		210
1/3-octave filter	$\Delta f = 0.231 \,(f_c)$		210
1/10-octave filter	$\Delta f = 0.069 \,(f_c)$		210
damping factor	$d_f = \ln (A_1/A_2)$	2.13	83
decibels			
intensity	$dB = 10 \log_{10} (I_x/I_r)$	4.4	127
inverse square law	$dB = -20 \log_{10} (d_i/d_r)$	8.4	257
pressure	$dB = 20 \log_{10} (p_x/p_r)$	4.7	135
narrow-band filter	$SPL_{nb} = SPL_{wb} - 10 \log_{10} (\Delta f_{wb}/\Delta f_{nb})$	6.12	217
wide-band filter	$SPL_{wb} = SPL_{nb} + 10 \log_{10} (\Delta f_{wb}/\Delta f_{nb})$	6.13	218

TERM	EQUATION	NO.	PAGE
doppler effect			
toward observer	$f' = f(s/s - s_s)$	8.18	297
away from observer	$f' = f(s/s + s_s)$	8.19	297
exponents			
Law I	$X^a \times X^b = X^{a+b}$		103
Law II	$X^a / X^b = X^{a-b}$		103
Law III	$(X^a)^b = X^{ab}$		104
force	$F = ma$	1.4	21
restoring force	$F_r = -kx$	1.8	26
inertial force	$F_i = F_r$	2.1	62
frequency			
and period	$f = 1/T$	1.12	32
of vibrating string	$f = 1/2L\sqrt{t/m}$	2.10	73
harmonic distortion	$\sqrt{\dfrac{V_2^2 + V_3^2 + ... + V_n^2}{V_1^2 + V_2^2 + ... + V_n^2}} \times 100$	7.1	245
Hooke's law	$F_r = -kx$	1.8	26
impedance	$Z = \sqrt{R^2 + (X_m - X_c)^2}$	2.18	90
inverse square law	$I \propto 1/(d_i/d_r)^2$	8.3	256
in decibels	$dB = -20 \log_{10}(d_i/d_r)$	8.4	257
logarithms			
Law I	$\log ab = \log a + \log b$		116
Law II	$\log a/b = \log a - \log b$		117
Law III	$\log a^b = b \log a$		117
Law IV	$\log 1/a = -\log a$		117

TERM	EQUATION	NO.	PAGE
mass reactance	$X_m = 2\pi fm$	2.14	87
mean square amplitude	mean square $= A^2/2$	2.7	67
momentum	$M = mc$	1.9	28
newton per square meter	$1 \text{ N}/\text{m}^2 = 10 \text{ dynes}/\text{cm}^2$	1.6	24
pascal	$1 \text{ Pa} = 1 \text{ N}/\text{m}^2 = 10 \text{ dynes}/\text{cm}^2$	1.7	24
period			
and frequency	$T = 1/f$	1.11	32
of pendulum	$T = 2\pi\sqrt{L/G}$	1.13	32
pressure	$p = F/A$	1.5	23
pressure spectrum level	$L_{ps} = SPL_{wb} - 10 \log_{10} (\Delta f_{wb}/\Delta_o f)$	6.9	214
	$= SPL_{wb} - 10 \log_{10} \Delta f_{wb}$	6.10	214
rectified average			
full-wave	$FW_{avg} = 2A/\pi = A(0.636)$	2.8	69
half-wave	$HW_{avg} = A/\pi = A(0.318)$	2.9	69
reverberation time	$T_{60} = k(V/A)$	8.15	290
root-mean-square amplitude	$rms = A/\sqrt{2}$	2.4	66
	$= A(0.707)$	2.6	66
spectral envelope			
sawtooth wave	$dB = 20 \log_{10} (1/h_i)$	5.1	168
	$= -20 \log_{10} h_i$	5.2	168
square wave	$dB = 20 \log_{10} (1/h_i)$	5.1	168
	$= -20 \log_{10} h_i$	5.2	168
triangular wave	$dB = 20 \log_{10} (1/h_i^2)$	5.3	174
	$= -40 \log_{10} h_i$	5.4	174

TERM	EQUATION	NO.	PAGE
speed	$s = d/t$	1.1	19
speed of sound	$s = \sqrt{\dfrac{E}{\rho}}$	1.16	36
string resonant frequencies	$f = \dfrac{1}{2L}\sqrt{t/m}$	2.10	73
	$f_0 = s/2L$	8.12	279
	$f_n = ns/2L$	8.13	279
tube resonant freqencies			
(open-closed)	$F_1 = s/4L$	8.6	273
	$F_2 = 3s/4L$	8.7	274
	$F_3 = 5s/4L$	8.8	274
	$F_n = [(2n)-1]s/4L$	8.9	275
(open-open) **or** **(closed-closed)**	$F_1 = s/2L$	8.10	276
	$F_n = ns/2L$	8.11	276
wavelength	$\lambda = s/f$	2.12	78
work	$W = Fd$	1.10	29

Index